# Pathology of
# Sharp Force Trauma

# Pathology of
# Sharp Force Trauma

## Professor Peter Vanezis

OBE MB, ChB, MD, PhD, FRCPath, FRCP(Glasg), FFFLM, FCSFS, FAFMS (UK), DMJ (Path)

Professor Emeritus, Queen Mary University of London;
Principal, Academy of Forensic Medical Sciences;
Formerly Regius Professor of Forensic Medicine and Science, University of Glasgow

Contributor:

## Dr Andrew Peter Vanezis PhD, MB, ChB, MRCP(UK), BSc.

Consultant Interventional Cardiologist Trent Cardiac Centre,
Nottingham City Hospital

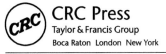

**CRC Press**
Taylor & Francis Group
Boca Raton London New York

CRC Press is an imprint of the
Taylor & Francis Group, an **informa** business

First edition published 2021
by CRC Press
2 Park Square, Milton Park, Abingdon, Oxon, OX14 4RN

and by CRC Press
6000 Broken Sound Parkway NW, Suite 300, Boca Raton, FL 33487-2742

© 2022 Peter Vanezis

CRC Press is an imprint of Informa UK Limited

*British Library Cataloguing-in-Publication Data*
A catalogue record for this book is available from the British Library

ISBN: 978-1-498-76862-7 (hbk)
ISBN: 978-0-367-72298-2 (pbk)
ISBN: 978-0-429-27246-2 (ebk)

Typeset in Minion Pro
by Deanta Global Publishing Services, Chennai, India

# Contents

## Contents

# Contents

# Note on Coverpiece – 'Knife Angel'

The Knife Angel, a 20 ft. high sculpture, was specifically designed to create social change by helping to raise better awareness of how violent and aggressive behaviour affects our communities, by educating and encouraging youth to renounce violence as a means to solve problems, and by acting as a memorial for those lives lost to these unnecessary actions. Clive Knowles, the Chairman of the British Ironwork Centre in 2014, developed the idea for its creation and the artist Alfie Bradley created the iconic sculpture. The Angel's construction involved the use of 100,000 confiscated and surrendered knives, donated by all 43 Police Constabularies in the United Kingdom.

# Acknowledgements

I would like to extend my thanks to many who have assisted and encouraged me throughout the time it has taken to complete the book. In particular, I would like to thank Mark Listewnik and his team at Taylor Francis who have supported and been patient with me at all times, despite many delays on my part before completion of the text.

I also thank my son Andrew Peter Vanezis for agreeing to write the section on iatrogenic and related injuries. I believe that it is appropriate for a clinician who understands and encounters such issues in routine practice to contribute on this topic. He is ideally placed to do so as an interventional cardiologist.

My thanks also go to Mr Dean Jones and his deputy Mr Martin Allix, both of the Home Office Forensic Pathology Delivery Board, for their advice and assistance in attaining permission from United Kingdom Police Forces for the publication of numerous images derived from autopsy cases.

I am also indebted to the many publishers of journals who have given permission for reuse of images. They have all been acknowledged alongside their respective image in the text. Particular thanks are due to the British Ironwork Centre for the inspiration to use the image of the "Knife Angel" as the cover to my book.

My thanks are also extended to my personal assistant Mr Adam Konstanciak for his help with the production of images and other technical assistance.

Undoubtedly, this book would not have been completed without the encouragement of my wife, Dr Maria Vanezis, who has worked with me in the past on a number of other forensic projects. I thank her for her unwavering support at all times.

# About the Author

**Peter Vanezis OBE** is Professor Emeritus of Forensic Medical Sciences at the William Harvey Research Institute, Queen Mary University of London. He began his career in forensic medicine at the London Hospital Medical College in 1974 in the department headed by Professor James Cameron. He became Reader and Head of the Forensic Department at the Charing Cross and Westminster Medical School in 1990, following which he was appointed Regius Professor of Forensic Medicine and Science in 1993 at the University of Glasgow. He was awarded the OBE in 2000 for leading the British Forensic team in the investigation of mass graves in Kosovo. After establishing a forensic pathology unit at the Forensic Science Service in 2003, he was appointed to the new chair of Forensic Medical Sciences at Queen Mary University of London where he pursued academic activities until his retirement in 2018. He continues his interest in forensic medical education and research through his Academy of Forensic Medical Sciences.

Professor Vanezis has a number of broad interests in the forensic medical sciences including human identification and human rights abuses. His previously published texts include *Pathology of Neck injury, Essential Forensic Medicine* and *Suspicious Death—Scene Investigation* as well as contributions to a number of forensic textbooks.

## Contributor

**Dr Andrew Vanezis** undertook his undergraduate medical training in Edinburgh, graduating in 2007. During this time he also obtained an intercalated BSc in Parasitology and Zoology. He embarked on a PhD at the University of Leicester under the tutelage of Professor Sir Nilesh Samani and successfully gained his degree in 2017; his thesis is titled "Remote Ischaemic Conditioning and its Effect on Maladaptive Cardiac Remodelling Following Myocardial Infarction." His training in Cardiology continued in the East midlands and included a fellowship in Edmonton, Canada, where he performed a number of complex coronary interventions. He has recently been appointed as an Interventional Cardiology Consultant at Nottingham City Hospital.

Dr Vanezis has a strong interest in chronic total occlusion percutaneous coronary intervention (CTO PCI). He also has a passion for teaching, instructing on a number of Advance Life Support (ALS) courses and running numerous teaching sessions for junior doctors and medical students. In addition, Dr Vanezis has a keen involvement in running and taking part in high quality clinical trial work including running the DREAM study, a multi-centre randomised controlled trial assessing the efficacy of remote ischaemic conditioning in modulating adverse left ventricular remodelling post-myocardial infarction.

# Preface

The idea of writing a book on sharp force trauma from a pathology perspective was conceived many years ago although it is only now that this aspiration has been fulfilled with the production of this monograph. Despite many authors, including myself, having contributed many chapters in forensic text books on the subject, the pathology of this manner of injury, as far as I am aware, has not been previously published as a single substantive text in the English language, despite the sad fact that knives and other sharp implements used as weapons, is such a common phenomenon in our society.

In fact, in many countries, with the exception of those where firearms are readily available, sharp force trauma, and in particular the use of knives, is the most common method of homicide and a frequent source of morbidity seen in emergency departments. It is also extremely concerning to find that in the United Kingdom, as well as a number of other countries, there has recently been an alarming upsurge in the use of knives in gang-related assaults and in terrorist incidents.

Although the book is intended primarily for pathologists and clinicians who are involved in the examination of such injuries in the post-mortem room or in a hospital environment, it will also be of interest to other forensic scientists and advocates, particularly those dealing with the "cut and thrust" of courtroom examination. In addition to its practical use as a reference during the investigation of a case, the book is readily accessible to all doctors and medical students who have an interest in trauma and its management.

The reader will find that the text is generously illustrated with case examples, many of which are from those I have personally examined over a period of 40 years. Furthermore, I have also included post-mortem sharp trauma, as in dismemberment as well as artefacts which resemble wounds. The reader is also reminded of the need to consider iatrogenic and related injuries which are encountered from time to time. This section is written by a clinician specialist in this field who encounters such injuries on a regular basis in routine hospital practice.

The reader will note that I have illustrated the cover with the iconic sculpture of the *Knife Angel* which has been created by the British Ironwork Centre in Oswestry, Shropshire. The sculpture was formed using 100,000 knives which had been confiscated by police forces throughout the country. The work, conceived by Clive Knowles and sculpted by Alfie Bradley, is unquestionably a poignant tour de force, unique in concept and embodying profound empathy for victims of knife attacks and their loved ones. It is to the memory of all these victims and that I dedicate this book.

Peter Vanezis

# ▌ Chapter 1

# Introduction, Scope and Historical Perspectives

## ▌ Introduction

This textbook gives an account of sharp force trauma as seen in forensic pathology case work and includes the clinical setting where relevant, and how one informs the other in interpreting such trauma for medico-legal purposes. Its aim is for the reader to gain a comprehensive understanding of different aspects of such trauma, most importantly the manner in which the victim has died, whether homicide, suicide or accident, the type of weapon responsible, how it was used and other such areas that are useful to the investigation of such cases.

It is important at this stage to define what we mean by *sharp force trauma* and how different terms are used in referring to such injuries by pathologists and other medical practitioners. A concise and useful but not an entirely watertight definition, as will be readily appreciated by the experienced forensic practitioner is: *The application of force to produce an injury which results in a clear division or separation of the skin and underlying tissues.*

Sharp force trauma may be caused by all manner of implements with a sharp edge and/or pointed end, whether or not they have been produced for use as a weapon and include knives, broken glass, scissors and many others, to name but a few. Certain tools, such as axes or machetes, combine a sharp edge with heavy weight and produce injuries with both sharp and blunt impact elements. In particular, propeller injuries show a distinct pattern of clean cut injuries in soft tissue yet demonstrate bone fractures typical of blunt force injury. Indeed, sharp force trauma has been regarded by some such as Kroman (2010) to be a continuum of injury progressing from sharp to blunt, arguing that the current classification system for trauma is too restrictive.

Among the various types of sharp force trauma, I have also included:

- penetrating injuries caused by pointed objects which have a linear component. Such implements include arrows, nails, spears, stakes and many others,

- cutting, penetrating and other sharp force injuries resulting from medical intervention in a healthcare environment, such as might occur during surgical procedures, as well as needle stick and other sharp injuries,

- sharp injuries caused by domesticated and wild animals in the chapter on accidental injuries.

A number of different terms as shown below, are used in the description of the resulting wounds seen in sharp force trauma and confusion can easily arise if there is ambiguity about the exact meaning of the different types that are being referred to.

- The general public and even many medical professionals use the word *laceration* as a general term for when the skin is breached whether the injury is caused by sharp or blunt trauma (Milroy and Rutty 1997). It is important to emphasise at the outset that a laceration is the result of blunt trauma and is a crushing injury. The skin splits, especially when such impact is over a bony area such as the face. There is bridging of tissue and the surface in most cases is slightly abraded with some bruising around the edges and does not consist of clean cut edges, except on occasions when there is a rapid splitting of the skin over bone (see also Chapter 7). In addition, occasionally, in medical records, one sees the use of the word *cut* to describe any breach of the skin whether due to sharp or blunt force trauma which can also cause confusion when reviewing clinical notes.

- The term *stab wound* means that the implement has penetrated the skin and underlying tissues and has produced a wound in which its length of penetration (track length) is longer than the length of the wound on the skin surface.

- *Incised wound* is a term which some pathologists use, as an overarching general term to refer to all injuries produced by a sharp implement, whether they are longer on the skin surface or are stab wounds. Others reserve the term incised wound for an injury which is longer on the skin surface rather than longer in its depth and do not regard it as being synonymous with a stab wound. In this book, in common with most others, the term incised wound will be used synonymously with *cutting injury* or *sharp force trauma* when discussing sharp force trauma in general terms. However, when discussing the detailed morphology of the various types of wounds, incised wounds will refer to wounds which are longer on the skin rather than in depth.

- A *slash wound* is a term used for an incised wound which expresses the way the weapon is used. It particularly describes the sweeping motion of a knife across the body (Bleetman et al., 2003). It is not a blanket term for all wounds which are incised and is only used in the text when it is appropriate to do so.

- A *puncture wound* is also used by some authorities synonymously with stab wound when the latter appears pointed. Most authorities prefer to use the word puncture when referring to a wound that has a small pointed round appearance and caused by the pointed end of an implement. The wound may be either superficial or deep. Sometimes the word *punctate* is used when the mark appears like a tiny dot and is superficial.

- A *chopping wound* is used when sharp force trauma is caused by a heavy object with a sharp edge. The resulting incised skin and underlying soft tissue wound is accompanied by significant additional blunt force trauma.

- The term *perforating wound* should not be confused with one which is described as *penetrating*. The term perforation applies both to wounds which have passed all the way through the body or all the way through one or more organs of the body. A good example would be a stab wound entering the body and passing through the heart leaving an entry and exit wound through the organ. On the other hand, a penetrating injury implies that the object has not passed all the way through the organ, other anatomical structures or indeed the whole body.

# Historic Accounts

Sharp force trauma has always been a common method of injury since pointed and sharp implements existed. I have included some material that many readers may already be aware of including the interesting recent findings in the exhumation of Richard III and a brief description of seppuku (hara-kiri) because of its importance in Japanese historical culture. I have consciously omitted the Whitechapel murders of 1888 as these are universally known to readers, and there are many texts available expounding the latest theories on the identity of "Jack the Ripper" or "Rippers."

## Archaeological Finds

There are many examples from early archaeological finds of examples of human remains found with injuries that have been caused by sharp trauma.

Early man, being a hunter-gatherer, used sharp-edged weapons for hunting and as utility tools for various purposes including attacking any apparent enemies. Flohr et al. 2015 report one of the earliest finds from the Bronze Age site in the Tollense valley, Germany, of a human humerus with an embedded flint arrowhead. When the arrowhead lesion was examined using micro-CT it showed no signs of healing confirming that it was a peri-mortem injury.

*Otzi (Iceman)*

A celebrated find from the early copper age of forensic as well as archaeological interest is that of the mummy found in the Otzaler Alps between Austria and Italy (Figures 1.1 and 1.2) It is one of the chronologically oldest discoveries of human remains which

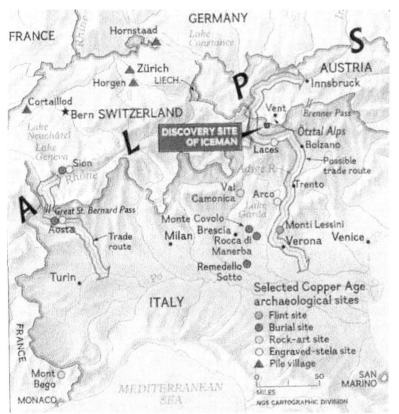

◀ **Figure 1.1** The body in the Otzaler Alps was between the Tisen and Hauslabjoch mountains of the Southern Tyrol near the Similaun Glacier, on the Austrian-Italian border, 3,210 metres above sea level and 92 metres into the Italian territory. (Public domain)

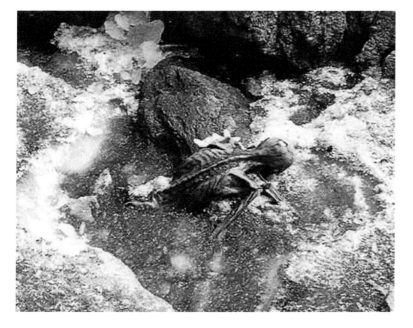

◀ **Figure 1.2** His head and upper back were seen emerging from the residual glacier in a rocky gully. (Public domain)

led to worldwide interest and extensive study. The mummy who came to be known as Otzi the Iceman, was found in a glacier on the Italian side of the Alps on 19 September 1991, by two climbers, Erika and Helmut Simon. His excellent state of preservation and good condition of the surrounding artefacts have given scientists the opportunity to study him and his environment in depth, which clearly has placed him as one of the most important archaeological findings of the late twentieth century. Initially the remains were thought to be of forensic interest although it was soon evident from the artefacts surrounding the body that it was of great archaeological significance (Figure 1.3).

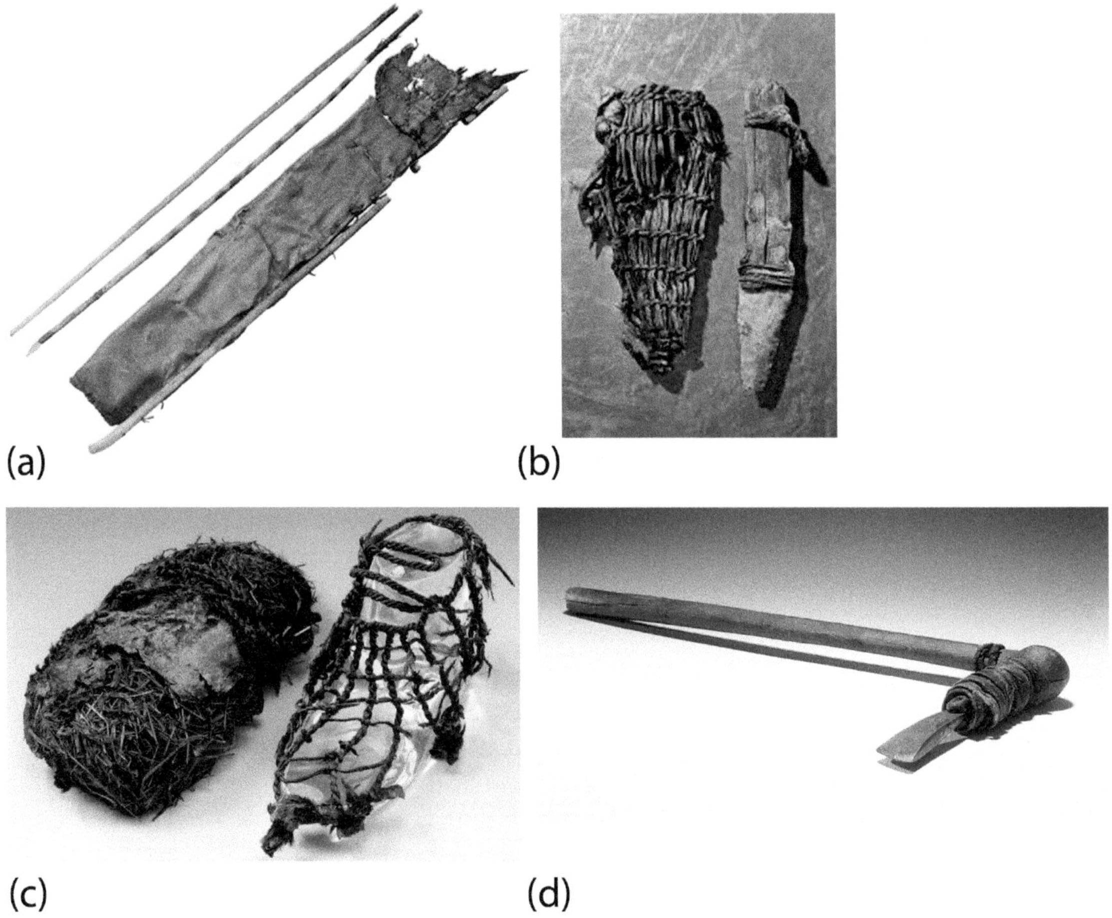

▲ **Figure 1.3** Among a number of artefacts found (clockwise) were (a) a quiver with arrows; (b) a flint knife; (c) remnants of footwear; and (d) a copper axe. (Public domain)

He was originally taken to the Forensic Institute at Innsbruck University as he was thought to be a modern case of sudden death. However, it was very soon appreciated, from artefacts associated with the body, that they were dealing with an archaeological find of tremendous importance that, had it not been for climate change, would probably never have been discovered.

Carbon-14 dating from body and plant remains, confirmed in three laboratories, revealed that he was from the early copper age dating back to 5,300 years.

How the Iceman had met his death was of interest to everyone and continues to be a matter of some debate. Much of the argument involved the findings on radiographs and CT scans which showed images which resembled an arrow tip. The arrow tip appeared to be situated in muscle tissue between the left scapula and pleural cavity above the level of the scapular spine. The scapula has a defect along its lateral border which resembles a fracture site. There is also a corresponding defect in the skin to indicate point of entry of the arrow (Figures 1.4, 1.5 and 1.6).

A possible trajectory is from the left side in an upward direction (shot from lower level or while he was crouching). Nevertheless, the question of whether the arrow had caused death remains an open one. There undoubtedly would have been blood loss which could have contributed to his death from secondary complications weakening him sufficiently to die at a later time. However, although the author of this text participated with other colleagues in an external examination of the body within the Bolzano Museum, which I must say was very informative, it became clear that an invasive autopsy would not be attempted as it would have been too destructive (Dickson et al. 2003). Even a local dissection of the left shoulder, which may have gone a long way in resolving the issue, was not permitted. Therefore, without scientific proof, the cause of his

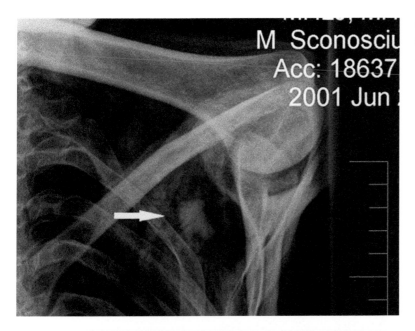

◀ **Figure 1.4a** Radiograph showing AP view with arrowhead (arrow). (Public domain)

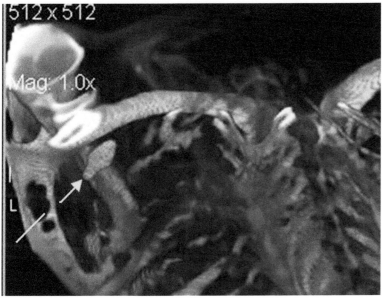

◀ **Figure 1.4b** CT scan of left shoulder showing defect in scapula and arrowhead (trajectory indicated by arrow). (Public domain)

5

death will remain, at least for the foreseeable future, a matter of some speculation.

## Homer's Iliad

One of the very earliest accounts of trauma from sharp as well as blunt implements can be found in Homer's epic poem the *Iliad* which was composed around 800 BC (Figure 1.7).

It gives a very graphic account of the various injuries suffered by combatants in the battle which occurred between the Achaeans and Trojans towards the end of the siege of Troy. Many masters captured the images in sculpture and fine art as we see in the painting by Rubens depicting Achilles slaying Hector outside the gates of Troy with a spear to his neck to avenge the death of his friend Patroclus (Figure 1.8). The following is an English translation by Alexander Pope (1688–1744) of Homer's *Iliad* which gives an account of Hector's death (*Complete Works of Alexander Pope* 1903):

> *So shone the point of great Achilles' spear.*
> *In his right hand he waves the weapon round,*
> *Eyes the whole man, and meditates the wound:*

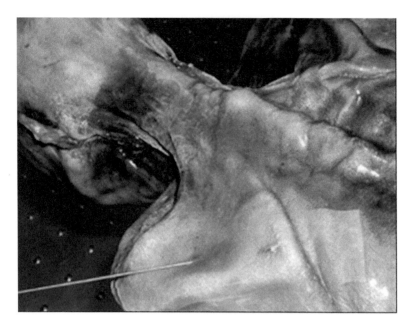

◀ **Figure 1.5a** Left scapula showing defect in skin with probe, thought to be the entry wound of the arrow. (Public domain)

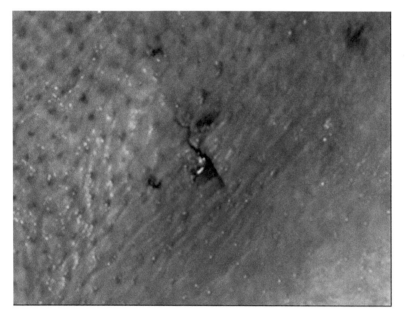

◀ **Figure 1.5b** Close-up of wound. (Public domain)

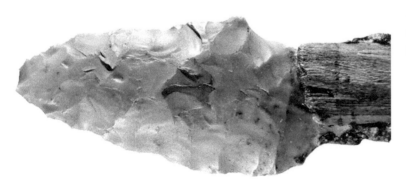

◀ **Figure 1.6** Flint arrowhead similar to that shown in Figure 1.4. (Public domain)

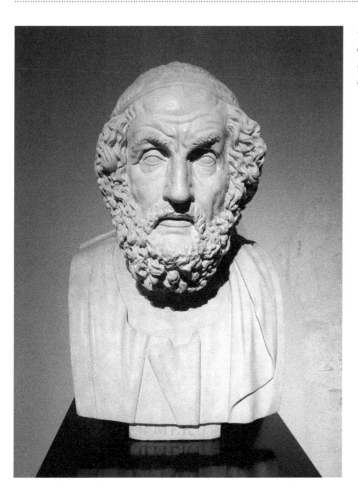

◀ **Figure 1.7** Replica of the Naples bust of Homer, made by Gaetano Rossi in 1875. (Wikipedia. User: Carole Raddato used per Creative Commons 2.0)

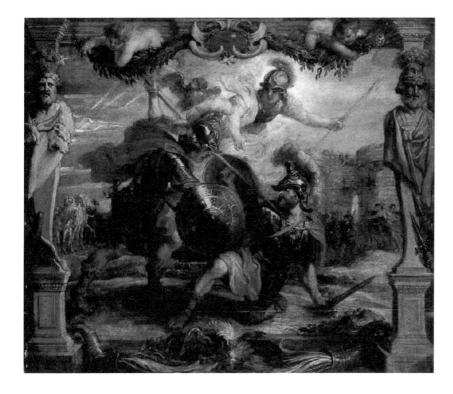

◀ **Figure 1.8** Achilles Slays Hector. Peter Paul Rubens (1630–1635). (Public domain)

*But the rich mail Patroclus lately wore,*
*Securely cased the warrior's body o'er.*
*One place at length he spies, to let in Fate,*
*Where 'twixt the neck and throat the*
*  jointed plate*
*Gave entrance: thro' that penetrable part*
*Furious he drove the well-directed dart:*
*Nor pierc'd the windpipe yet, nor took the*
*  power*
*Of speech, unhappy! from thy dying hour.*
*Prone on the field the bleeding warrior lies,*
*While thus, triumphing, stern Achilles cries:*
*'At last is Hector stretch'd upon the plain,*
*Who fear'd no vengeance for Patroclus slain':*

Apostoloakis et al. (2010) found 54 consecutive thoracic injuries described in the *Iliad* and the most common weapon used was the spear (63%), stones (7.4%), the arrow or sword (5.5%). The injuries proved fatal in 38 of the 54 victims (mortality of just over 70%). Injuries to the upper extremities are described by Hutchison and Hirthler (2013) and the authors also compare the injuries seen to other sites on the body, including those found by Apostolakis et al. op.

cit. From the detailed description and anatomical knowledge shown by Homer in his epic poem, the latter authors postulate the possibility that he had medical skills and was either a physician or a nurse who cared for the warriors in the battlefield.

## Old Testament

There is a multitude of interesting historical accounts of violence, including sharp force attacks in the Bible. A number of these are depicted in medieval and renaissance art by many of the masters of that time. In the book of Judith,[1] the Old Testament relates how Nebuchadnezzer (605–562 BC) sent his general Holofernes to subdue the Jews by besieging them in Bethulia, a city on the southern verge of the Plain of Esdraelon. Judith, a widow, to exact revenge, goes into the camp of the Assyrians and captivates Holofernes by her beauty. She seizes her opportunity and finally takes advantage of the general's intoxication to cut off his head. The beheading of Holofernes is vividly depicted by the Renaissance artist Artemisia Gentileschi, c 1625 (Judith is seen holding the knife with her servant lending assistance (Figure 1.9).

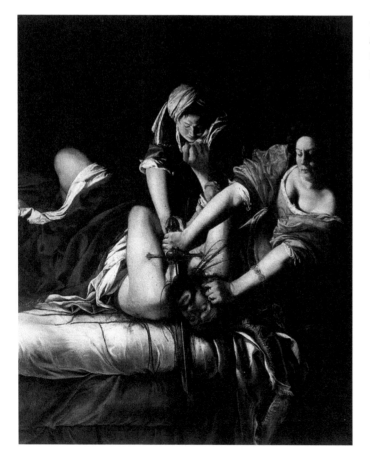

◀ **Figure 1.9** Judith slaying Holofernes by Artemisia Gentileschi, c.1612–1613 Museo e Gallerie Nazionali di Capodimonte, Naples. (Public domain)

## Two Caesars

Stabbing, throughout human history, has been a common method employed to assassinate a number of distinguished historical figures, such as the Roman emperors Julius Caesar (Figure 1.10) and Caligula (Figure 1.11) who both received multiple stab wounds.

### Julius Caesar

He was as assassinated at the age of 55 on the Ides of March (15 March) 44 BC. His death was mainly due to the resentment and opposition to his increasing role and power as a dictator of Rome rather than espousing the principle of the Republic which his political rivals wished to strengthen. A plot to assassinate him was hatched. Gaius Cassius Longinus, who was the moving spirit in the plot to murder him, and Marcus Junius Brutus, the symbolic embodiment of Roman republicanism, were both former enemies. It is said that there were 60 assailants and he was stabbed 23 times.

### Caligula

As one of the cruellest, most unbalanced and unpredictable tyrants of the Roman Empire, Caligula had a number of conspiracies plotted against him. In January AD 41, four months after his return to Rome from Gaul, Caligula was murdered at the Palatine Games by Cassius Chaerea, tribune of the Praetorian guard, Cornelius Sabinus and others. Caligula's wife, Caesonia, and his daughter were also put to death. He was succeeded as emperor by his uncle Claudius.

## Exhumation of Richard III

Richard III, King of England from 1483 to 1485, was the last King of the House of York and of the Plantagenet line (Figure 1.12). He was defeated and died at the Battle of Bosworth Field which was the last battle of the War of the Roses. Following his death, he was taken to the city of Leicester but his remains were lost until very recently following an archaeological excavation supported by the Richard III Society.

The discovery of Richard III's burial place in a car park in Leicester has been one of the most significant discoveries of the twenty-first century. Of relevant interest were the large number of wounds caused by medieval weapons with a sharp edge (Appleby et al. 2015). The investigators found peri-mortem injuries to the skull (Figure 1.13) and two to the postcranial skeleton. No healed injuries were identified. The injuries were consistent with those created by weapons from the later medieval period.

Three of the injuries – two to the inferior cranium and one to the pelvis – could have been fatal. It was also suggested from the wounds to the skull that Richard was not wearing a helmet, although the absence of

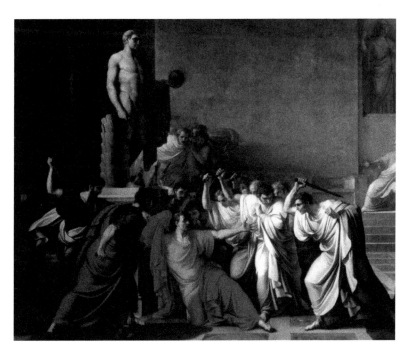

◀ **Figure 1.10** The Death of Julius Caesar 1798 (detail) by Vincenzo Camuccini (b. 1771, Roma, d. 1844, Roma) Oil on canvas, 400 × 207 cm Museo Nazionale di Capodimonte, Naples. (Public domain)

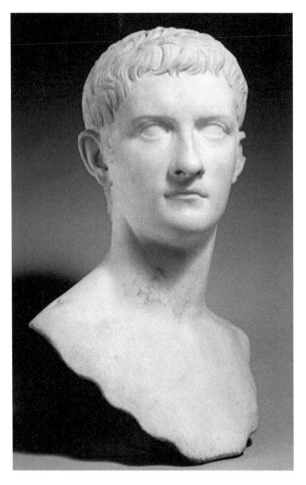

◀ **Figure 1.11** Gaius, known as Caligula (AD 12–41). Marble portrait bust of the emperor Metropolitan Museum of Art, New York. (Public domain)

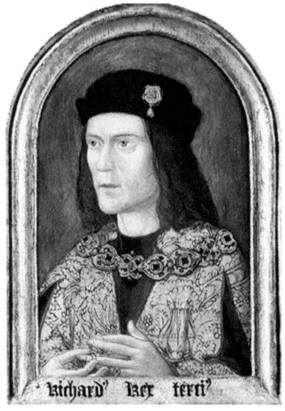

◀ **Figure 1.12** Richard III: The earliest surviving portrait of Richard III of England c.1520, formerly owned by the Paston family and now the Society of Antiquaries, London, since 1828. (Public domain)

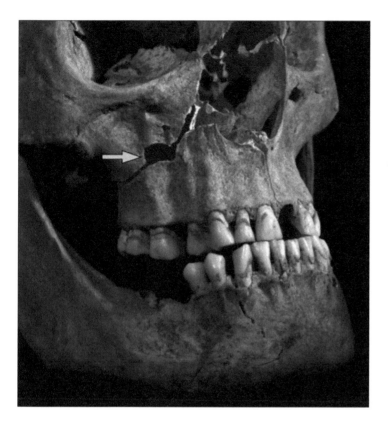

◀ **Figure 1.13** Maxilla and mandible. Arrow shows the penetrating injury to the right maxilla consistent with being caused by a dagger (Source: Courtesy Appleby J, Rutty GN, Hainsworth SV, Woosnam-Savage RC, Morgan B, Brough A, Earp RW, Robinson C, King TE, Morris M, Buckley R.(2015). Perimortem trauma in King Richard III: a skeletal analysis. Lancet, 385:253–9).

defensive wounds on his arms and hands suggests he was still otherwise wearing armour. Therefore, the potentially fatal pelvic injury was probably received post-mortem, meaning that the most likely injuries to have caused his death were the two to the back of the skull.

## Christopher Marlowe

Christopher Marlow was a well-known playwright and poet who lived at the time of Queen Elizabeth I (Figure 1.14).

It was popularly thought that his untimely death at the age of 29, was as a result of a tavern brawl, although this was not the case. It was well known that Marlowe led a very colourful and eventful short life, mixing with both rogues and the highest in Elizabethan society. The official story is that on the evening of 31 May 1593 Christopher Marlowe was stabbed to death by Ingram Frizer in the house in Deptford of a widow, Mrs Bull. There were two other men also present, Nicholas Skeres and Robert Poley[3] All three men were in the service of Sir Francis Walsingham who was Queen Elizabeth I's Secretary and "Spymaster"

(there is evidence that Marlowe had also been working as Walsingham's agent). Over the course of the day the four men had met, eaten and said to have played backgammon in Mrs Bull's house. Following a walk in the garden they had returned to the room when an argument broke out over the bill to be paid. As a result, Marlow sustained a fatal stab wound above the right eye from a dagger (Figure 1.15). The circumstances and motive for delivery of the fatal wound remain to this day a controversial matter entangled with the political machinations of the day. Indeed, Rowling (1999) states that the account given to the coroner at the inquest by the three men who were with Marlowe, was the only evidence heard, and therefore begs the question as to whether they were covering his killing for political reasons.

## Seppuku

In Japan, the historical practice of stabbing oneself deliberately in ritual suicide is known as *seppuku* (more colloquially hara-kiri, literally "belly-cutting" since it involves cutting open the abdomen) (Figure 1.16). The ritual is highly codified, and the person committing suicide is assisted by a "second"

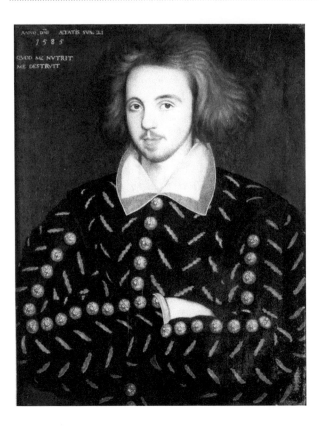

◀ **Figure 1.14** Portrait thought to be of Christopher Marlowe at the age of 21. Corpus Christi College Cambridge, UK. The inscription reads "Quod me nutrit me destruit,"[2] 1585. (Public domain)

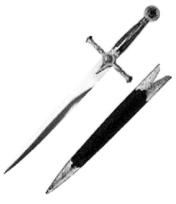

◀ **Figure 1.15** Dagger of the type worn by Elizabethan gentlemen and thought to have fatally wounded Christopher Marlowe. (Public domain)

who is entrusted to decapitate him cleanly (and thus expedite death and prevent an undignified spectacle) once he has made the abdominal wound. *Seppuku* (Japanese: "self-disembowelment") is also called hara-kiri, the honourable method of taking one's own life practised by men of the samurai (military) class in feudal Japan. Two forms of *seppuku* are recognised: voluntary and obligatory. Voluntary *seppuku* evolved during the twelfth century as a method of suicide and was used frequently by warriors who, defeated in battle, chose to avoid the dishonour of falling into the hands of the enemy. Occasionally, a samurai performed *seppuku* to demonstrate loyalty to his lord by following him in death or to protest against some policy of a superior or of the government, or to atone for failure in his duties (Encyclopaedia Brittanica 2019). The most recent case of *seppuku* was in 1970 by a well-known novelist and Nobel Prize nominee, Mishima Yukio. He disembowelled himself after he led a failed coup against his government and to demonstrate his opposition to the erosion of Japan's cultural identity loss of traditional values. Andrew Rankin's book published in 2011 is recommended for a detailed historical account of this practice.

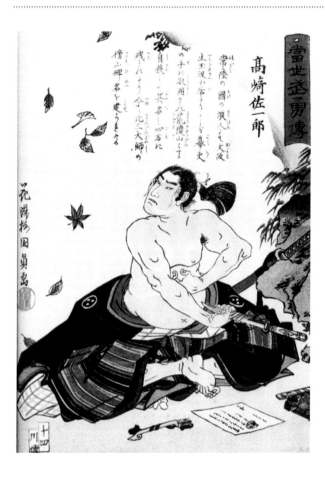

◀ **Figure 1.16** "Tousei buyuuden: Takasaki Saichirou." Ukiyo-e woodblock print of warrior about to perform seppuku. Original work by artist Kunikazu Utagawa (circa 1850s). (Public domain)

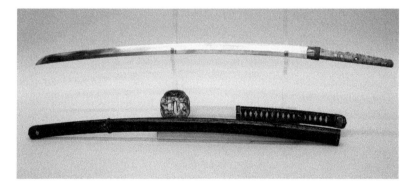

◀ **Figure 1.17** A nineteenth-century katana sword with a curved blade longer than 60 cm fitted with an uchigatana-style mounting and worn in a waist sash with the cutting edge facing up. Metropolitan Museum of Art. (Public domain)

*Testing the Katana Sword*

The samurai warriors in the development of their famed katana sword (Figure 1.17) tested its sharpness by experimenting on both animals and humans Kremer et al. (2008). The technique which began before 1600 in the Koto period involved testing the sword on humans and was called "tameshi-giri" or literally "test-cutting." They used the bodies of convicted criminals who had been executed by decapitation. They made a number of cuts in stipulated regions from which the pelvis was the most difficult to cut through, and the wrists and ankles, the easiest. The tests on humans continued until the mid-eighteenth century when sword cutting of the human body became prohibited.

## "Wound Man"

Finally, this chapter cannot end without noting a most interesting fifteenth-century depiction of a man with multiple wounds, including many from a variety of sharp-edged and other similar weapons

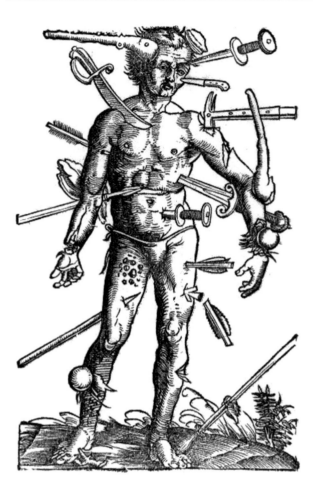

◀ **Figure 1.18** "Wound-man," woodcut, sixteenth century by Hans von Gersdorf, published by H. Schott, Strasbourg, 1517. (Public domain)

(Figure 1.18). Similar images have been produced by many artists to illustrate mediaeval surgical treatises depicting different types of injuries, how they were caused and their treatment (Hartnell 2016). This woodcut version of the "Wound man" is perhaps one of the best known and widely referred to from many similar examples. It is contained within the sixteenth-century textbook *Feldbůch der Wundartzney,* or *Fieldbook of Surgery,* written by Hans von Gersdorf and published in Strasbourg in 1517. The text remained widely used throughout Europe for many years.

## Notes

1. The Book of Judith is considered deuterocanonical and is in the Septuagint (earliest translation of the Greek translation from the Hebrew scriptures) and is included in and the Catholic and Eastern Orthodox versions of the Old Testament of the Bible, but excluded from Jewish texts and assigned by Protestants to the Apocrypha.
2. Tr. "What nourishes me, destroys me."
3. Poley had been heavily involved in preventing the assassination of Queen Elizabeth I, known as the Babington plot of 1586 whose goal was to place Mary Queen of Scots on the throne thus restoring the Catholic monarchy. It led to the execution of Mary Queen of Scots when it was discovered that she consented to the assassination.

# References

Apostolakis E, Apostolaki G, Apostolaki M, ChortiM. (2010). The reported thoracic injuries in Homer's Iliad. *J. Cardiothoracic Surg*, 5, 114.

Appleby J, Rutty GN, Hainsworth SV, Woosnam-Savage RC, Morgan B, Brough A, Earp RW, Robinson C, King TE, Morris M, Buckley R.(2015). Perimortem trauma in King Richard III: a skeletal analysis. *Lancet*, 385, 253–259.

Bleetman A, Watson CH, Horsfall I, Champion SM. (2003). Wounding patterns and human performance in knife attacks: optimising the protection provided by knife-resistant body armour. *J Clin Forensic Med*, 10, 243–248.

Dickson JH, Oeggl K, Handley LL (2003). The iceman reconsidered. *Sci Am*, 288, 70–79.

Flohr S, Brinker U, Schramm A., Kierdorf U, Staude A, Piek J, Jantzen D, Hauenstein K, Orschiedt J. (2015). Flint arrowhead embedded in a human humerus from the Bronze Age site in the Tollense valley, Germany - A high-resolution micro-CT study to distinguish antemortem from perimortem projectile trauma to bone. *Int J Paleopathol*, 9, 76–81.

Gersdorff, Hans von. Feldtbůch der Wundartzney: newlich getruckt und gebessert. Strassburg: Hans Schotten zům Thyergarten (1517). Source: https://www.nlm.nih.gov/exhibition/historicalanatomies/gersdorff_bio.html.

Hartnell J. (2016). The Many Lives of the Medieval Wound Man. Essays, The Public Domain Review. https://publicdomainreview.org/2016/12/07/the-many-lives-of-the-medieval-wound-man/ (accessed September 2019).

Hutchison RL, Hirthler MA (2013). Upper extremity injuries in Homer's Iliad. *J Hand Surg Am*, 38, 1790–1793.

Kremer C, Racette S, Schellenberg M, Chaltchi A, Sauvageau A. (2008). Tameshi-giri, or Japanese sword test-cutting: a historic overview. *Am J Forensic Med Pathol*, 29, 5–8.

Kroman A. (2010). Rethinking bone trauma: a new biomechanical continuum based approach. *Proceedings of the 62nd Annual Meeting of the American Academy of Forensic Sciences*; Feb. 22–27; Seattle, WA. Colorado Springs, CO: American Academy of Forensic Sciences, 355–356.

Milroy CM, Rutty GN (1997). If a wound is "neatly incised" it is not a laceration. *BMJ*, 315 (7118), 131.

Pope, Alexander (1903). *The Complete Poetical Works*, ed. by Henry W. Boynton. Boston and New York: Houghton, Mifflin & Co. Translations from Homer, The Iliad. Book XXII The Death of Hector.

Rankin A (2011). *Seppuku: A History of Samurai Suicide*, 1st ed., Kodansha International, Tokyo; London.

Rowling JT. (1999). The death of Christopher Marlowe. *J R Soc Med*, 92, 44–446.

Seppuku. *Encyclopaedia Brittanica*, https://www.britannica.com/topic/seppuku (accessed September 2019).

# ▌ Chapter 2
# Knife Crime – Epidemiology, Impact on the Community and Legislation

## Crime Trends Involving Knives and Other Sharp Implements

### Incidence

It should be understood and obvious to all, that in many countries, a high violent crime and homicide rate, is driven by the availability and use of firearms, with knives much further down the list as the type of weapon used. Nevertheless, in many European countries and elsewhere in the world where firearms are not so easily to hand, the use of knives and other sharp weapons is responsible for a large, if not the largest, proportion of homicide or serious crime-related injury. The global homicide rate has been falling steadily over the last 25 years. The rate in 1993 was 7.4 per 100,000 population compared to 6.1 in 2017. For further details, the reader is referred to the UNDOC (United Nations Office on Drugs and Crime) publication (2019).

The incidence in young people has been reported on by Sethi et al. (2010) where they discuss the common nature of knife crime as the third leading cause of death and a leading cause of disability among people aged 10–29 in the 53 countries of the WHO European Region. They describe the multifactorial reasons for such crime and put forward proposals for improving the situation.

*Incidence in the United Kingdom*
In the United Kingdom, over the long term, the chances of being a victim of crime has fallen considerably. In adults, 4.7% were victims of violent crime in 1995 decreasing to 1.7% in the year ending March

2018 (ONS 2019). However, police-recorded crime data does show a genuine increase in some higher-harm violent offences.

Although all homicides have increased recently, this remains a low-volume crime. The total number of homicides recorded by the police rose by 8% (to 739 offences). However, recent trends are affected by the recording of exceptional incidents with multiple victims such as the terrorist attacks in London and Manchester. Despite these attacks, there has continued to be an upward trend in homicides since March 2014, indicating a change to the long-term decrease over the previous decade. Over the last year, police figures from 43 forces indicated a rise in some higher-harm violent offences involving the use of weapons. In offences involving a knife or sharp instrument there was a 7% rise to June 2019 (Figure 2.1).

The latest figures for the year ending September 2019 continued to show a 7% rise in offences involving knives or sharp instruments with a total of 44,771 offences. This is 46% higher than when comparable recording began (year ending March 2011) and the highest on record (ONS Crime statistics 2020). The use of a knife or other sharp instrument was the most common form of homicide at 40%, a similar proportion to the previous year. Further information on how offences involving a knife or sharp instrument vary by police force area can be found in the Office of National Statistics Statistical bulletin for Crime in England and Wales (ONS 2020 op. cit.) as well as in previous releases.

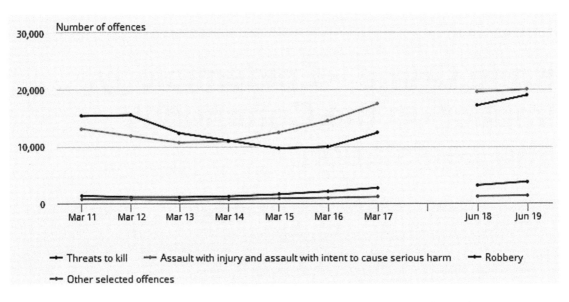

▲ **Figure 2.1** Rising trend in crimes involving knives or sharp instruments, driven by increases in assaults with injury or assaults with intent to cause serious harm and robberies. England and Wales, year ending June 2019 (ONS Crime statistics 2019). (Public domain)

# Impact of Knife Crime on Communities and on the Healthcare Burden

The rise in this type of crime is supported by admissions data for NHS hospitals in England which have shown an increase in admissions for assault by a sharp object in the year to March 2018. In the previous decade Nair et al. (2011) surveyed all patients who attended a North London Teaching Hospital between 1 January 2006 and 31 December 2008. In their series there was a gradually increasing number of stabbings among individuals in the under-20 age groups and reduced numbers in the 20–30 and above age groups. Their hospital is based in Haringey – a district of London with an age structure younger than the national average. The higher youth stabbings appear to reflect the increased gang culture and possession of penetrating weapons among young people. This is especially important in the locality where there is a history of social tension between the communities. Other factors have also been implicated in youth stabbings including increased underage drinking, drug use, exposure to violence in the media and the advent of violent gaming software. Many people have blamed the media and supermarket sales of cheap alcoholic beverages for the increased "binge drinking" cultures seen in the younger population (Simon 2008).

More recently Ashton (2019) commented on the various issues which have given rise to the increase in knife crime in the young and in particular emphasised the outcomes from the complex interactions between economics, social climate and the response by the media and state institutions. To tackle the problem, Concha-Eastman (2001) based in Columbia, proposed a holistic model encompassing structural and institutional factors as well as other facilitating problems such as the use of alcohol and drugs and the availability of weapons. Ashton (op. cit.) commended the public health work of Concha-Eastman and his colleagues who over the years have been instrumental in producing a dramatic decrease in homicides in Cali, one of the worst affected cities, where the rate in 1995 of 100/100,000, was reduced to 47.3/100,000 in 2001.

Lam et al. (2019) carried out a retrospective study of data from the emergency department at a major trauma centre in West London of patients below 18 years that had sustained a stabbing injury between March 2015 and July 2017. They focused on socioeconomic status measured using the 2015 English index of multiple deprivation (Department for Communities and Local Government, 2015). Incident postcode and home postcode were matched to an index of multiple deprivation decile, with one being the most deprived. Their study strongly indicated that there is a strong association between paediatric stabbings and areas of high deprivation and recommended that future research could be directed to intervention in such areas. As with the above authors, they highlight the importance of investment in social infrastructure and tackling the multifactorial aetiology that drives social deprivation.

It has been estimated that the annual cost to the National Health Service for all violent injury against adults is £2.2 billion per year (Bellis et al. 2008). In relation to knife crime patients treated by Emergency trauma services, the United Kingdom has witnessed a rising incidence particularly in London. Pallett et al. 2014 noted that between 1997 and 2005 the number of people admitted to hospital with an injury caused by a "sharp object" increased by 30%. Furthermore, in England and Wales during 2011–2012 there were 200 homicides, 246 attempted murders and 4,490 admissions to hospital due to a sharp object were officially recorded.

Based on the Trauma Audit and Research Network (TARN) database, the costs of penetrating trauma per patient in England and Wales have been estimated at many thousands of pounds per patient. The Department of Health in 2012, advocated a public health approach to violence prevention for England. The Health Development Agency recommended that a health needs assessment, begins with establishing the size and nature of the problem. For knife injuries, a comprehensive understanding of the type of person injured, when and how, is therefore required in order to inform future evidence-based violence prevention strategies. No national routine surveillance system exists for all knife injuries. The TARN has data entry

criteria for the most serious cases including hospital admission for longer than 72 hours. Hospital Episode Statistics (HES) also records national data but is limited by formal admission to hospital data only. Detailed descriptive studies from ad hoc surveys based in UK Emergency Departments (ED) have previously been published but are limited by non-standardised case definitions of *penetrating trauma* and *sharp objects*. Common perceptions among ED practitioners are that these injuries are substantially more prevalent than reported within existing systems, and that true *assaults* are often concealed and described as *accidents* to avoid police involvement. In addition, selective high-profile media and political attention to mortality cases alone, risks not accurately understanding true prevalence trends.

Attempts have been made at various times to reduce knife crime including the use of knife amnesties. The Home Office organised a five-week national knife amnesty in 2006, during which period 89,864 knives were handed in. The Centre for Crime and Justice Studies in their most recent report (Grimshaw and Ford 2018) have cast doubt on its success in reducing knife-carrying and knife-related offences, noting this figure constitutes less than 1% of the knives that could be used, assuming that every household in England and Wales possesses at least one kitchen knife. The amnesty also appeared to have a limited impact on crime levels. For example, the Metropolitan Police Service did notice a reduction in knife-enabled offences five weeks into their operation, but six weeks after the end of the operation these had returned to pre-operation levels (Eades et al. 2007). It appears from the available evidence that amnesties on their own are unlikely to dissuade persistent offenders from carrying knives.

# Legislation in the United Kingdom

In many countries there is legislation enacted specifically in relation to knives which limits or forbids the carrying of these implements and similar sharp objects which might be used as lethal weapons. This chapter describes current legislation in the United Kingdom, much of which is very similar to knife crime prevention legislation in other countries.

## Outline of the Relevant Acts Concerning Knives and Other Offensive Weapons

*Prevention of Crime Act 1953*
This act prohibits the carrying of any offensive weapon in a public place without lawful authority

or reasonable excuse. A public place includes private premises to which the public have access. An offensive weapon is defined as any article made or adapted for use for causing injury to the person, or intended by the person for such use.

## Restriction of Offensive Weapons Act (ROWA) 1959

This act prohibited the manufacture, sale, hire or offer for sale or hire, and importation of flick knives and gravity knives.

## Criminal Justice Act (CJA) 1988

This act created an offence of having an article with a blade or point in a public place without good reason or lawful excuse. An exemption applies to folding pocket knives with a blade of less than three inches: CJA 1988 also prohibited the manufacture, sale, hire, offer for sale or hire of a range of weapons specified in the Criminal Justice Act 1988 (Offensive Weapons) Order 1988. These are mainly items designed to cause serious injury, for example knuckledusters, hand claws and certain Martial Arts equipment, or those which can be easily concealed, including swordsticks.

## Offensive Weapons Act 1996

This act amended the 1988 Act to prohibit the sale of knives and certain articles with a blade or point to persons under 16.

## Knives Act 1997

This act created offences relating to the unlawful marketing of knives as suitable for combat, or in ways likely to stimulate or encourage violent behaviour. It also extended the power to stop and search in anticipation of violence contained in the Criminal Justice & Public Order Act 1994. Section 60 of the Criminal Justice & Public Order Act 1994, as amended by the Knives Act 1997 – contains a power under which an officer of inspector rank or above could, in certain circumstances, authorise police officers within a given area to stop and search for offensive weapons.

## Violent Crime Reduction Act 2006

This act makes further provisions and amendments to raise the minimum age to buy a knife from 16 to 18.

# Specific Provisions Made in Legislation Relating to Knife Crime Prevention

- Section 1 of the Prevention of Crime Act 1953 and section 139 of the Criminal Justice Act 1988 respectively provide for offences of having an offensive weapon in a public place without lawful authority or reasonable excuse and having an article with a blade or sharply pointed in a public place without lawful authority or good reason. A public place also includes private premises to which the public have access.

- Section 139A of the Criminal Justice Act 1988 provides that it is an offence to have an article within either of the above offences on school premises.

- Sections 139 and 139A of the Criminal Justice Act 1988 apply to any article which has a blade or point except a folding pocket knife unless the cutting edge of its blade exceeds 7.62 centimetres (3 inches).

- Section 1 of the Prevention of Crime Act 1953 provides that an offensive weapon is any article made or adapted for use for causing injury to the person, or intended by the person having it with him for such use by him or by some other person.

- Since the introduction of the Violent Crime Reduction Bill in 2005, further provisions and amendments were made in 2006 to raise the minimum age to buy a knife from 16 to 18 and increase the maximum sentence for carrying a knife from 2 to 4 years. In addition, teachers were given more power to search pupils for weapons. However, it is disturbing to find that, according to Vaughan (2019) reporting in The Independent newspaper, more than 1,000 children were caught carrying knives in schools in 2018 – with the youngest aged just 4. Weapons seized by police included machetes, hunting knives, a samurai sword and even a highlighter pen which had its nib changed to a blade. He also noted the figures obtained by Channel 5 News under Freedom of Information laws, which showed that a total of 1,144 knife possession offences in schools, where the suspect was a child, were recorded in England, Scotland and Wales in 2018. The number more than doubled over the past five years, among the 36 forces in England and Wales that provided comparable data, soaring from 372 in 2014 to 968 in 2018.

- The Knife Act 1997 created offences relating to the unlawful marketing of knives as suitable for combat, or in ways likely to stimulate or encourage violent behaviour. It also extended the power to stop and search in anticipation of violence contained in the Criminal Justice & Public Order Act 1994. It is illegal to

  - sell a knife to anyone under 18 (16- to 18-year-olds in Scotland can buy cutlery and kitchen knives) unless it is a knife with a folding blade 3 inches long (7.62cm) or less

  - carry a knife in public without good reason – unless it's a knife with a folding blade 3 inches long (7.62cm) or less

  - carry, buy or sell any type of banned knife

  - use any knife in a threatening way (even a legal knife)

  - lock knives. They are not classed as folding knives and are illegal to carry in public without good reason. Lock knives:

    - have blades that can be locked and refolded only by pressing a button

    - can include multi-tool knives – tools that also contain other devices such as a screwdriver or can opener.

## Good Reasons for Carrying a Knife or Weapon in Public

One of the essential aspects of knife legislation is for the possessor of a knife to demonstrate that he/she has a good reason for the knife being in their possession. The provision for this legislation is explicit in the Criminal Justice Act (CJA) 1988, Section 139 being the most important:

"It is an offence for any person, without lawful authority or good reason, to have with him in a public place, any article which has a blade or is sharply pointed except for a folding pocket-knife which has a cutting edge to its blade not exceeding 3 inches" [CJA 1988 section 139(1)].

The phrase "good reason" is intended to allow for "common sense" possession of knives, so that it is legal to carry a knife if there is a bona fide reason to do so. Examples of bona fide reasons which have been accepted include a knife required for one's trade (e.g. a chef's knife), as part of a national costume (Figure 2.2) or for religious reasons (e.g. a Sikh Kirpan). In this case, "public place" is meant as anywhere accessible to the public. Also, knives should only be carried to and from and used at the location where they are needed. For example, leaving a knife in a car for use when you go fishing would be illegal. It should be taken back into the house each time you use the car (other than to go fishing).

In *DPP v Gregson* – QBD (Div Ct) (McCowan LJ, Popplewell J), 21 July 1992 it was ruled that a defendant who had forgotten that he had in a public place an article (a knife with a fixed four-inch blade) to which s 139 of the Criminal Justice Act 1988 applied, could not rely on forgetfulness as constituting the defence under s 139(4) that "he had good reason . . . for having the article with him."

The special exception which exists in the Criminal Justice Act 1988 (s139) for folding knives (pocket knives) is another "common sense" measure accepting that some small knives are carried for general utility. However, even a folding pocket knife of less than 3 inches (76mm) may still be considered an offensive weapon if carried or used for that purpose. It was a long-held common belief that a folding knife must be non-locking for this provision to apply. The case law is found in a Crown Court case, *Harris v DPP*; *Fehmi v DPP* – QBD (Div Ct) (McCowan LJ, Popplewell J), 21 July 1992 in which it was ruled that a folding knife having a pointed blade of less than 3 inches and capable of being secured in an open position by a locking device was not a "folding pocketknife" within the meaning of s 139(2) of the Criminal Justice Act 1988, and carrying it in a public place was therefore an offence. To be a folding pocketknife, the blade must be readily foldable simply by the folding process. The knife was not in that category because it required the pressing of a button.

A lock knife for all legal purposes, is the same as a fixed blade knife. A folding pocket knife must be

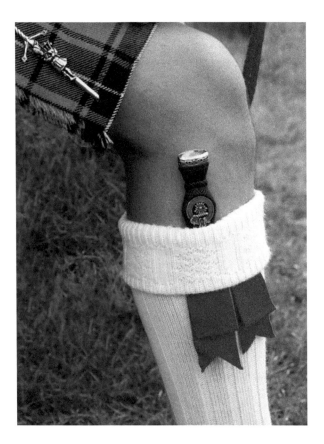

◀ **Figure 2.2** Dress Sgian Dubh with Gemstone and Clan Crest (Courtesy, The Scotland Shop, Greenknowe, Berwickshire).

**22**

readily foldable at all times. If it has a mechanism that prevents folding, it is a lock knife (or for legal purposes, a fixed blade) The Court of Appeal (*R v Desmond Garcia Deegan 1998*) upheld the Harris ruling stating that "folding was held to mean non-locking". No leave to appeal was granted.

Although English law insists that it is the responsibility of the prosecution to provide evidence proving a crime has been committed, an individual must provide evidence to prove that they had a bona fide reason for carrying a knife (if this is the case). Whilst this may appear to be a reversal of the usual burden of proof, technically the prosecution has already proven the case (prima facie) by establishing that a knife was being carried in a public place.

## Age Restriction

British law also covers age restriction on the sale of knives in the Criminal Justice Act 1998:

"It is an offence for any person to sell to a person under the age of 18 any knife, knife blade, razor blade, axe or any other article which has a blade or is sharply pointed and which is made or adapted for causing injury to the person" [CJA 1988 section 141A]. British courts have in the past taken the marketing of a particular brand of knife into account when considering whether an otherwise legal folding knife was carried as an offensive weapon. A knife which is marketed as "tactical", "military", "special ops", etc., could therefore carry an extra liability. The Knives Act 1997 now restricts the marketing of knives as being offensive weapons and thus it is much more unlikely that such marketing could be used as evidence against a defendant. In practice, this law makes it highly unlikely that most shops would sell a knife to someone younger than 18.

## Illegal Knives

In the UK, the main knife legislation is found in the Criminal Justice Act (CJA) 1988. However certain types of knife are banned under the Restriction of Offensive Weapons Act (ROWA) 1959, the relevant section of the latter being Section 1.

"It is an offence for a person to manufacture, sell, hire or offer for sale or hire or expose or have in his possession for the purpose of sale or hire, or lend or give to any person:

A) any knife which has a blade which opens automatically by hand pressure applied to a button, spring or other device in or attached to the handle of the knife, sometimes known as a "flick knife" or "flick gun";

or,

B) any knife which has a blade which is released from the handle or sheath thereof by the force of gravity or the application of centrifugal force and which, when released, is locked in place by means of a button, spring, lever, or other device, sometimes known as a "gravity knife" [ROWA 1959 S 1(1)].

[ROWA 1959 S 1(2)] also makes it illegal to import knives of this type. As a result, it is (almost) impossible to obtain possession of such a knife without either committing or abetting an offence. Note that the above legislation does not refer to possession of such knives other than possession for the purpose of sale or hire. It is therefore not illegal per se to merely possess such a knife. This law is aimed primarily at knives designed with features specific to fighting/assault rather than use as a tool.

*Banned Knives in the United Kingdom*

- butterfly knives (also known as "balisongs") – a blade hidden inside a handle that splits in the middle

- disguised knives – a blade or sharp point hidden inside what looks like everyday objects such as a buckle, phone, brush or lipstick

- flick knives (also known as "switchblades" or "automatic knives") – a blade hidden inside a handle which shoots out when a button is pressed

- gravity knives

- stealth knives – a knife or spike not made from metal (except when used at home, for food or a toy)

- zombie knives – a knife with a cutting edge, a serrated edge and images or words suggesting it is used for violence

- swords, including samurai swords – a curved blade over 50cm (with some exceptions, such as antiques and swords made to traditional methods before 1954)

- sword-sticks – a hollow walking stick or cane containing a blade

- push daggers

- shurikens (also known as "shaken," "death stars" or "throwing stars")

- kusari-gama – a sickle attached to a rope, cord or wire

- kyoketsu-shoge – a hook-knife attached to a rope, cord or wire

# References

Ashton J. (2019). Tackling violence as a public health issue. *J R Soc Med.* 112, 164–165.

Bellis MA, Hughes K, Anderson Z, Tocque K, Hughes S. (2008). Contribution of violence to health inequalities in England: demographics and trends in emergency hospital admissions for assault. *J Epidemiol Commun Health.* 62, 1064–1071.

Concha-Eastman A. (2001). Violence: a challenge for public health and 'Health For All'. *J Epidemiol Commun Health.* 55, 597–599.

Criminal Justice Act 1988. https://www.legislation.gov.uk/ukpga/1988/33/section/139 (Accessed June 2017).

Criminal Justice Act 1988 (Offensive Weapons) Order 1988 http://www.legislation.gov.uk/uksi/1988/2019/made (accessed January 2020).

Criminal Justice & Public Order Act 1994. http://www.legislation.gov.uk/ukpga/1994/33/contents (accessed January 2020).

Department for Communities and Local Government. The English index of multiple deprivation (IMD) 2015 – guidance. https://assets.publishing.service.gov.uk/government/uploads/system/uploads/attachment_data/file/464430/English_Index_of_Multiple_Deprivation_2015_-_Guidance.pdf (accessed January 2020).

Department of Health (2012). Protecting people Promoting health A public health approach to violence prevention for England. www.gov.uk/government/publications/a-public-health-approach-to-violence-prevention-in-england

Eades C, Grimshaw R, Silvestri A, Solomon E (2007). Knife crime: a review of evidence and policy, 2nd ed., London: Centre for Crime and Justice Studies, p. 27.

Grimshaw R, Ford M. (2018). Young people, violence and knives - revisiting the evidence and policy discussions. Justice Policy Review Focus Issue 3. Centre for Crime and Justice Studies, The Hadley Trust. UK.

Harris v DPP 1 All ER 562, [1993] 1 WLR 82, 96 Cr App Rep 235, 157 JP 205 (1992).

Lam C, Aylwin,C, Khan M. (2019). Are paediatric stabbings in London related to socioeconomic status? *Trauma*. 21, 310–316.

Nair MS, Uzzaman MM, Al-Zuhir N, Jadeja A, Navaratnam R. (2011) Changing trends in the pattern and outcome of stab injuries at a North London hospital. *J Emergencies, Trauma,Shock*. 4, 455–460.

Office for National Statistics. (2019). The nature of violent crime in England and Wales: year ending March 2018.

Offensive Weapons Act 1996. http://www.legislation.gov.uk/ukpga/1996/26/contents (accessed January 2020).

Office of National Statistics. Statistical bulletin. Crime in England and Wales: year ending. June 2019 (and previous releases). Release date 23rd January 2020. https://www.ons.gov.uk/peoplepopulationandcommunity/crimeandjustice/bulletins/crimeinenglandandwales/yearendingoctober2019 (accessed March 2020)

Office of National Statistics. Statistical bulletin. Crime in England and Wales: year ending. September 2019 (and previous releases). Release date 23rd January 2020. https://www.ons.gov.uk/peoplepopulationandcommunity/crimeandjustice/bulletins/crimeinenglandandwales/yearendingseptember2019 (accessed March 2020)

Pallett JR, Sutherland E, Glucksman E, Tunnicliff M, Keep JW. (2014). A cross-sectional study of knife injuries at a London major trauma centre. *Ann R Coll Surg Engl*. 96, 23–26.

Prevention of Crime Act 1953 (Section 1). https://www.legislation.gov.uk/ukpga/Eliz2/1-2/14/section/1 (Accessed June 2017).

R- v - Desmond Garcia Deegan [1998] EWCA Crim 385, [1998] Crim LR 562, [1998] 2 Cr App R 121

Restriction of Offensive Weapons Act (ROWA) 1959 http://www.legislation.gov.uk/ukpga/Eliz2/7-8/37/section/1 (Accessed June 2017).

Sethi D, Hughes K, Bellis M, Mitis F, Racioppi F (2010). World Health Organization, Europe. European Report on Preventing Violence and Knife Crime among Young People. WHO Regional Office for Europe, Copenhagen, Denmark. http://www.euro.who.int/__data/assets/pdf_file/0012/121314/E94277.pdf?ua=1

Simon M. (2008). Reducing youth exposure to alcohol ads: targeting public transit. *J Urban Health* 85, 506–516.

The Knives Act 1997. https://www.legislation.gov.uk/ukpga/1997/21/contents (Accessed June 2017).

United Nations Office on Drugs and Crime (UNODC) (2019). Global study on homicide https://www.unodc.org/unodc/en/data-and-analysis/global-study-on-homicide.html (accessed on 1st October 2019).

Vaughan H. (2019). Knife crime: children as young as four among hundreds caught with blades at school. Independent newspaper, 23rd August 2019.

Violent Crime Reduction Act 2006. http://www.legislation.gov.uk/ukpga/2006/38/contents (accessed January 2020).

# ▌Chapter 3
# Types of Knives and the Dynamics of Sharp Force Trauma

Although many types of implements are capable of causing sharp force trauma, undoubtedly the most common type of implement associated with forensic work is the knife. Accordingly, this chapter will give an account of the structure of different types of knives and the dynamics of the trauma they produce.

Although the focus, particularly in this chapter, will be on the knife, the importance of other sharp-edged implements will be described throughout the book in the context of the type of situations in which they occur and injuries that are caused.

## Types of Knives – Historical Perspective

Knives have existed since man started making tools at least since 2.6 million years ago (Smithsonian, National Museum of History, 2020) and are recognised as one of the most important tools to help him/her survive. The knife has an important role in all aspects of culture from food preparation to combat, as well as building and construction. It can be adapted in shape and size according to the basic materials available at each time. With the passage of time, fire enabled the melting and use of metals to forge stronger blades compared to their older stone counterparts.

In Neolithic times cutting implements were in the form of flakes of flint, quartz or obsidian (a form of volcanic glass produced from felsic larva). They had either a single or two cutting edges and some were pointed in order to facilitate a stabbing action (Figure 3.1). In addition to their usefulness as a tool for cutting in general, they were also used as weapons in hunting and killing animals

Tapered knives throughout history have had either one or two cutting edges and some, which were used as weapons in hunting, also had pointed tips to be more efficient at stabbing. Unlike modern knives, the blade and handle were one solid piece. Today the knife has evolved into a much more technological implement consisting of blades which are fixed or folding and made from advanced materials such as iron, steel, copper, bronze and titanium.

The use of pointed knives for eating had been recognized for some time as dangerous since they could readily be used for stabbing someone, for example, during a disagreement at the dining table and elsewhere. As a result, in 1669 King Louis XIV of France decreed "illegal" all pointed knives on the street or used at the dinner table, and ordered all knife points to be ground down, like those similarly used today, in order to reduce violence (Patrick and Thompson 2009; Hern et al. 2005).

## Modern Knives

There is a huge variety of knives manufactured today and it is beyond the scope of this book to give an exhaustive description of these. For those readers who wish for further detailed information, there are innumerable websites that can readily be accessed, carrying information on knives of all types and their uses.

Knives can be categorised based on either their shape or function and in this text I will describe those that are encountered in forensic casework. They can be categorised into broadly generic types based on their construction and anatomical features or by their function.

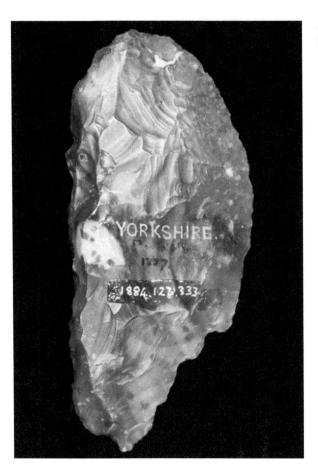

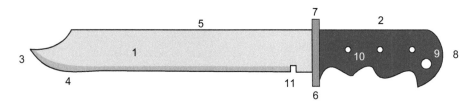

▲ **Figure 3.2** Common parts of the modern knife. (Source: Author)

# Knife Parts

The modern knife, in general terms, has a number of parts as numbered below and shown in Figure 3.2.

1. the *blade*

2. the *handle*

3. the *tip* tapering to the *point* – the end of the knife used for piercing

4. the *edge* – the cutting surface of the knife extending from the point to the heel

5. the *spine* – the thickest section of the blade; on a single-edged knife, the side opposite the edge; on a two-edged knife, more towards the middle

6. the *ricasso* – the flat section of the blade located at the junction of the blade and the knife's hilt or guard

---

* This prehistoric flint knife, with a curved edge and straight back, is probably Neolithic in date. Its recorded provenance, "Yorkshire", is unspecific, but the faded number in black ink, "1337", matches with a manuscript source dating from 1874 in which Pitt-Rivers recorded a "triangular flint knife or arrowhead" in his collection. Pitt-Rivers was a Yorkshireman by birth, and returned there throughout his life; so the object could have been acquired by him any time before 1874, in the first 47 years of his life. Quoted from http://excavatingpittrivers.blogspot.com/2014/08/prehistoric-yorkshire.html

7. the *hilt* or *guard* – the barrier between the blade and the handle which prevents the hand from slipping forward onto the blade and protects the hand from the external forces that are usually applied to the blade during use

8. the *butt* – the end of the handle utilised for blunt force

9. the *lanyard hole*– for a strap to secure the knife to the wrist

10. the *rivets (pins)* for securing the tang in the handle slabs

11. the *choil* allows the knife to be sharpened all the way to the tang.

## Handle

The handle, used to grip and manipulate the blade safely, may include a tang, a portion of the blade that extends into the handle. Knives are made with partial tangs (extending part way into the handle, known as "stick tangs") or full tangs (extending the full length of the handle, often visible on top and bottom). The handle may include a bolster, a piece of heavy material (usually metal) situated at the front or rear of the handle. The bolster, as its name suggests, is used to mechanically strengthen the knife. A variety of materials are used to construct a knife handle which is often textured or grooved for a better grip. Some of the most commonly used materials include wood, Kraton (synthetic rubber replacement made by Kraton Polymers) leather, injection moulding from higher-grade plastics, stainless steel and Micarta. The latter is composed of canvas, paper, linen, carbon fibre, fibre glass and other thermosetting plastics, and due to its durability and stability, is an extremely popular option.

## Blade

The blade edge can be plain or serrated or a combination of both. Single-edged knives may have a *reverse edge* or *false edge* occupying a section of the spine. These edges are usually serrated and are used to further enhance function. In terms of the overall construction, the blade may be in a fixed position in relation to the handle or able to fold into the handle.

A fixed blade knife is one in which the blade does not fold and extends most of the way into the handle. This type of knife is typically stronger and larger than a folding knife. Activities that require a strong blade, such as hunting or fighting, typically rely on fixed blade knives.

A folding or pocket knife is one that has a pivot between handle and blade, allowing the blade to fold into the handle. Most folding knives are small working blades (pocket knives are usually folding knives (Figure 3.3). Some folding knives have a locking mechanism: The most traditional and commonplace lock is the *slip-joint*. It consists of a back spring that wedges itself into a notch on the tang on the back of the blade. In some, a small knob or thumbscrew, allows the user to open the knife quickly with one hand.

**27**

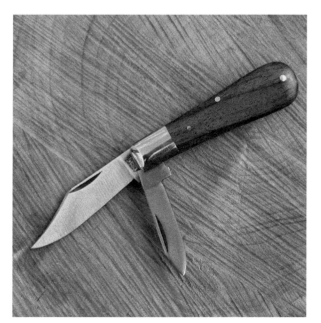

◀ **Figure 3.3** Two-bladed folding knife (Public domain)

In assessing the characteristics of a knife blade it should be appreciated that there are many different designs of blade, possessing a large variety of shape and size depending on the knife's function, as stated above. The knife illustrations that follow show a number of current blade types that may be encountered. As the reader will see, it is by no means exhaustive but demonstrates those commonly seen (Figures 3.4–3.13).

## Knife Types by Function

- In general, knives are either working *everyday use blades*, or *fighting knives*. The term *hunting knife* is used loosely to mean any standard straight blade sheath knife that is at least somewhat geared towards real hunting use. There are, however, some types of knives that are made specifically for hunting practices.

- Many other knives are designed for all types of domestic and outdoor use. In particular, utility or multi-tool knives, which may contain several blades to facilitate their use, have proved to be very popular.

- Large agricultural and fighting knives such as the kukri and the machete are common in Africa and Asia.

- Another type of knife, only very occasionally seen in modern forensic practice, includes the dagger which is a short bladed weapon designed for stabbing rather than cutting.

The pathologist will be required to assess the type and dimensions of the implement which caused injury whenever this is possible: thus estimation of blade width and length, sharpness of the cutting edge and, if a stab wound is present, the characteristics of the non-cutting edge if the knife has only a single cutting side. The characteristics of the guard or the ricasso, may be visible, indicating entry of the complete length of the blade. The term hilt is also commonly used and refers to the enlarged section of the handle and protected by the guard which in turn protects the hand from an opponent's knife or sword.

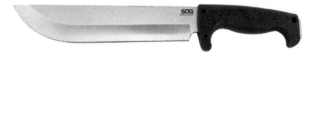

◀ **Figure 3.4** *A normal or straight back blade* has a curving edge and flat back. A dull back allows the wielder to press down with the thumb to get leverage and concentrate force; it also makes the knife heavy and strong for its size. The curve concentrates force on a small point, making cutting easier. (Public domain)

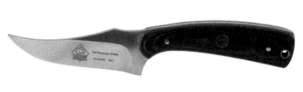

◀ **Figure 3.5** A curved, *trailing-point knife* has a back edge that curves upward. This lets a lightweight knife have a larger curve on its edge. Such a knife is optimised for slicing, skinning or slashing. (Public domain)

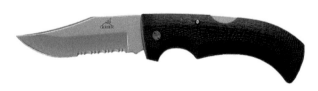

◀ **Figure 3.6** A *clip-point blade* is like a normal blade with the back "clipped" or concavely formed to make the tip thinner and sharper. The back edge of the clip may have a false edge that could be sharpened to make a second edge. The sharp tip is useful as a pick, or for cutting in tight places. The Bowie knife has a clipped blade and clip-points are quite common on pocket knives and other folding knives. (Public domain)

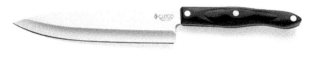

◀ **Figure 3.7** *A drop-point blade* has a convex curve of the back towards the point. It handles much like the clip-point though with a stronger point less suitable for piercing. Swiss army pocket knives often have drop-points on their larger blades. (Public domain)

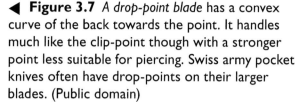

◀ **Figure 3.8** *A spear-point blade* is a symmetrical blade with a spine that runs along the middle of the blade. The point is in line with the spine. Spear-points may be single-edged (with a false edge) or double-edged or may have only a portion of the second edge sharpened. Pen-knives are often single-edged, non-spined spear-points, usually quite small, named for their past use in sharpening quills for writing. Some throwing knives may have spear-points but without the spine, being only flat pieces of metal. (Public domain)

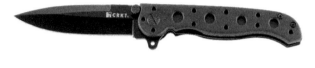

◀ **Figure 3.9** *A needle-point blade* is a symmetrical, highly tapered, twin-edged blade often seen in commando knives. Its long, narrow point offers good penetration but is liable to breakage if abused. The design may also be referred to as a stiletto or (slender variety of) dagger due to its use as a stabbing weapon albeit one very capable of slashing as well. (Public domain)

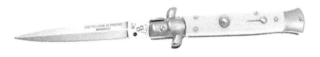

◀ **Figure 3.10** *A spay-point knife* (once used for spaying animals) has a single, mostly straight edge that curves strongly upwards at the end to meet a short, dull, straight clip from the dull back. With the curved end of the blade being closer to perpendicular to the blade's axis than other knives and lacking a point, making penetration unlikely. (Public domain)

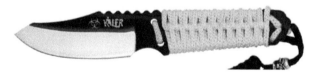

◀ **Figure 3.11** A Westernised *tanto style* knife has a somewhat chisel-like point that is thick towards the point (being close to the spine) and is thus quite strong. It is superficially similar to the points on most Japanese long and short swords (katana and wakizashi). (Public domain)

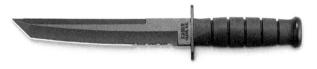

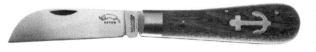

◀ **Figure 3.12** *A sheepsfoot* knife has a straight edge and a straight dull back that curves towards the edge at the end. It gives the most control, because the dull back edge is made to be held by fingers. (Public domain)

29

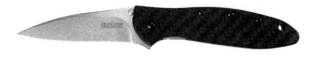

◀ **Figure 3.13** *A Wharncliffe blade* is similar in profile to a sheep's foot but the curve of the back edge starts closer to the handle and is more gradual. Its blade is much thicker than a knife of comparable size. (Public domain)

# Dynamics

Dynamics, in the context of sharp force trauma, refers to a complex interaction of variables to produce injury. This chapter will discuss the issues arising that need to be considered and assessed by pathologists and others involved in the investigation of such injuries and by those involved in the design of protective clothing used against knife assaults.

In assessing the dynamics, which affect the force of impact of a weapon and thus the potential severity of inflicted trauma, it is important to consider:

- The types of forces involved in different kinds of impacts

- The mechanism of producing various types of sharp force trauma

- The resistance offered to impacts from types of clothing, skin, subcutaneous tissue, bone muscle and organs.

## Forces Involved in Stabbings and Other Sharp Force Trauma and Influencing Factors

*Introduction*

The pathologist is frequently required to assess the amount of force used in stabbing, in order to assist with establishing the intent of the attacker. However, it is difficult to quantify biomechanical measurements that are made in a laboratory, with the real-life situation of a dynamic event, which is then presented to a pathologist in the autopsy room. Most pathologists (apart from a few that prefer not to be drawn to give a view on the matter) express their opinion in a subjective manner, employing non-validated scales of 1–10 or categories such as slight, moderate or severe, or by using analogous phraseology such as likening the stab to a *hard punch*. Furthermore, its estimation may well not equate with the severity of the wound itself in terms of the length of its

track or organs injured. It is evident that, all other conditions being equal, (and such equality may be difficult to demonstrate in each case) that an impact with greater force is much more likely to produce a more severe injury than an impact of lesser force. Nolan et al. (2018) in an attempt to evaluate the use of a scale, such as that based *on mild, moderate or severe* carried out studies using a dynamometer to measure the peak forces achieved by adult male and female volunteers by stabbing skin simulants and porcine samples with knives and screwdrivers. They concluded that it was inappropriate to use a subjective scale and suggested that four areas should be investigated by the pathologist in relation to the force required: the radius of the tip of the weapon, minimal force required for penetration, the sex of the assailant and whether the penetrating force necessary to penetrate the skin is greater than can be produced by the assailant.

The difficulty in quantifying force for a sharp implement to penetrate human tissue as well as clothing, adds to the problem faced by the forensic pathologist as to whether a knife wound was caused with intent (and the degree of intent), or whether the victim fell or ran onto a knife. The ability to measure force objectively, rather than what currently routinely amounts to a subjective impression as stated by Nolan et al. (op. cit.), would assist in reducing the doubt regarding the alleged accidental cases and assist in assessing the effort and speed of repetition of the blows in multiple stabbings.

In the clinical setting it should also be appreciated that unnecessary deaths still occur in cases where the stab wound track length and the severity of trauma to the underlying structures is not fully appreciated by clinicians treating a victim. Knowledge of the various factors involved in the production and severity of different injuries in different locations of the body would assist doctors to rapidly and effectively assess injury severity and commence appropriate treatment.

Despite, therefore, the difficulty of expressing the magnitude of the force involved as described above, it is essential that both pathologists in the mortuary and clinicians dealing with acute emergencies, appreciate the various factors which are instrumental in the causation and degree of severity of injuries in any assault by a sharp weapon. These factors itemised below need to be taken into account and carefully assessed in the overall estimation of force and its relationship to the severity of injury.

- *Intrinsic properties of the knife:* Shape and sharpness of the knife blade; weight of the knife

- *Delivery of blow by the assailant and assailant type:* Velocity of the thrust, including follow through on impact; type of thrust (whether over arm or under arm); trained or untrained assailant, gender, age and state of health

- *Movement of the knife up to the point of impact with the skin which is affected by the victim:* Clothing; properties of the skin; movement of victim

- *Movement of the knife after penetration of the skin to its point of termination in the body:* Resistance offered by bone; resistance offered of soft tissue and organs; movement of victim, assailant and knife.

In other words, in the assessment of force, consideration should take account of the multifactorial nature of the assault from the movement of the knife up to the point of impact with the skin and from the skin to the point of termination within the body.

*Delivery of the Weapon to the Body and Stabbing Techniques Used*

Furthermore, both these two phases must be considered in conjunction with the properties of the knife as well as the way the assailant delivers the blow, in terms of speed and direction. In relation to the speed of a knife on entry, Miller and Jones (1996) found from their study in which they investigated the differences in the magnitude of force involved with four different stabbing actions (long and short overarm and long and short underarm) that long overarm motion produced greater entry speeds than the corresponding short overarm delivery. This is because the longer overarm motion allows extra speed to be built up over the longer path of the knife. The underarm delivery produces less speed than the overarm methods. Examples of overarm and underarm stabbing actions with the position of the knife in the hand are shown in Figures 3.14 and 3.15.

The technique in which a knife is used plays an important part not only on the amount of force

31

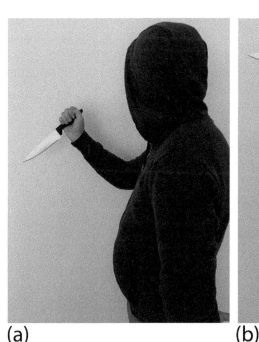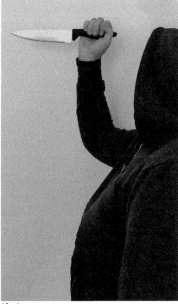

(a) (b)

◀ **Figure 3.14** (a) Short and (b) long overarm action showing position of hand with knife blade protruding from the ulnar aspect of the palm and little finger. (Source: Author)

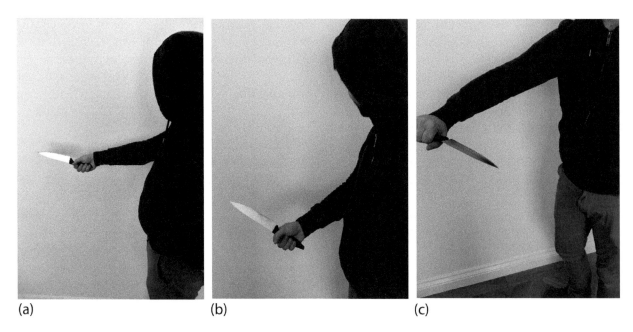

(a)  (b)  (c)

▲ **Figure 3.15** (a), (b) and (c) Underarm positions of hand with knife blade protruding from the radial side of the palm at the thumb and forefinger. The underhand deliveries produce less speed than the overarm methods. (Source: Author)

delivered to the victim (Miller and Jones, 1996; Horsfall, 2005) but also on the follow-through mechanics after impact. Thus the expertise of the weapon user is an important consideration and recent work has highlighted how weapons are used by a trained user (Carr et al. 2019; Mahoney et al. 2017). The various grips of a knife used by trained users to deliver a quick and targeted impact have been described by Carr et al. (op. cit) and some of these are shown in Figures 3.16–3.19.

*Skin Resistance and Underlying Tissue*

Before means were available to accurately assess the dynamics of stabbing, observers were of the view that once the skin had been pierced, then, unless the knife impacted against bone, there was virtually no resistance offered by the internal soft tissues including the major organs (Knight 1975). Later work by a number of researchers have given us a more accurate assessment of the situation and indeed the appreciation that we are dealing with a more complex scenario than previously appreciated (Chadwick et al. 1999, Horsfall et al. 1999).

The mechanical properties of human skin have been studied by numerous authors but attention has largely been focussed on the elastic response (tensile strength) prior to failure, using skin simulants. Ankerson et al. (1999) used pig skin as a simulant in experiments. They employed tensile tests to identify suitable skin simulants with synthetic chamois and pigskin as candidate materials. Quasi-static penetration experiments were also performed in which a knife blade penetrated a skin simulant target (Ankerson et al. 1998). Pigskin was found to be much stronger than chamois under tensile load yet the puncture resistance was almost identical for the two materials.

It appears that once the skin has been pierced, significant resistance may be offered by the internal organs and other soft tissues. This is not merely of academic interest. Once the knife has impacted on the skin and even after piercing it, there still needs to be a firm hand on the knife to push the weapon further into the body because it has been slowed down by the resistance offered by the skin.

O'Callaghan et al. (1999) in their experiments to investigate skin and other human tissue resistance, constructed an instrumented knife using a piezo-electric force transducer (Brüel and Kjær type 8200) which was sandwiched between the handle and blade. Any force produced between the handle and the blade was transmitted to the transducer which produced an output in the form of charge (C); the amount of charge produced being proportional to the applied force (tension or compression). The study involving stabbing of amputation specimens and

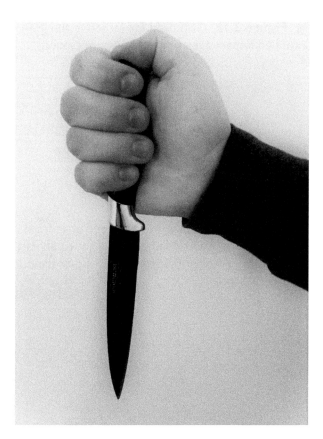

◀ **Figure 3.16** Knife gripped with the thumb capping the end of the handle to prevent it slipping back on to the hand. (Source: Author)

◀ **Figure 3.17** Grip used to throw a knife which can also serve for putting body weight behind the knife in a stabbing action to assist penetration of clothing. (Source: Author)

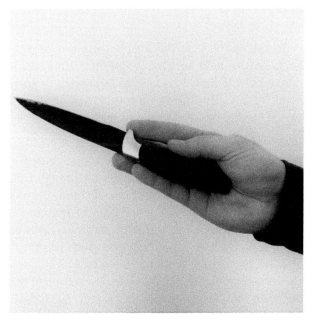

cadaveric tissue and results were recorded for stabs made into the tissues of the thigh to a depth of 10 cm (to the hilt of the knife) and through various combinations of dissected tissues which included

- skin, subcutaneous fat and muscle

- subcutaneous fat and muscle

- muscle only

- subcutaneous fat only.

They found that skin provided the greatest resistance to penetration, the mean penetration force being 49.5 N. However, considerable secondary resistance forces not previously recognised were found when

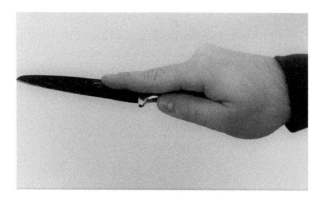

**Figure 3.18** Grip used for targeting the intended impact area more accurately. (Source: Author)

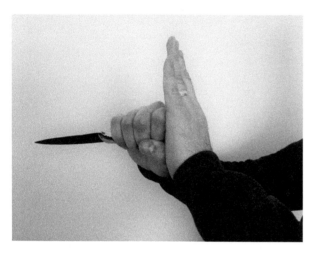

**Figure 3.19** Grip with reinforced push from the other hand with added body weight to enable penetration of heavy clothing or soft body armour. (Source: Author)

the knife was stabbed into the tissues underlying the skin. The resistance of subcutaneous fat to penetration was found to be low in comparison with that of skin and muscle. They showed that subcutaneous fat resists penetration until a force of magnitude 2 N is attained, implying that deep penetration of fat tissue means very little in terms of force.

The diminished resistive force involving underlying tissues may be easily overcome by the follow-through of an assailant performing a stabbing action and can be considered inconsequential for this situation. However resistive force of various soft tissues is of importance when considering penetration due to a projectile, e.g. when a knife is thrown. Since force is directly proportional to energy, the kinetic energy possessed by the projectile is absorbed by the resistive force of the underlying tissues which will result in a reduced depth of penetration.

In an accidental stabbing or where a knife has been thrown, one would expect there to be less penetration into the body. In the case of accidental stabbing, it is much more likely that once resistance is offered by the skin, there would not be a follow-through thrust as in a deliberate movement. To produce such a further

deliberate movement, the weapon would need to be anchored or held firmly. To produce impalement onto a knife there would need to be enough momentum by the victim moving towards the knife, and it would need to be fixed firmly in some way.

In a study carried out by O'Callaghan et al. (2001) in relation to a case involving a stab wound caused by glass, they emphasised that the follow-through from a firm grip which would have force behind it, would exceed the threshold for penetration of muscle and leave the impression that no further force was required. A thrown object as opposed to one which was firmly gripped, has a finite amount of energy which is used up in overcoming the resistance to penetration of skin and then muscle to a much lesser extent. As energy is related to the product of force applied over a distance, its energy will diminish the deeper it penetrates until it stops. In other words, the main resistance will be by the skin to cause significant loss of its kinetic energy and because there would be no follow-through, the penetration into the body may not be deep because of the further resistance of the internal tissue.

Testing was carried out by Muggenthaler et al. (2013) to assess which of three possible ways, based on witness statements, had caused a 3-cm-deep stab wound to a woman's neck. These were (a) by the knife having been thrown from a distance of about one metre, (b) accidentally slipping from the hand or (c) with the knife being held whilst stabbing. They carried out experiments to assess which was the most likely by using the knife in question and four comparable knives. The victim was represented by a pig carcass. Four male and three female subjects performed test throws which were documented by video recordings, and measurements of the penetration depth were noted. Six of the seven subjects were able to generate stab wounds by throwing the knives, whereas a knife accidentally slipping from the hand never caused a stab wound in the tests.

*Knife Throwing*

Knife throwing has its roots in prehistoric times when early man used throwing sticks to hunt animals. The throwing stick, widely considered one of the first weapons to be used by prehistoric man, is similar to the boomerang used by Aborigines in Australia. After man began to make metal objects the technology was soon used to make deadlier weapons, including metal knifes. Throwing knifes almost immediately became a practical, supplemental weapon and warriors began to carry them into battle as backup weapons.

During the nineteenth century, the sport of knife throwing began to grow in popularity. Competitions were designed to find out who had the most skill and accuracy. Soon circuses began to feature knife throwing acts (Figure 3.20). There have been very occasional accidental injuries seen in knife throwing when part of a performance act, on television and in various places of entertainment. The most famous knife-throwing stunt is called *The Wheel of Death*. This involves strapping the knife thrower's assistant, usually an attractive girl, to a large wooden wheel, which is then spun around. The knives are thrown as the girl continues to spin on the wheel.

*Intrinsic Properties of Knife Blades and Penetration Force*

From work carried out by Nı´ Annaidh et al. (2013, 2015), examining the individual characteristics of knife blades, it can be seen that the tip angle is the most important characteristic dimension, having the largest variation in penetration force over the chosen range. Because the tip angle and the tip radius are the regions that make the first contact with the skin, these two dimensions appear to be dominant. They also found that once the blade indents beyond that distance, it is the tip angle that becomes the dominant dimension (Figure 3.21).

35

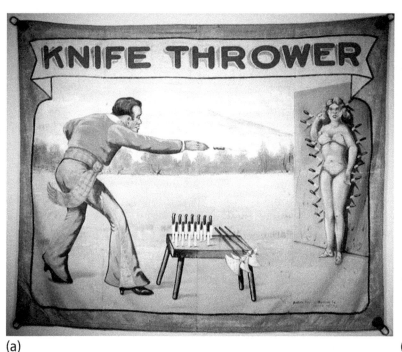

(a)

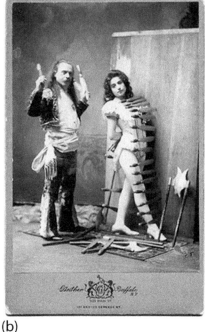

(b)

▲ **Figure 3.20** (a) Vintage poster of knife throwing circus act. (b) Victorian antique cabinet photo of knife thrower and female assistant (Public domain).

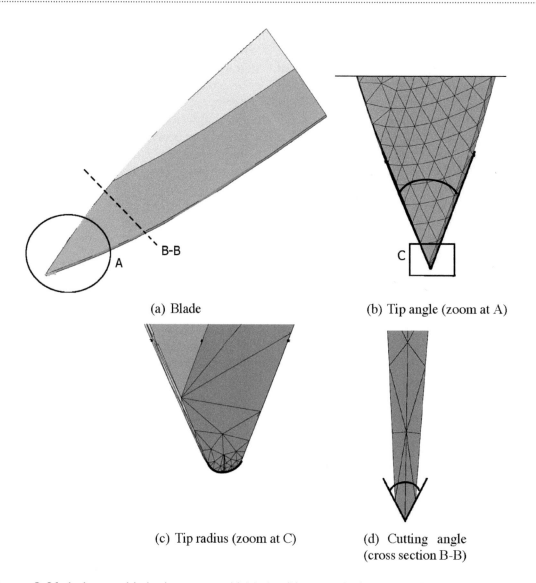

(a) Blade  (b) Tip angle (zoom at A)

(c) Tip radius (zoom at C)  (d) Cutting angle (cross section B-B)

▲ **Figure 3.21** Indicative blade dimensions (a) blade, (b) tip angle (zoom at A), (c) tip radius (zoom at C), (d) cutting angle (cross-section B-B). (Source: Courtesy Annaidh AN, Cassidy M, Curtis M, Destrade M, Gilchrist MD (2013). A combined experimental and numerical study of stab-penetration forces. Forensic Sci Int., 233:7–13.)

The authors (Ní Annaidh et al., op. cit.) incorporated the results of their stab-penetration simulations into a "stab metric" which aims to predict the minimum penetration force for a given blade. Multiple linear regression techniques were used to fit the data to a statistical model.

A total of 30 different simulations with varying blade dimensions were modelled and the evaluated model was given by the following equation:

$$\text{Penetration Force} = 15{:}45 + 0.016\ \text{TR} + 0{:}69\ \text{TA} + 0.16\ \text{CA}$$

where TR is the blade tip radius in micrometres, TA is the blade tip angle in degrees and CA is the cutting

angle in degrees. The penetration force has dimensions of Newtons in this form of the equation. This model has been used to quantify the effect of blade geometry on the magnitude of force and could be used to predict the minimum force required by a given blade to penetrate bare skin.

Their tests also included consideration of other important elements in the estimation of force of penetration including

• *Presence of clothing*: Stab-penetration tests were carried out on polyurethane at 100 mm/min with various layers of clothing present. For the four types of clothing tested (cotton, tracksuit, fleece and denim), they found an increase in

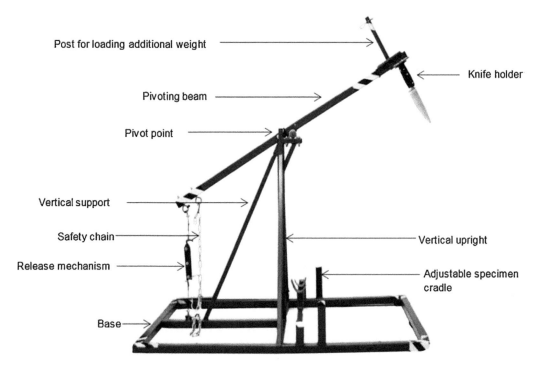

Post for loading additional weight

Knife holder

Pivoting beam

Pivot point

Vertical support

Safety chain

Vertical upright

Release mechanism

Adjustable specimen cradle

Base

▲ **Figure 3.22** Device with labelled components for analysing forces in knife attacks. Safety mechanisms designed to prevent accidental release of pivoting beam and a trigger mechanism allows remote release. (Source: Courtesy Humphrey C, Kumaratilake J, Henneberg MA (2016). Stab in the dark: Design and construction of a novel device for conducting incised knife trauma investigations and its initial test. Forensic Science International 262, 276–281.)

penetration force varying from 10% for cotton to 50% for denim for a single layer of clothing. Adding additional layers of clothing has an accumulative effect on the penetration force.

- *Knife blades v non-blade implements:* They compared the penetration force of knife blades to the non-blade implements in their experiments and found that the much blunter objects they used (scissors, flat head screwdriver, Phillips screwdriver) could exceed 300% of the penetration force of a sharp-bladed implement. In addition, it was found that the blunt implements failed to puncture the skin or polyurethane at 1m/s, and simply rebounded off with no visible damage to the material.

- *Speed of attack:* Similarly, the influence of the speed of attack was investigated by examining a range of test speeds varying from quasi-static (50 mm/min) to dynamic (up to 9.2 m/s). They found that the test speed had a statistically significant effect on the penetration force (P = 0.002).

More recently, Humphrey et al. (2016) constructed a device to analyse the characteristics and forces involved in knife attacks, particularly incised wounds (Figure 3.22). The mechanical variables (e.g. force, angle, knife geometry) involved in knife attacks were considered in order to design and construct a suitable device, which allowed these variables to be systematically controlled and varied. They included a pivoting arm and instrumented knife holder. The arm had an adjustable angle and weight so that knives could be operated at different calculated forces. They investigated the repeatability of incised knife trauma and produced findings which appear promising.

*Stab Protection from Body Armour Systems*
Stabbing assaults against police and prison officers and in close combat military conflict, have necessitated the development of protective stab-resistant armour systems. Stab threats can be classified into two categories: puncture and incised (slash). Stab attacks generate high loads; to defeat them armour needs to be of a certain thickness and stiffness. Commercially, a number of stab-resistant materials are available. Metal ring mesh (also called "chain mail") is frequently used for cut protection in commercial applications such as meat packing, and have

also been incorporated into some stab-resistant vests. These ring meshes, however, do not provide puncture resistance. Other commercial designs utilise layers of titanium foil, which offer both cut and puncture resistance. However, both the foil and mesh solutions are relatively heavy and offer little ballistic resistance.

The specification for the level of protection of the modern knife-resistant body armour, which is issued to the Police is designed to prevent serious injury or death, was derived from tests which simulated the energies generated by human stabbing attempts with test blades. The maximum permissible depth of penetration of a blade through armour into the human body was arrived at by CT and ultrasound studies (Bleetman and Dyer (2000); Connor et al. (1998); Croft (2003).

In clinical practice, slash wounds are much more commonly encountered than stabbing, yet little consideration has been given to the type and distribution of knife wounding to the body in determining the areas of the body which require protection from such wounds. Slash attacks produce much lower loads, and armour designed to defeat them can be far lighter and more flexible. Stab-resistant armour will defeat slash attempts, but slash-resistant armour will not offer protection against stabbing. By providing more coverage to the body for anti-stab and anti-slash protection the wearer will have a garment that offers good protection against both types of injury (Bleetman et al. 2003).

# References

Ankersen J, Birkbeck AE, Thomson RD, Vanezis P (1999). Puncture resistance and tensile strength of skin simulants. Pro*c Inst Mech Eng H.* 213: 493–501.

Ankerson J, Birbeck A, Thomson R, Vanezis P (1998). The effect of knife blade profile on penetration force in flesh simulants. *Technol Law Insur.* 3, 125–128.

Annaidh AN, Cassidy M, Curtis M, Destrade M, Gilchrist MD (2015). Toward a Predictive Assessment of Stab-Penetration Forces. *Am J Forensic Med Pathol.* 36, 162–166.

Annaidh AN, Cassidy M, Curtis M, Destrade M, Gilchrist MD (2013). A combined experimental and numerical study of stab-penetration forces. *Forensic Sci Int.* 233, 7–13.

Bleetman A, Dyer J. (2000). Ultrasound assessment of the vulnerability of the internal organs to stabbing: determining safety standards for stab-resistant body armour. Injury. 31(8), 609–612.

Bleetman A, Watson CH, Horsfall I, Champion SM. (2003). Wounding patterns and human performance in knife attacks: optimising the protection provided by knife-resistant body armour. *J Clin Forensic Med.* 10, 243–248.

Carr DJ, Godhania K, Mahoney PF. (2019). Edged weapons awareness. *Int J Legal Med.* 133, 1217–1224.

Chadwick EK, Nicol AC, Lane JV, Gray TG. (1999). Biomechanics of knife stab attacks. *Forensic Sci Int.* 105, 35–44.

Connor SE, Bleetman A, Duddy MJ. (1998). Safety standards for stab-resistant body armour: a computer tomographic assessment of organ to skin distances. *Injury.* 29(4), 297–299.

Croft J. (2003). PSDB body armour standards for UK police Pt 3. Knife and spike resistance PDSB St Albans Herts

Hern E, Glazebrook W, Beckett M. (2005). Reducing knife crime. *BMJ.* 330, 1221.

Horsfall I, Watson CH, Champion SM, Prosser PD, Ringrose T. (2005). The effect of knife handle shape on stabbing performance. *Appl Ergon.* 36, 505–511.

Horsfall I, Prosser PD, Watson CH, Champion SM. (1999). An assessment of human performance in stabbing. *For Sci Int.* 102, 79–89.

Humphrey C, Kumaratilake J, Henneberg MA. (2016). Stab in the dark: Design and construction of a novel device for conducting incised knife trauma investigations and its initial test. *Forensic Sci Int.* 262, 276–281.

Mahoney PF, Godhania K, Carr DJ. (2017). Investigating the use of concealable and disguised knives. *Police J: Theory, Practice Principles.* 91, 139–149.

Miller SA, Jones MD. (1996). Kinematics of four methods of stabbing: a preliminary study. *Forensic Sci Int.* 82, 183–190.

Muggenthaler H, Drobnik S, Hubig M, Niederegger S, Mall G (2013). Experimental throws with a knife to clarify a case of domestic violence [article in German]. *Arch Kriminol.* 231, 46–54.

Nolan G, Hainsworth SV, Rutty GN. (2018). Forces generated in stabbing attacks: an evaluation of the utility of the mild, moderate and severe scale. *Int J Legal Med.* 132, 229–236.

O'Callaghan PT, Jones MD, James DS, Leadbeatter S, Evans SL, Nokes LD (2001). A biomechanical reconstruction of a wound caused by a glass shard--a case report. *Forensic Sci Int*. 117, 221–231.

O'Callaghan PT, Jones MD, James DS, Leadbeatter S, Holt CA, Nokes LDM. (1999). Dynamics of stab wounds: force required for penetration of various cadaveric human tissues. *Forensic Sci Int*. 104, 173–178.

Patrick BK, Thompson J. (2009). *An Uncommon History of Common Things*. Washington, D.C.: National Geographic.

Smithsonian National Museum of History. (2020). Early Stone Age Tools. http://humanorigins.si.edu/evidence/behavior/stone-tools/early-stone-age-tools (Accessed March 2020).

# ■ Chapter 4
# Scene Examination in Cases of Sharp Force Trauma

## What is Meant by the Crime Scene?

The scene where a body is discovered is often referred to as the "crime scene" and to give the location such a designation is appropriate, but it should be understood that where a body is found may not be where death occurred or where the incident or crime occurred which led to death. It is not unusual therefore for forensic investigators to have to assess a number of possible "crime scenes," taking into consideration the circumstances in which the body is discovered. Most commonly, the place where the person is killed is the same as where the body is found. In one study (Vanezis 1996a) this was found to be the case in 471 of 634 deaths (74 %) (Table 4.1). On the other hand, it is not uncommon to find that a person is stabbed in a particular location and then is able to walk, or even run off only to be discovered lifeless elsewhere.

In one particular case seen by the author, although the circumstances are not uncommon, an 18-year-old male had been stabbed at the back of a public house (bar). He then staggered down the road, leant on a car, which showed a few blood stains. He then continued a further 10 metres where he collapsed and died. It was initially thought that he had emerged from the house adjacent to where he was found (Figure 4.1a,b).

Physical activity after a stabbing which proves to be fatal, including injury to the heart or great vessels, is common and there are many examples of walking or running away following an assault, or even to carry on engaging with the assailant for some time before collapsing and dying (Franchi et al., 2016; Karger et al. 1999). In the case reported by Franchi et al., the victim, a 15-year-old boy, was seen on CCTV beginning to chase the assailant and was active for 38 seconds before collapsing with a stab wound to the heart (see also Chapter 6).

## Use of CCTV Cameras

Nowadays CCTV cameras in private premises and public areas, such as town centres and streets, airports, on public transport and high roads are commonplace. It is therefore not surprising that many incidents are witnessed in this way as in the case above. Indeed, Grega et al. (2016) point out that London, with over 8 million inhabitants, has an estimated 900,000 cameras of which the police have access to 60,000, more than any other European and US city. In 2009, Scotland Yard used CCTV recordings during the investigation in 95% of murder cases.

In the United States, after installing cameras in a number of major cities, since 2007 there has been a 35–60% decrease in the number of crimes committed in monitored areas. A further important aspect of the use of CCTV cameras, which is the main focus of Grega et al.'s paper, is based on maximising the efficiency of such cameras in crime detection by proposing algorithms for alerting human camera operators to the automatic detection of persons carrying dangerous weapons, in particular knives or firearms.

**Table 4.1** Interrelationship between the scene of the fatal incident, death and discovery of the body

| The Scene | | | | |
|---|---|---|---|---|
| Where the incident occurred | Where death occurred | Where the body was discovered | n | % |
| Same | Same | Same | 471 | 74 |
| Different | Same | Same | 123 | 20 |
| Same | Same | Different | 36 | 6 |

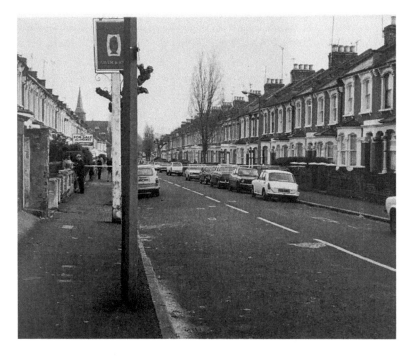

◄ **Figure 4.1a** Cordoned-off area seen where the deceased is found, from the direction of the public house.

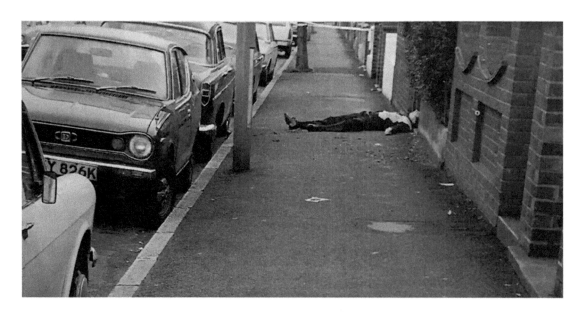

▲ **Figure 4.1b** The deceased is seen in the protected area from the other direction.

# Scene Management

## General Considerations

A scene in which the deceased is discovered and has sustained sharp force wounds is usually associated with significant blood on and around the body and requiring careful assessment of the quantity and the distribution of the blood together with other scene findings to assist in attempting to reconstruct the events leading to death. It is therefore vital that the scene and/or scenes be identified and protected to allow uninterrupted examination by the investigating team and prevent or minimise contamination by uninvited persons.

As part of the multidisciplinary forensic team, the pathologist will work alongside colleagues to assess the body and its environment as well as assisting in the collection of evidence. Reconstructing the circumstances in which a person has died when they are discovered at a scene, requires a number of important initial questions which need to be addressed. They include, whether or not the deceased died at the location in which they were found and how (the manner) the deceased came to their death – in other words, is it a case of homicide, suicide or accident? In a number of instances, although the police are very anxious for some initial guidance by the pathologist to assist them with their investigation, it is not always possible to give any clear answers in a specific way regarding the manner of death or the type of weapon used. I have experienced cases where, because there had been a large amount of blood and sometimes with clothing and other material covering the wound sites, it had made differentiation between different types of wounds such as stab or firearm injuries difficult or even masked the wound completely. Since the scene is not the place for the pathologist to carry out a detailed examination for obvious reasons of contamination, the safest approach is to keep one's own counsel until the post-mortem examination in the mortuary has been carried out.

Scenes are so varied that one can only categorise them in very broad terms. The examination of each type of scene frequently requires a different approach, with the attendance of appropriate forensic expertise. The senior investigator when assessing a scene will decide on the approach and the various types of experts that might be required. This will depend on the location, type of incident, number of deceased, health and safety aspects, urgency of examination and climatic conditions.

Satisfactory management of a scene involves a number of important actions that need to be carried out.

- If a person has been reported missing, the circumstances may dictate searching for a body which may have been concealed in a particular location. This frequently involves substantial resources both in manpower and machinery, occasionally of a highly specialised nature. In such circumstances, particularly if burial is suspected, an archaeologist will be able to advise on methods of locating graves and assist in the recovery. A number of different techniques are available in practice or appear promising but not yet used operationally on a routine basis. The use of cadaver dogs is one of the oldest methods for successfully detecting human remains, not just in burials but also in major catastrophes (Migala and Brown, 2012). Other techniques commonly used include geophysical surveys employing different methods including the use of ground-penetrating radar (Salsarola et al. 2015). A pathologist will also be able to advise on the possible condition of the remains that are being sought, taking into account the likely post-mortem interval together with environmental factors.

- Discovery of a body and preliminary assessment will be made to ascertain whether there are suspicious circumstances or overt evidence of a criminal act. The person making the discovery, who in many cases is a member of the general public, may cause contamination, move an obviously dead body or attempt resuscitation where inappropriate.

- The most urgent and prime consideration on finding someone who is apparently lifeless is to maintain life if there is any chance that the victim may still be alive. Thus a doctor or paramedic may enter a scene to try and revive an injured person before any precautions are taken to prevent contamination of the body and its immediate environment.

**43**

- Ascertaining whether or not there is, or might be, criminal involvement in the victim's death is in some cases a straightforward matter, and advice may be initially sought from the clinical forensic medical examiner who had been called to certify the fact of death. If the death is one that requires the assistance of a forensic pathologist, then usually he/she will be contacted and informed of the circumstances so as to give advice to the police. It should be appreciated that there are other deaths which require special examination of the scene, which may not involve a criminal offence but may nevertheless be in the public interest for an investigation along such lines, e.g. deaths in custody.

- Having ascertained that a forensic investigation is required, a senior officer will be appointed with the formation of a scene team, including relevant specialists. On arrival at the scene the senior investigating officer (SIO) and his/her team will carry out a preliminary assessment, draw up a plan of action, set up an incident room and assemble the scene team.

- The first action that will be taken will be to ensure that the scene is secured to protect it from intruders. It is extremely important that access to the scene is limited and takes into account the need to prevent contamination and/or the loss of vital evidence. This includes securing a wide perimeter around the scene. In an indoor scene as opposed to outdoors, the limits are well defined. Aerial cover such as a tent over the body or even a marquee if one is dealing with multiple deaths, to prevent unauthorised photography of the scene and the deceased from long distance, high vantage points or from light aircraft. Once the scene is secured then the senior investigating officer with the advice of the scene team will decide the best way to approach a scene to minimise disturbance.

- Only personnel authorised to be at a scene by the investigating officer should attend, with access being restricted to a small but well-trained group of professionals. Each scene team member will be carrying out their own particular role and must be aware of each other's tasks and especially the need for preservation and collection of different types of evidence by the various specialist examiners. It is imperative that protective clothing be worn to protect the examiner from materials at the scene and also to protect the scene from the examiner.

- It is necessary to photograph the scene from an early stage to provide a record of the position of items within a room for example, so that that any subsequent movements of furniture can be recognised. Sometimes furniture or other items are moved by a paramedic attempting resuscitation or by the person who found the body.

In cases involving the use of a weapon, as in sharp force trauma, there will inevitably be a search for the responsible instrument, whether it be a knife or other type of sharp-edged instrument. In homicide cases, where the assailant flees the scene, the weapon in question is usually, but not always, removed and in many cases deposited elsewhere. Such a situation was seen in the case of a drug abuser murdered in a squat and the knife used deposited at a nearby school gate (Figure 4.2). In domestic cases, if a kitchen knife is used it might be cleaned by the assailant and placed back in a drawer or disposed of. In one case seen by the author, the perpetrator was less than meticulous in hiding the knife, by leaving it in a sink with blood stains still on the blade; the drawer from where it had been taken, remained half open (Figure 4.3). In cases involving street violence, it is nearly always removed from the scene and in many cases thrown away, usually within a short distance of the assault.

## Health and Safety

It is essential to ensure the safety of the team working at the scene and wherever possible certain circumstances and locations require care and assessment as to their safety and possible risk to the scene team.

- An obvious example is a building which has been on fire and has been rendered structurally unsafe, buildings subjected to other forms of disruption such as in an explosion.

- There may have been the release of noxious substances into the environment such as in certain industrial incidents involving chemicals or radiation.

44

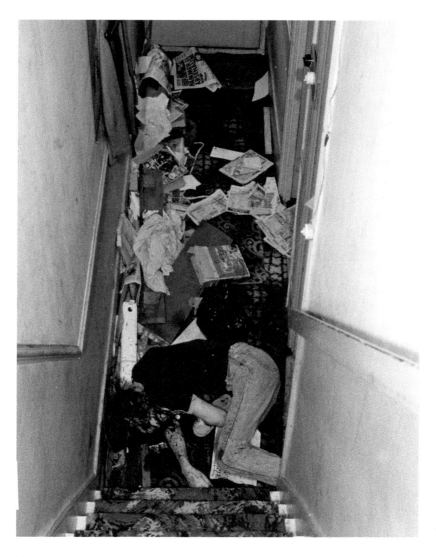

▲ **Figure 4.2a** Male drug abuser found stabbed in the hallway of a squat.

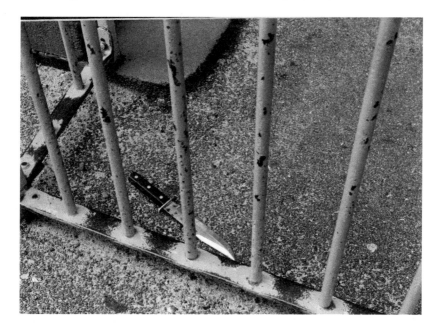

▲ **Figure 4.2b** The perpetrator has discarded the knife used by the gates of a nearby school.

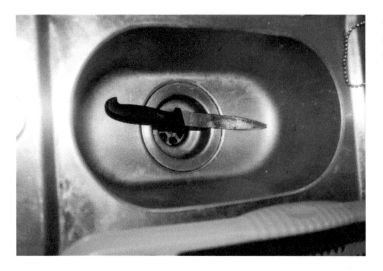

◄ **Figure 4.3a** Kitchen knife left in the sink with blood smearing on the blade after a domestic homicide.

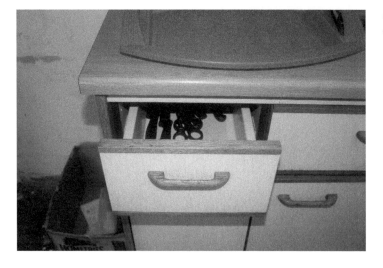

◄ **Figure 4.3b** The drawer from which it had been taken is open.

- Another type of scene which poses a real risk of causing death to the investigators is an atmosphere where the air is irrespirable e.g. a mine shaft. Special breathing equipment will be required in such circumstances.

- Occasionally, booby traps may have been laid at a scene to cause injury to the investigators and to prevent them from carrying out their tasks particularly in situations where there is civil disturbance.

- The terrain where a body is discovered may be relatively inaccessible and hazardous. For example, recovering bodies from a mountainous terrain in an air crash where the investigators will need to be adequately acclimatised to lower oxygen saturation in the atmosphere at high altitudes.

- Careful consideration should be given to the risk of infection from microbial agents such as HIV of Hepatitis B or C which may be present in body fluids or from blood contaminating discarded hypodermic syringes and needles in death scenes involving intravenous drug abuse. The risk is minimal provided protective clothing is worn and the examiner is careful when moving the body where there may be an excess of blood or other fluids associated with it. It should also be noted that the risk of infection from the exhumation of human remains is minimal, unless internment has been recent and death has resulted from an epidemic disease such as cholera (Morgan et al. 2006).

- Attack by predators may also be a risk where there are venomous snakes or wild animals in the vicinity.

## Climatic Conditions

The weather conditions prevailing at the scene may dictate the approach that needs to be adopted for investigation at the location.

- Adverse conditions may require the body to be moved to the mortuary as soon as possible. If this cannot be done, appropriate steps such as erecting a tent, should be taken to protect the body from the elements.

- In a particularly hot environment, decomposition would be rapidly accelerated and the body should be removed at the earliest opportunity for autopsy.

## Location of Body

The location may be in a building or enclosed within a structure, such as a residence or workplace. It is essential to understand the connection, if any, between the location and the deceased, i.e. if the location is the deceased's residence.

Domestic disputes are a common cause of fatal stabbings; and in some series stabbing occurs, most commonly, in the victim's own home. Rogde et al. (2000), from a series of 141 homicides from two Scandinavian capitals, Oslo and Copenhagen, found that 78% of all females were killed in their own home, while this was the case for 49% of males. This is hardly surprising as many of the victims are known to their assailants; and knives in a household, particularly from the kitchen drawer, are close to hand to be used as weapons. Among the victims killed in their own home, 51% of the females and 35% of the males shared this home with the offender (most often their spouse) (Figure 4.4). By contrast, 21% of males were killed outdoors compared to only 6% of females.

In a further case the male victim was found collapsed outside the entrance to an address which was close to where he lived. There was a trail of blood from his flat to where he collapsed. Resuscitation attempts were carried out, including a clamshell thoracotomy but the deceased died from a stab wound to the neck and had also suffered a number of other injuries (Figure 4.5).

An outdoor scene may be either an urban or countryside environment and in a number of situations involves some degree of concealment, particularly in homicide cases where there has been an attempt to dispose of the body. Occasionally a body is disposed of by burial and there may well be the need to locate the deceased.

The author was part of a team which investigated the case of a fully clothed body of a woman that was discovered in a shallow grave next to a lime tree (Figure 4.6). She had been missing for five years. Her identification was based on medical records including the use of facial superimposition. The length of internment in the grave was calculated from the lime tree root lengths and their rings growing through her. It is believed that this was one of the first cases where this technique was employed. The botanist was accurate to within one season from the five years from when she had been missing. Since then there have been a number of publications in the forensic literature which have demonstrated the usefulness of examination of tree roots and other associated plant growth as a means of estimating the length of internment (Quatrehomme et al., 1997; Margiotta et al., 2015). The cause of her death was established by close examination of her clothing and skeletal remains. Examination of her lace blouse, particularly on the inner aspect clearly demonstrated two tears, although more were suspected, that appeared to have been caused by a knife. Examination of her rib cage confirmed a fracture to the fourth left rib anteriorly, fifth rib below showing complete severance and a small cut on the inner aspect of the sixth rib. All were in line and were typical of a thrust of a sharp implement such as a knife into the chest (Figures 4.7 and 4.8). From the damage seen to the fourth rib, it was reasonable to assume that the knife used had entered up to the hilt with the assailant's hand also making contact against the chest delivering the blow as if by a hard punch. The skeletonised chest was devoid of soft tissues but this did not deter the Court from making the correct assumption that vital organs would have been seriously injured (Vanezis et al. 1978).

A further case seen by the author which illustrates the importance of a thorough scene examination is that involving a missing 14-year-old schoolgirl who had been abducted and murdered by her stepfather (Vanezis1996b). He had been sexually abusing her since she was an 8-year-old child. He was convicted of her murder before her body was found. Whilst in prison, and from conversations with other prisoners,

47

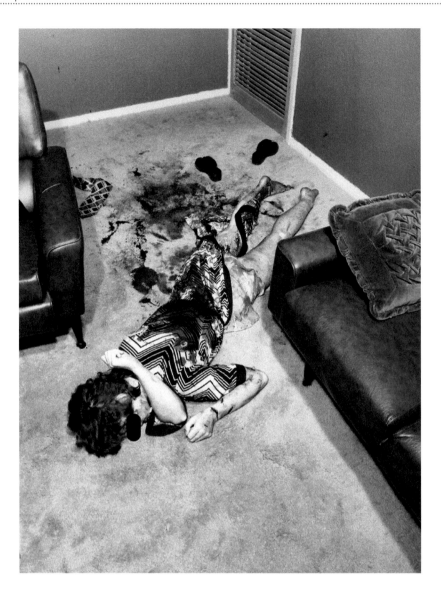

**▲ Figure 4.4** The deceased was found stabbed in the lounge by her husband.

it emerged that she did not die in a car crusher, as he had originally asserted, but he had killed her by other means and had deposited her body in a disused Victorian cemetery in North London. Most of her remains were eventually found, partially covered by dense vegetation after they had been scattered by predators to different parts of the periphery of the cemetery (Figures 4.9, 4.10 and 4.11). Identification was confirmed by her mother from her clothing found separately but nearby (cardigan, skirt and shoe) as well as a ring, watch and necklace. Assessment of the remains by an anatomist and dentist found her age to be consistent with that of the missing girl. In addition, examination of clothing and skeletal remains by a forensic scientist and myself revealed findings demonstrating that she had

been stabbed which included a diagonal clean cut on a portion of one of the left ribs. On her cardigan there were five tears typical of having been caused by a knife as well as a number caused by animal teeth. The knife tears were to the front left part of the cardigan. A further six tears were seen on the left sleeve indicating that she had tried to defend herself.

A body found in, or near, water begs the question in cases of sharp force and other types of injury, whether or not the individual had been killed and deposited into a river, sea or other body of water. The injuries need to be assessed as to whether they are ante-mortem or post-mortem. If they are ante-mortem were they responsible for causing death or did the deceased, despite suffering injuries before death, die from drowning or some other cause

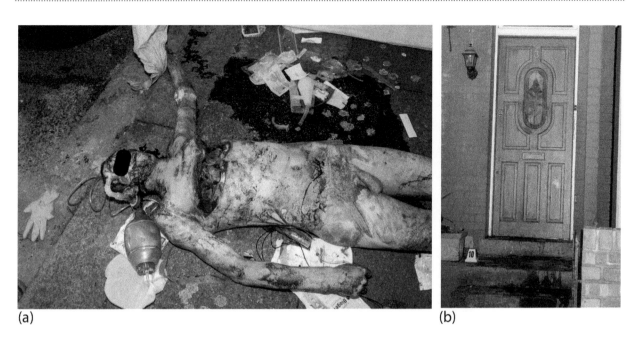

(a)  (b)

▲ **Figure 4.5** The victim (a) is on the ground at the foot of the steps of the front door (b) which show substantial amounts of blood. A clamshell thoracotomy has been carried out and medical equipment as well other items from medical intervention have been left on and around the deceased.

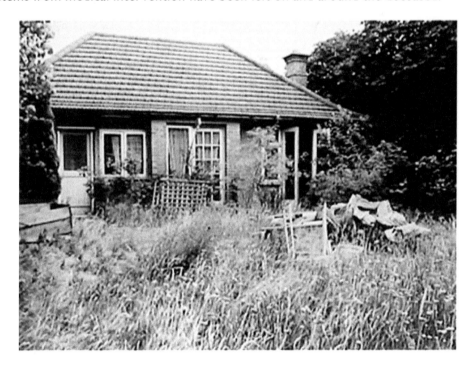

▲ **Figure 4.6a** Back garden of house where deceased had been buried.

associated with water. Such cases may well provide serious challenges for the investigators. A number of issues need to be resolved such as where the deceased entered the water in relation to where they were found. The use of diatomaceous examination may provide some insight into this aspect of the investigation, although results should be treated with caution (Coelho et al. 2016). They emphasise the importance of the creation of a diatom database at different regions and at different seasons to assist the investigator with identifying potential points of entry into water.

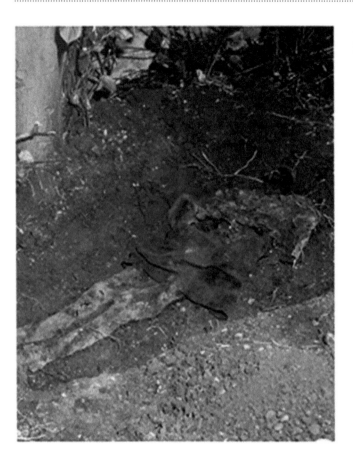

▶ **Figure 4.6b** Partly dug grave showing human remains.

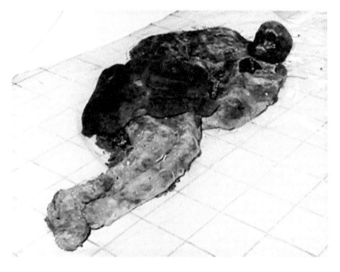

▶ **Figure 4.6c** Fully clothed, skeletonised remains, with some adipocere present in the legs.

A number of complex suicides have been reported using more than one method of self-injury including, very rarely, self-stabbing followed by drowning.

The first complex suicide involving multiple stab wounds followed by drowning was reported by Kaliszan et al. 2013. The victim, a young man, was seen walking into the sea partially submerged. He had at some stage stabbed himself in the chest and abdomen a number of times before disappearing under the water. A post-mortem examination revealed emphysema aquosum which is typical of drowning. He left some of his personal belongings on the beach. Suicide was clearly determined on the basis of the circumstantial evidence prior to death, where he was found and the distribution of the wounds on his trunk. Peyron et al. (2018) report a case of a man found in a river with 18 stab wounds, which presented a serious challenge in assessing whether the deceased had died from his wounds or from drowning and whether or not they were

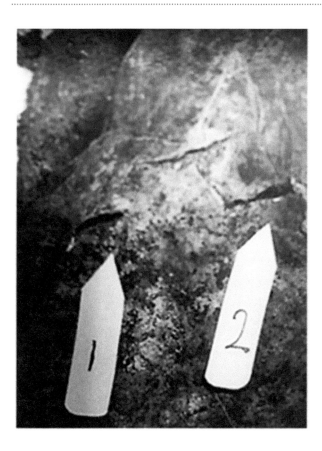

◀ **Figure 4.6d** Tears in blouse from knife.

◀ **Figure 4.6e** Root growing through blouse.

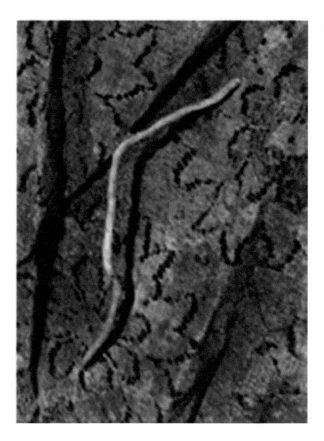

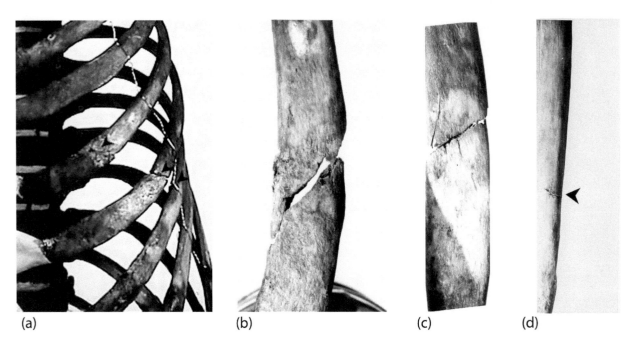

(a)　　　　　　　　(b)　　　　　　　　(c)　　　　　　　　(d)

▲ **Figure 4.7** (a) Left anterior rib cage showing the location of damage caused by stabbing to the fourth, fifth and sixth ribs (arrows). Detail of the ribs show (b) rib 4 which is fractured. (c) Rib 5 is severed and (d) the sixth rib is cut on the inner aspect (arrow). All are indicative of a forceful overarm stabbing action.

**52**

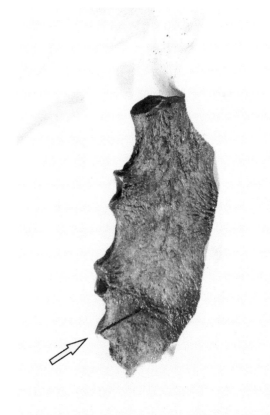

◀ **Figure 4.8** Stab wound to lower right side of the body of the sternum (arrow).

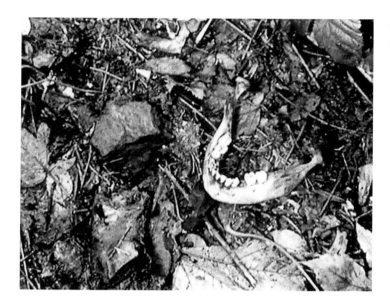

◀ **Figure 4.9a** Mandible found separately from other scattered remains.

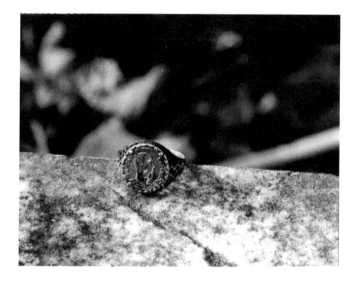

◀ **Figure 4.9b** Ring found nearby.

self-inflicted or homicidal. He had been stabbed in the chest and was found to have a haemothorax and lung injuries. However, the post-mortem and histological examination revealed that the death was *consistent with a death caused by drowning.* They were not certain of the manner of death although a police investigation concluded that the death was a suicide.

In the case of a deceased found by the seashore – or indeed close to any body of water, such as a riverbank – the question will arise as to whether the person died at the site of discovery or had been previously in water. This is not always an easy question to answer and will depend very much on the investigation of the circumstances and post-mortem findings.

Such a question arose when a 60-year-old man was found partly covered by seaweed by some rocks close to a harbour wall. Initially it was not known whether he had entered the water from one of the ships just outside the confines of the harbour or fallen over from the harbour wall. The post-mortem examination revealed a stab wound to his left upper arm and an incised wound to the back of his head and to the palm of his right hand. There were superficial friction marks, indicative of contact with stones from the harbour wall near where he had been found. Following local enquiries, it was established that a man, later identified as the deceased had been involved in a knife fight with two men. During the fight, he had lost his balance, fallen over the harbour wall and drowned.

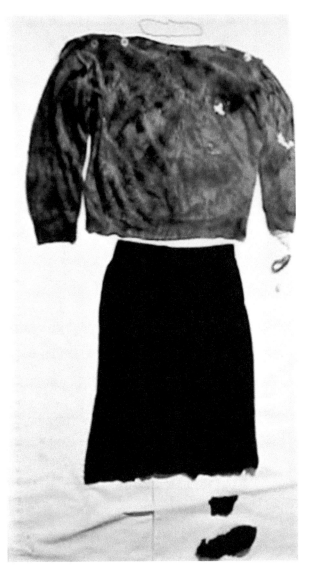

◀ **Figure 4.10a** Garments and other objects worn.

In addition to some of the locations discussed above, there are many other types of locations such as the street, commonly seen in cases of gang violence, or in other public places including bars, night clubs and elsewhere (see also section on CCTV cameras).

## Position of the Body

The position of the body may be of assistance in many cases to resolve both the manner of death (whether homicide accident or suicide) and help reconstruct the scenario and ascertain the locus where wounding had occurred and whether or not the deceased had died in the same area where injured, or had moved elsewhere, either when still alive by the victim moving themselves after injury, or being moved after death. It is crucial for the pathologist to document the position of body and ascertain whether it had been moved prior to his/her attendance at the scene and reasons for doing so. There are a number of legitimate reasons why a body may be moved from its initial position:

- movement by someone e.g. relative to check for signs of life.

- for resuscitation purposes.

- to collect evidence which may otherwise be lost or become contaminated.

- to secure/make the scene safe.

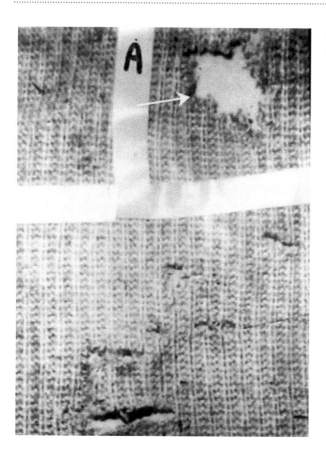

◀ **Figure 4.10b** Close up of tears on left side of cardigan.

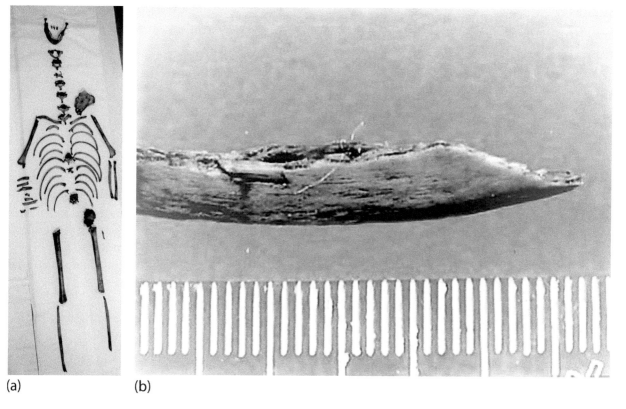

(a)        (b)

▲ **Figure 4.11** (a) Partial skeleton recovered and (b) Section of a rib identified with a diagonal cut caused by a sharp implement. On the shaft there can also be seen animal marks most probably caused by animals.

## Blood Distribution

The handling of the scene, the blood distribution and the collection of trace evidence are, on the whole, tasks that are addressed by forensic scientists and police personnel although with respect to blood distribution there are some areas of shared expertise between the biologist and the pathologist. In one case seen by the author, the blood on the blade of the knife was wiped from the blade on to a shirt which had been covering a radiator, giving an impression of the width of the blade and sharpness of its tip (Figure 4.12).

The appearance of blood needs to be assessed in relation to the position of the body and in particular to any wounds that are found. The pattern of distribution of such blood stains may indicate whether they were produced during life or after death. Care must be taken to assess the distribution and quantity of blood with regard to whether or not movement of the body has taken place prior to carrying out scene examination, for example for resuscitation. Such movement may cause large quantities of blood to flow from major stab wounds. The blood in these cases originates from within the body cavity and, particularly with chest wounds, large quantities may spill out on to the floor on turning the body over.

Examination of the blood stain patterns at the scene gives an insight into the actions and activities of victim and assailant, and may be of particular value in assessing the direction of travel of blood spots, their velocity on impact and distance travelled (Figure 4.13). Forensic scientists, experienced in blood distribution patterns, will use their experience, together with experimental testing and published work, to interpret different patterns in order to estimate site of attack and number of impacts. The size and orientation of stains, from spots to splashes, is indicative of the type and location of the attack.

By the very nature of many sharp weapons, most cases of homicidal sharp force injury require close contact between the perpetrator and the victim. As such, important trace evidence (hairs, fibres, fluids) that might potentially link a suspect to the crime might be present on the victim or at the scene. If the attacker sustains injuries during the attack, the suspect's blood and/or hair may also be present at the scene. With certain sharp force homicides, a sexual assault may have preceded or coincided with the sharp force attack. An examination of the scene may be helpful in identifying seminal fluid or other trace evidence.

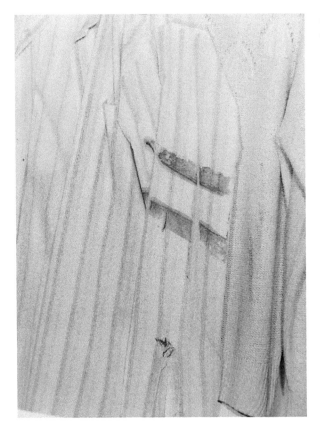

◀ **Figure 4.12** Blood staining on shirt caused by wiping the blade used in stabbing.

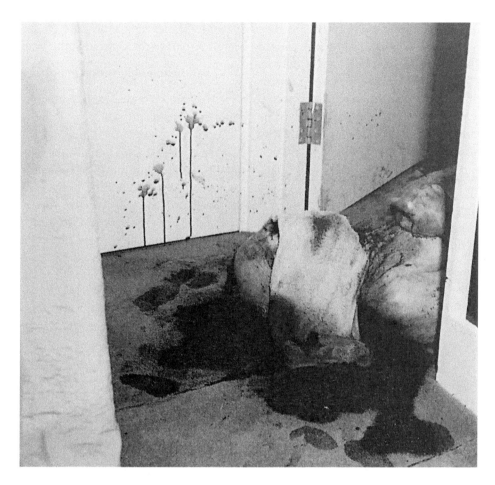

57

▲ **Figure 4.13** Arterial blood spurts from the left common carotid artery seen on the door, opposite the left side of the face and neck. Observe the extensive pooling of blood from his wounds and the foot print marks from blood surrounding the deceased's head.

Tissue damage to a body, which may be of a very extensive nature, can be produced by pets with no other access to food when acting as predators and locked in a house with their owner (Rossi et al. 1994). At first sight such injuries may resemble incised or puncture wounds.

# Homicide or Suicide?

There are a number of considerations that the investigator must address when dealing with a stabbing, where the possibility of suicide has been raised. Although it should be generally appreciated that in some cases, the issue of the manner of death may never be resolved satisfactorily, there are a number of useful features of the scene, which, when considered together with other circumstances and autopsy examination, lead one to the opinion that the injuries were self-inflicted. Most suicidal stabbings occur in private, and a substantial number in the bedroom of their own home (Start et al. 1992, Karlsson 1998). The weapon in nearly all cases is still at the scene and usually very close to the deceased, occasionally still in the hand or within the stab wound. One must be mindful of the possibility that a well-meaning relative has removed the implement in question from the scene. There is little disturbance of the scene, in marked contrast to the vast majority of homicidal scenes. Frequently a door is locked from inside to ensure privacy. Careful examination of the clothing at the scene, before removal of the body to the mortuary, may reveal that garments have been lifted or moved aside to stab through the exposed skin rather than through clothing (see Chapter 13). The presence of tentative wounds is another very helpful indicator of self-infliction (Vanezis and West 1983), but they should not be confused with signs of torture caused before killing a victim. In such cases there may be other signs at the scene to assist. The use of a mirror to view oneself just prior to death is also well recognised (Riddick et al. 1989) and was also observed by the author of this chapter in a middle-aged male who incised his own neck.

A suicide note or similar message, either handwritten (Patel 1971), or on a computer, mobile phone or other recording/electronic device is helpful if present and authenticated. Patel found that written evidence in suicides was found in less than 50% of cases.

Gerbeth emphasised the caution that is necessary in his paper published in 2013 in which he discussed the mistakes that might be made in the assessment of cases thought to be suicide.

These are listed as:

- Assuming the case is a suicide based on the initial report.

- Assuming "the suicide position" at the crime scene.

- Not handling "the suicide" as a homicide investigation.

- Failure to conduct victimology.

- Failure to apply the three basic investigative considerations to establish if the death is suicidal in nature:

  - The presence of the weapon or means of death at the scene.

  - Injuries or wounds that are obviously self-inflicted or could have been inflicted by the deceased.

- The existence of a motive or intent on the part of the victim to take his or her own life.

- Failure to properly document any suicide notes.

- Failure to take each factor to its ultimate conclusion.

It is known that occasionally the manner of death may be suicide but may be disguised as a homicide by the victim, thus adding more complexity to the investigation. Such a case was reported by Pelletti et al. (2017) of a 72-year-old woman who was found dead in her bedroom with a 4 cm vertical stab wound in the abdomen. A bloodstained knife was found in the top drawer of her bedside table. The clothes worn by the victim were undamaged. A bloodstained vest and a sweater with incisions at the front of the garments were found far from the victim in the bathroom and in the bedroom, respectively. Bloodstains were found in every room of the apartment. The evidence found during the forensic examination and, in particular, the bloodstain pattern, indicated that her death was a result of a suicide disguised as a homicide, with the victim being capable of some minutes of purposeful activity prior to her death.

In addition to the above, the occurrence of a homicide disguised as a suicide should always be borne in mind. A case in my experience involved a 44-year-old woman who was found in her bed at home lying on her back and dressed in pyjamas. She had a large kitchen knife protruding from her chest. The room was undisturbed. There was a suggestion of mental issues, but no previous evidence of self-harm. She had no defensive injuries, or for that matter any hesitation marks. Initially the case was thought to be one of suicide, although it eventually transpired that she was killed by her husband with a single stab wound and the knife left inserted in the wound (see also the case of Sultan Abdul Aziz described in Chapter 10).

# Retrospective Scene Visit

It should also be appreciated that the body may have been removed to hospital before, or soon after death, and hence cannot be viewed in situ at the scene. Nevertheless, much valuable information is frequently gained by a retrospective visit to the scene. Some would even argue that on occasions, a visit after, rather than before the post-mortem examination, may be more beneficial to the pathologist, bearing in mind that he will have thoroughly assessed injuries and other significant marks at autopsy and as a result be better placed to accurately reconstruct events leading to death and/or advise as to the type of instrumentation causing trauma. In addition, there are occasions when, because of prevailing climatic conditions, or poor lighting, it is necessary to return to the scene at a later stage, in some cases after the autopsy has been completed.

# References

Coelho S, Ramos P, Ribeiro C, Marques J, Santos A. (2016). Contribution to the determination of the place of death by drowning - A study of diatoms' biodiversity in Douro river estuary. *J Forensic Leg Med.* l (41), 58–64.

Franchi A, Kolopp M, Coudane H, Martrille L. (2016). Precise survival time and physical activity after fatal left ventricle injury from sharp pointed weapon: a case report and a review of the literature. *Int J Legal Med.* 130, 1299–1301.

Gerbeth VJ (2013). The seven major mistakes in suicide investigation. *Law & Order.* 61, No. 1, January.

Grega M, Matiolański A, Guzik P, Leszczuk M. (2016). Automated detection of firearms and knives in a CCTV image. Sensors (Basel). Published online 2016 Jan 1. doi: 10.3390/s16010047

Kaliszan M, Karnecki K, Tomczak E, Gos T, Jankowski Z. (2013). Complex suicide by self-stabbing with subsequent drowning in the sea. *J Forensic Sci.* 58, 1370–1373.

Karger B, Niemeyer J, Brinkmann B. (1999). Physical activity following fatal injury from sharp pointed weapons. *Int J Legal Med.* 112, 188–191.

Karlsson T (1998). Homicidal and suicidal sharp force fatalities in Stockholm Sweden. Orientation of entrance wounds in stabs gives information in the classification. *Forensic Sci Int.* 93, 21–32.

Margiotta G, Bacaro G, Carnevali E, Severini S, Bacci M, Gabbrielli M. (2015). Forensic botany as a useful tool in the crime scene: Report of a case. *J Forensic Leg Med.* 34, 24–28.

Migala AF, Brown, SE (2012). Use of human remains detection dogs for wide area search after wildfire: a new experience for TexasTask Force 1 Search and Rescue resources. *Wilderness Environment Med*, 23, 337–342.

Morgan O, Tidball-Binz M, van Alphen D (Eds). (2006), Management of Dead Bodies after Disasters: A Field Manual for First Responders. Pan American Health Organization: Washington D.C.

Patel NS (1971). A study on suicide. PhD thesis, University of London.

Pelletti G, Visentin S, Rago C, Cecchetto G, Montisci M. (2017). Alteration of the death scene after self stabbing: a case of sharp force suicide disguised by the victim as a homicide? *J Forensic Sci.* 62, 1395–1398.

Peyron PA, Casper T, Mathieu O, Musizzano Y, Baccino E. (2018). Complex suicide by self-stabbing and drowning: a case report and a review of literature. *J Forensic Sci* 63, 598–601.

Quatrehomme G, Lacoste A, Bailet P, Grévin G, Ollier A. (1997). Contribution of microscopic plant anatomy to postmortem bone dating. *J Forensic Sci.* 42, 140–143.

Riddick L., Mussel G., Cumberland GD (1989). The mirror's use in suicide. *Am J Forensic Med. Pathol.* 10, 14–16.

Rogdea S, Hougen HP, Poulsen K (2000). Homicide by sharp force in two Scandinavian Capitals. *Forensic Sci Int.* 109, 135–145.

Rossi ML Shahrom AW, Chapman RC, Vanezis P. (1994) Post-mortem injuries by indoor pets. *Am J For Med and Path.* 15, 105–109.

Salsarola D, Poppa P, Amadasi A, Mazzarelli D, Gibelli D, Zanotti E, Porta D, Cattaneo C. (2015). The utility of ground-penetrating radar and its time-dependence in the discovery of clandestine burials. *Forensic Sci Int.* 253, 119–124.

Start RD, Milroy CM, Green MA (1992). Suicide by self-stabbing. *Forensic Sci Int* 56, 89–94.

Vanezis P. (1996a). General principles of scene examination, Chapter 1, pp. 8–10, in *Suspicious Death Scene Investigation*, Eds. Vanezis P and Busuttil A, Arnold, London.

Vanezis P. (1996b). Scene location and associated problems, Chapter 5, p. 77, in Suspicious Death Scene Investigation, Eds. Vanezis P and Busuttil A, Arnold, London.

Vanezis P, Sims BG, Grant J. (1978). Medical and scientific investigations of an exhumation in unhallowed ground. *Med Sci Law.* 18, 209–221.

Vanezis P and West IE (1983). Tentative injuries in self-stabbing. *Forensic Sci Int.* 21, 65–70.

# Further Reading

Geberth, VJ (2015). *Practical homicide investigation: tactics, procedures, and forensic techniques.* 5th ed., CRC Press, Inc., Boca Raton, Florida.

# ◼ Chapter 5
# The Post-Mortem Examination in Sharp Force Trauma Deaths

## Aims of the Autopsy

As every forensic pathologist knows, the post-mortem examination of the body may well begin with attendance at the scene where the body is discovered. Findings from the scene will be included in the autopsy report, much of which is taken up with the examination in the mortuary, together with the results of further medical/scientific investigations carried out, such as histology, toxicology and other necessary ancillary tests.

As is generally known, the purpose for carrying out an autopsy, whether it be for medico-legal purposes or for clinical audit is to have a better understanding of all the factors that lead to that person's death and wherever possible to gain insight into the prevention of deaths in similar circumstances. The discussion in this chapter, however, will primarily focus on dealing with cases involving sharp force trauma as well as essential basic practice principles expected of forensic pathologists. There will also be some discussion of new autopsy techniques in terms of their applicability to the assessment of sharp force injuries.

For a general and detailed description of autopsy practice, there are a number of excellent text books available and I have listed two at the end of the chapter to which the reader who wishes to seek further information should refer. The reader may also wish to consult standard recognised guidance published both nationally and internationally. In the United Kingdom, The Royal College of Pathologists Autopsy Guidelines series, which is updated regularly and accredited by NICE (National Institute for Clinical Excellence), is a good starting point (RCPath 2020).

As with any autopsy, the pathologist aims to answer and advise the police on a number of questions pertaining to death, namely:

- the manner: whether homicide, suicide, accident, natural or undetermined;

- the mode (mechanism or method): such as asphyxia or heart failure;

- the underlying cause of death: such as stab wound to the heart;

- advise on reconstruction of events and other relevant issues from post-mortem findings.

In cases where sharp force trauma is involved, there are a number of important issues which need to be considered during the autopsy by the pathologist to assist the investigation team. A resolution to many of these will only be achieved by performing a thorough examination and working closely with the team at all stages. These include the following:

- *Whether the injuries are due to sharp force trauma or are a combination of different types of injury.* One of the initial problems which may need to be addressed particularly where the types of trauma are mixed (blunt and sharp) is which injuries are incised wounds and which are lacerations (see chapters 1 and 7). A combination of sharp and non-sharp trauma is not unusual and the pathologist will need to evaluate how and at what stage each type was caused.

- *The effect of post-mortem changes such as putrefaction, on the appearance of ante-mortem injuries and the production of defects after death resulting from decomposition and /or animal predation* (see Chapter 12).

- *Whether injury resulted from an intentional assault by another person, or was caused as a result of self-harm or by accidental means.* As stated above, the manner of death may need to be clarified. It is essential for the pathologist, to consider the post-mortem findings together with the circumstances in which the deceased was found, bearing in mind that in such cases a cautious approach must be taken. Each such case should be dealt with as a suspected crime until there is overwhelming evidence of suicide or an accidental manner of death (see Chapter 10).

- *Whether conclusions can be drawn from the number, distribution and pattern of the injuries.* A great deal can be gleaned regarding the number and distribution of wounds. In highly charged emotional situations, seen particularly in victims that are intimately involved with the other person, there is a tendency to find more wounds on a victim than if they were only slight acquaintances or strangers. Being under the influence of alcohol and/or drugs as well as the involvement of mental issues, may also produce a more intense assault (see Chapter 6).

- *The severity of the trauma.* In addition to the number of injuries seen externally on the victim, the internal examination will demonstrate the extent of the severity of trauma suffered. The pathologist will be expected to assess the degree of injury and where possible assist with the amount of force required to produce such injuries. The effects of such trauma, whether single or multiple, on the cause of death will need to be considered. The severity of trauma may also reflect the amount of physical activity which the victim might be capable of after a fatal wounding. Such activity may include walking or running for a number of seconds, even for a few minutes, before collapsing (see Chapter 4). The pathologist will need to evaluate such activity in light of the victim's injuries to assess whether the activity is consistent with the trauma seen.

- *The type of implement that may have been used.* The pathologist in collaboration with the police needs to consider the type of weapon used and its size in general terms wherever possible, taking into account the morphology of the wounds seen both in terms of shape and size (see below).

- *Whether more than one implement was used.* This question may arise if there are more than one assailants with weapons. The pathologist may well find this question challenging, bearing in mind the variable sizes and shapes of wounds that may be produced by a single knife.

- *The characteristic features (morphology) of the injuries.* A detailed account of the characteristics of wounds is essential and may assist with identification of the type of instrument, how it was used and with what force (morphology of wounds is discussed in detail in Chapter 7).

- *The direction from which an injury was inflicted* whether from the deceased's left side, front or back and how the direction was affected by the dynamics (movements) between the victim and the attacker.

- *Length of stab-wound tracks within the body.* This information may assist the pathologist to some extent in estimating the length of a blade although in some situations such an estimation could be misleading.

- *The direction of tracks within the body.* The direction will indicate how the knife has travelled within the body and give some insight to the possible organs injured.

- *The organs and other structures injured.* The pathologist will examine each organ, noting the extent of structures damaged within organs and assess the effect on the victim.

- *Whether other factors such as medical intervention are relevant.* Any issues which may involve medical intervention in some way need to be discussed in the first instance with the relevant medical personnel prior to the autopsy, together with the examination of the medical records, and if necessary, medical staff should attend the autopsy.

- *The period of time over which the assault was carried out.* The pathologist may be able to give some guidance as to the period of time over which the injuries were inflicted, taking into account their number, type and distribution.

- *Whether death resulted from complications following the initial trauma.* The pathologist may need to examine a victim of sharp force trauma some days, weeks, months and occasionally years after an attack and be required to assess whether the initial injury or injuries were responsible for death. These issues are discussed in detail in chapter 8.

# Scene Examination

The pathologist may be invited to examine the deceased at the scene where the body is found. Scene examination is described in detail in chapter 4. On many occasions, however, the body for various reasons, (including the body being taken initially to hospital from the scene), is delivered directly to the mortuary for examination by the pathologist. In such a situation a retrospective visit to the scene may prove useful and assist in the evaluation of some of the post-mortem findings.

# Examination in the Mortuary

## Arrival and Storage Prior to Autopsy

The body is conveyed to the mortuary after it has been placed within a body bag, at the scene or at the hospital with suitable identification details on the outside. The bag should be sealed with a device that cannot be tampered with until ready to be opened in the mortuary. Prior to placing the body in a bag, in most instances where the deceased is not in a hospital environment, the hands, head and feet are protected by covering them with plastic bags. Unfortunately, where there has been significant bleeding, blood may well contaminate the covered areas and this can be a particular problem with head injuries. In addition, when undertakers are removing the body from a scene, care should be taken not to cause post-mortem injuries bearing in mind that the deceased may be in a tight and uneven environment. The pathologist must be made aware of any injuries caused in this way. Once the body has arrived at the mortuary, it will then either be placed within a chill refrigerator at around 4 degrees centigrade until the pathologist is able to carry out the autopsy or placed initially on the mortuary table if the pathologist is attending soon after the arrival of the deceased. In cases where the time of death may be an issue, the body is not refrigerated in order to allow core body temperature (most commonly rectal) and ambient readings to be taken.

## Briefing to Pathologist

There will then follow a discussion between the pathologist and the investigating officer or one of his/her team, usually with other necessary personnel in attendance, to give an account to the pathologist of the circumstances as they are aware of at the time. Clearly, accounts given may change and the pathologist should therefore always keep an open mind at all times during his/her examination. If and when further relevant information comes to light, the pathologist should be prepared to modify, qualify or even radically alter their view in the light of new evidence. It is important, however, that the pathologist considers such evidence in a timely manner and that it is properly documented, as part of their preparation of the pathological evidence.

## Identification Prior to the Autopsy

As part of the briefing process and discussion with the mortuary staff, the pathologist will have the identity of the victim made known to him/her. In criminal cases identification of the victim will be confirmed later by one or more of the three primary methods; DNA, dental or fingerprints. The pathologist will also check that the name band, body bag label and description of the body all match and are consistent with being from the same person. In Scotland, in homicide cases, because of the requirement for corroboration in suspicious deaths, two next of kin identify the deceased directly to two pathologists who will be conducting the autopsy (Crown Office, Procurator Fiscal Service 2015).

## Radiographic Imaging

Before an autopsy is carried out, a decision needs to be made if there is a requirement for imaging, whether it be conventional radiography, CT scanning or MRI. It is now becoming commonplace for the use of PMCT and to a lesser extent, MRI, prior to the post-mortem examination. Thomsen et al. (2009) carried out a study in their institute to assess whether PMCT was beneficial and whether it outweighed the costs and extra work involved. They compared their findings in 20 cases, comparing the radiological with the autopsy findings. They concluded, as is agreed by most authorities, that in forensic cases all types of imaging are a good adjunct to the traditional examination, and benefit from the combined cooperation of forensic and radiology expertise.

The importance of imaging in enabling the examination for the presence and distribution of air or fluids (haemothorax, pneumothorax and air embolism) prior to dissection of the body, cannot be overstated and this is particularly the case with penetrating trauma. Furthermore, imaging before proceeding with the internal examination in relation to assessing wounds and their tracks should also be considered wherever possible because of the potential for producing artefacts during dissection. Thali et al. (2002) describe the case of a penetrating knife wound to the aorta. They were able to locate the tip of the knife with Computed Tomography and subsequent two- and three-dimensional reconstruction. Tracts may well be disturbed and misaligned once dissection of the body begins. In such circumstances therefore, a CT scan prior to commencement of the autopsy might assist with the assessment of the track length and direction (Schnider et al. 2009), although those who have measured tracts using Multi Slice Computerised Tomography (MSCT) with Contrast Medium (CT) feel that such imaging has limitations insofar as tracts appear irregular and unpredictable within body cavities compared to viewing and assessing the length with the naked eye, and with the careful use of a probe (Bolliger et al. 2014; Fais et al. 2016). In a situation, however, where the knife is in situ, a CT scan will be extremely useful in allowing a more accurate assessment of the angle of entry of the knife and the length of the track (Winskog 2012) (Figure 5.1). In the case of suicide from a stab wound to the heart described in a 57-year-old

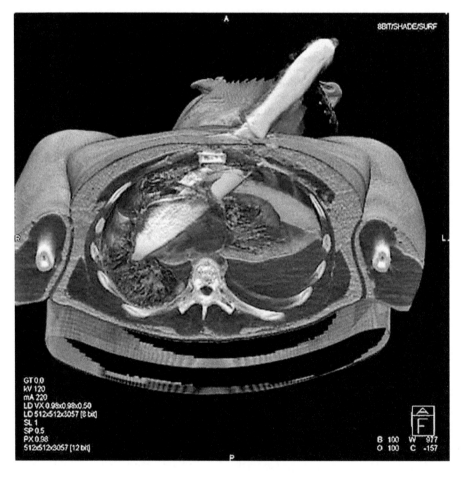

▲ **Figure 5.1** 3-D CT scan reconstruction showing the angle of the knife and shifting of the heart and lungs to the right side of the thorax (Source: Winskog C (2012). Precise wound track measurement requires CAT scan with object in situ: how accurate is post-mortem dissection and evaluation, Forensic Sci. Med. Pathol. 1, 76–77; Used with permission and courtesy *Forensic Science, Medicine, and Pathology*, Springer).

male by Ruder et al. (2011) assessment of the wound track proved difficult with non-contrast CT showing a track lateral to the heart, but demonstrated the correct direction was when CT angiography was carried out. Shifting of the position of the heart and lungs from haemothorax or pneumothorax or transportation of the body may all further make CT scan interpretation challenging.

Occasionally the tip of a knife or a piece of glass may be embedded in the body and this may be easily visualised with appropriate radiographic views. Kawasumi et al. (2012) reported two cases of homicide victims that had broken pieces of a weapon in their skull, in one case the tip of a kitchen knife, and the tip of an ice pick in the other. Post-mortem MSCT demonstrated the metal fragments in the skull of the victims. In both cases, pieces of metal had broken off the weapon and had become embedded in the skull. It goes without saying, that from the safety perspective, knowledge of the location of such fragments prior to dissection of the body may prevent any accidental injury to the prosecutor (Figure 5.2).

## Photography

At all stages during the autopsy, photography will be taken to ensure thorough documentation of all the findings both positive and negative. Photography will begin with the body within the bag and then full-length views, before and after removal of clothing then external and internal views as the autopsy proceeds (Figures 5.3, 5.4 and 5.5).

It is essential to photograph details of blood stains and their distribution on the body and clothing as well as any equipment related to medical intervention such as intravenous lines, oro-pharyngeal airway, naso-gastric tube, chest and abdominal drainage, dressings and so on. Much useful information may be gained from documenting and examining such detail, prior to undressing, cleaning blood and other material from the body as well as removing medical intervention equipment if present.

All images should be briefly described by the pathologist to the photographer to enable the images to be appropriately titled as to what is being shown and its location. This will facilitate the identification of all images at a later stage when they may be referred to in court or reviewed by another pathologist. Furthermore, prior to taking a close-up view of a particular area of interest it will be necessary, to take a view from further away so that the location of the image is made obvious. It also goes without saying that photographs should be accompanied by scales (Figure 5.6). The importance of accurate placement of scales and other essential requirements for

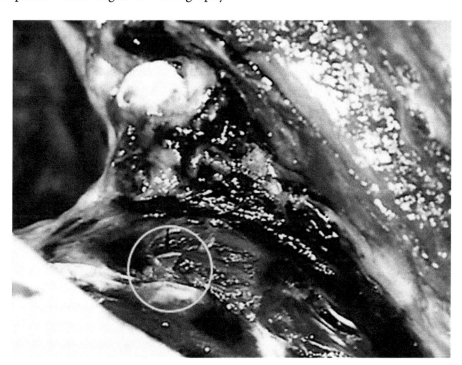

▲ **Figure 5.2** Left side of neck with broken tip of knife embedded in the cervical vertebra (circled).

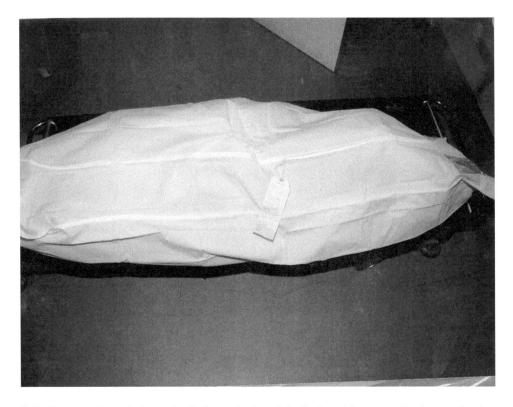

▲ **Figure 5.3** Deceased sealed in a body bag which is labelled and has a zip lock attached.

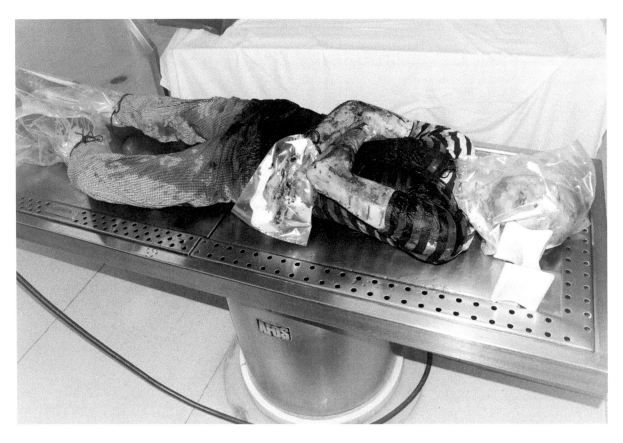

▲ **Figure 5.4** Dressed body with head, hands and feet bagged for protection from contamination.

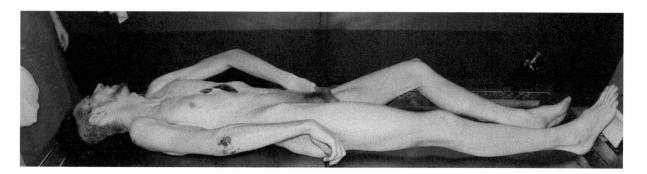

▲ **Figure 5.5** Body undressed and washed.

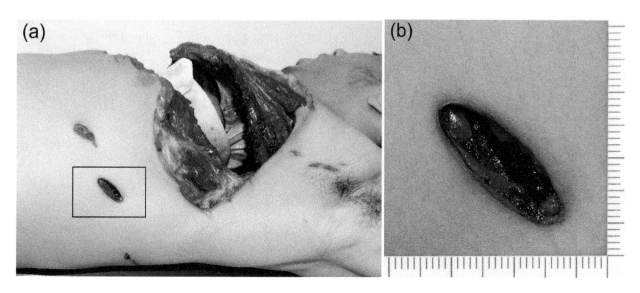

▲ **Figure 5.6** (a) View of the left side of a body to show the location of the wound which is shown in the close up image in (b).

photographing wounds and other marks on a person are discussed by Evans et al. (2014).

## The External Examination

The external examination of the body will comprise a number of stages, from a full, general description of the clothed body (if the body has not been undressed) to a detailed examination of all external findings.

### Examination of Clothing

Examination of the clothing will include the blood distribution which will be of assistance in assessing the position of the victim whilst the assault was taking place as well as how their position may have changed. In other words, to provide assistance with the dynamics of the assault. The arrangement of clothing may well be of importance, particularly in cases which might involve sexual assault. The clothing can then be removed and examined further to look for cuts or tears caused by sharp force or by other means during an assault, such as pulling and tearing. All the clothing must be photographed with scales, defects measured and their shapes described.

### Examination of the Body

Once the body is undressed, a full external examination can proceed with special attention being paid to the photography of various wounds and a detailed description of the wound characteristics shape, orientation, regularity, location on the body, as well as consideration of other types of injuries which may be present, e.g. bruises and grazes caused during an assault. Once again, the undressed body should be photographed before cleaning blood and other material from it, and attention paid to any blood stain distribution, pattern or amount seen. Occasionally there may be evidence of a recognisable pattern in blood of a hand or foot or other object and such findings should be photographed with a scale.

*Description of Injuries*

The deceased may have any number of wounds ranging from a single stab wound to very many (occasionally over a hundred stab wounds are seen). Where there are many wounds grouped together it is more practical to give the dimension of the range of their length, e.g. from 1 to 2.5 cm, as well as the area over which they are distributed, in addition to the region in which they are found. Furthermore, to also label each wound separately in such circumstances may easily cause confusion and

clutter up the photographs taken (Figure 5.7). The important principle to aim for is clarity of images. Furthermore, one must bear in mind that labelling wounds either numerically or alphabetically in photographs to match with descriptions should be prefaced in the report with a caution that the number or letter ordering should not be assumed (as might occasionally be the case) by some, that the sequence of the numbers or letters refers to the order in which the injuries were caused.

Wounds should be clearly described according to their surface characteristics and their location should be described in terms of the distance from fixed anatomical points as shown in Figure 5.8. An

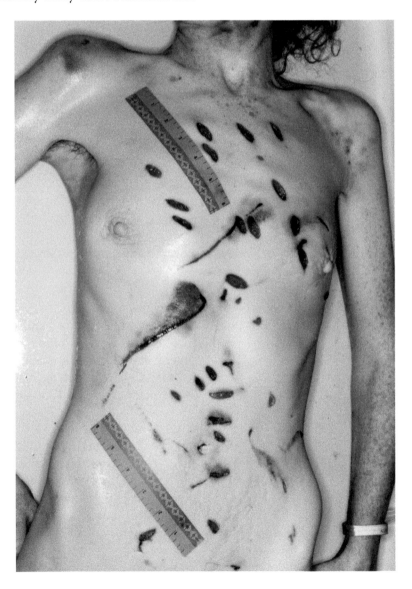

▲ **Figure 5.7a** Multiple stab wounds are present on the trunk. In such circumstances it is preferable to measure the size of the groups of wounds that are close to each, and give a range for the size of the wounds.

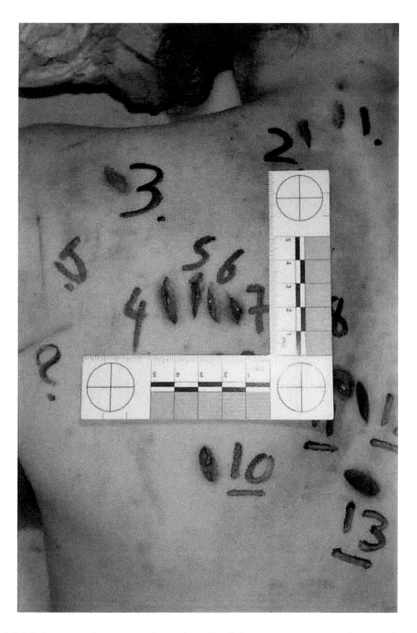

▲ **Figure 5.7b** Multiple wounds are numbered with a felt tip pen giving a cluttered appearance and additionally a scale is obscuring a number of the wounds.

annotated body diagram showing the locations of wounds is useful to the pathologist when writing his/her statement and is frequently required to be viewed by the court to assist in clarifying the presented evidence.

In addition, care should be taken to photograph a wound as it appears on the body. It may appear slit-like or narrow when aligned to Langer's lines or gaping when crossing them (see Chapter 7). It is also important to appreciate that when the edges of a gaping wound are approximated it is usually easier to assess the ends of the wound, whether, pointed or square. Furthermore, notches or other forms of

discontinuity in wounds can be more accurately assessed as can the overall length of a wound. I have always found that careful apposition of the wound edges using clear adhesive tape which does not cause any unwanted highlights to obscure the production of a clear image of the wound when photographed, is ideal. It is not good practice to use one's fingers to approximate wounds with the digits appearing on the images. (Figures 5.9 and 5.10).

Defensive injuries are frequently found and these are described in detail in Chapter 9. In terms of their identification, they can easily be missed if they are within crease lines, for example within the palm of

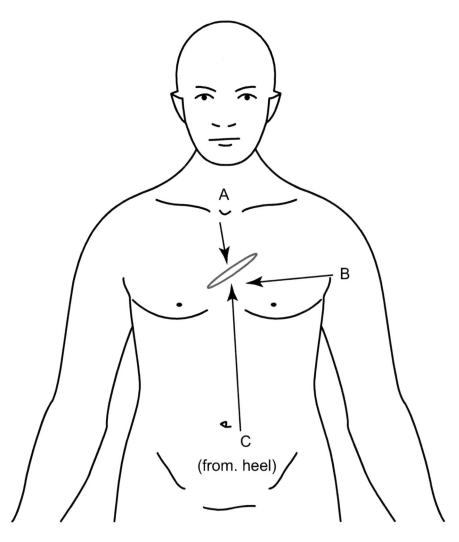

**▲ Figure 5.8** Diagram of the front of the body showing position of a stab wound to the chest and fixed anatomical landmarks to assist with the description of the location of the wound. Thoracic inlet (A), Left Axilla (B) to the mid stab wound; note that with significant stab wounds, their heights are also measured above the heel (C). This measurement may assist in assessing the relative positions of the assailant and victim and whether the impact was likely to be the result of overarm, underarm or horizontal thrust actions. (Source: Author)

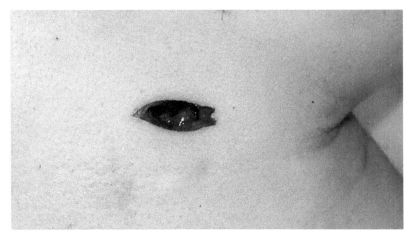

**◀ Figure 5.9a** Stab wound on right side of the neck which is gaping.

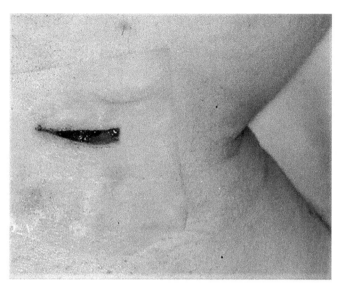

◀ **Figure 5.9b** In this view the wound edges have been approximated with the use of clear adhesive tape. The pointed and blunt ends are seen in both views, more square in (b).

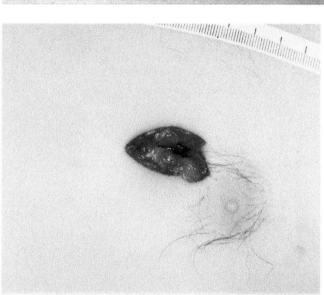

◀ **Figure 5.10a** Stab wound on chest showing gaping notched wound before the use of adhesive tape.

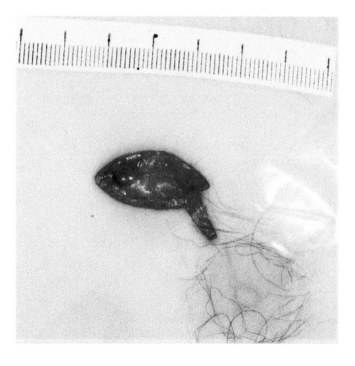

◀ **Figure 5.10b** The tape has approximated the notched component to allow a clearer view of its size and direction.

the hand. They can also be mistaken for streaks of blood, if any blood staining on the body is not carefully wiped away.

At the external examination stage, as well as documentation of the findings, relevant external samples are taken as necessary and retained as police exhibits in criminal cases, such as hair, nails, ano-genital swabs, wound swabs for trace evidence, buccal swab for DNA and other samples as necessary.

Medical intervention marks should be documented in full. Drainage wounds may resemble stab wounds or a clamshell thoracotomy may modify or obscure completely a wound; it is therefore important to consider the medical records in all cases.

# The Internal Examination

Although, in many cases the external examination will assist in reaching a preliminary view that death resulted from sharp force trauma, it is impossible to assess the extent of injuries seen on the external surface without a comprehensive internal examination of the body.

*General Assessment of Injuries*

The internal examination will allow the pathologist to assess:

- the degree of force that may have been used,

- the length of the wound tracks and their direction,

- the relative movements between assailant and victim (dynamics),

- which organs have been injured and the severity of such injury,

- the effects of such injuries on the mechanism of death, whether soon after injury or delayed, as well as giving rise to overall morbidity, or from complications that may arise leading to death at a later stage.

The effects of internal injury in different regions of the body are discussed in detail in Chapter 8; this chapter will deal with the general principles and procedure of the internal examination.

With sharp force trauma in particular, it is essential that before the internal examination is begun, the possible findings should be anticipated. Therefore, it is essential to ensure good radiographic imaging is proceeded with prior to dissection, to facilitate the detection of a number of important consequences of sharp trauma, such as air embolism, pneumo- or haemo-thorax.

*Testing for the Air Embolism*

Air embolism may occur in sharp force trauma or by therapeutic procedures such as operations in the head or neck region, and is caused by air being sucked into injured veins and the gas affecting the contractility of the heart, being found on the right side, pulmonary trunk and arteries. A chest radiography, or if available CT scanning where death has occurred very soon after the embolism will be best placed for diagnosis. It has to be borne in mind, however, that if the victim has survived for a number of hours, air will dissolve and not be visualised. Such an examination is equally of no use if decomposition is advancing, as air seen on images may be from post-mortem production of gases.

When the autopsy is being conducted, confirmation of the presence of air according to a number of current publications (Waters 2006; Burton and Rutty 2010; Spitz and Spitz 2006; Saukko and Knight 2015) follows a technique regarded as the procedure of choice, originally described by Richter (1905). The object of this technique is to prevent air entering the right heart whilst opening the thorax. This method involves the following steps:

- Leaving intact the skull, sternoclavicular joints, clavicles, and subclavian vessels.

- Cutting the ribs, exposing the heart and filling the pericardial sac with water.

- The right ventricle or pulmonary artery is then cut and the water is inspected to see if there are any bubbles.

Bajanowski et al. (1998) described the use of an aspirometer, for the detection, measurement and storage of gas from the heart ventricles. The gas is then analysed by gas chromatography.

For the diagnosis of air embolism, the amount of carbon dioxide in the embolised gas should be less than 15 vol% with a nitrogen gas content higher than 70 vol%, leading to a ratio of < 0.1 or < 0.2. The volume of oxygen is between 8 and 15%. When methane and hydrogen are detected, the embolism may be mixed with putrefactive gases.

*Testing for Pneumothorax*

Rutty and Burton (2010) describe the methods used at autopsy for the detection of a pneumothorax which include: Direct visual inspection without water and underwater techniques. Direct inspection involves careful dissection of the subcutaneous tissue and muscles of the thorax ensuring not to cut through the intercostal muscles. At this point an anterior intercostal muscle is carefully removed so as to enable a visual inspection of the parietal pleura to see if the lung is expanded and normally sited, indicating that there is no tension pneumothorax. With the underwater technique that is more commonly employed, the help of an assistant is necessary to hold up the skin that is reflected away from the rib cage. Water is filled into the intervening space and one of the intercostal spaces is punctured to allow any air to produce bubbles in the water. Care should be taken not to puncture any bullae in the lung which may give a false positive result. A modified and refined underwater procedure, which is occasionally used, employs the use of a wide bore hypodermic needle and syringe pushed into the intercostal space after being filled with water and to observe if any bubbles are seen in the syringe.

*Assessment of the Length of Wound Tracks*

The pathologist when examining the tracks of wounds will need to carry out a layered dissection of the soft tissue. As discussed above, CT may be useful as an adjunct to the examination, in measuring the length of a track, although it should not replace internal dissection.

One further important point to understand regarding tracks is that the *length* of a wound track is not synonymous with *depth of penetration* of a wound. The latter indicates how far a wound has penetrated into the body e.g. the chest cavity, whereas the former could be a tangentially impacted wound to the body which has penetrated only a few centimetres but nevertheless may have a much longer track.

*Assessment of Extent of Injury and the Effect of Surgical Intervention*

Assessment of the extent of injury to internal structures will allow the pathologist to have a better understanding of the severity of injury and the mechanism causing death in the overall assessment of the case. The presence of surgical intervention may on occasions cause difficulty in the interpretation of wounds; it is therefore vital to be aware of the clinical management of the case up to the time of death. The effect of clinical management should also be taken into consideration in terms of its influence on the outcome.

# Examination of a Possible Weapon

Examination of any implement such as a knife or other implement, if available should be brought into the mortuary suitably packaged in a tamper-proof evidence tube or container (Figure 5.11) so as to prevent contamination as well as any accidental injury if it is not properly packaged. It should not under any circumstances be examined prior to or during the autopsy to avoid any preconceived notions of whether it might be the knife that was used. It should only be viewed within its packaging to take measurements of the weapon and well away from the body, preferably in an anteroom. It goes without saying that there are absolutely no circumstances in which a suspected knife should be inserted into a stab wound "to see if it fits." The pathologist will only be able to state whether an implement is consistent with the injury caused and in such circumstances must always bear in mind the possibility of other knives of approximately similar dimensions having been used. Occasionally, where part of the knife, is bent, particularly near the tip, wounds may be produced which match such a defect. Of course if the tip of the knife is broken off and found within the body (see above), this can be mechanically matched to the rest of the blade.

# Briefing After the Autopsy

The pathologist after completion of the autopsy, will prepare a preliminary statement summarising his/her findings and will in most cases have a discussion with the senior investigating officer and others as appropriate, to update the investigative team. A preliminary report will need to be completed, summarising the findings and stated what further investigations are being carried out.

# Preparing the Autopsy Report

Following completion of the autopsy and following any further examination of the deceased if necessary

73

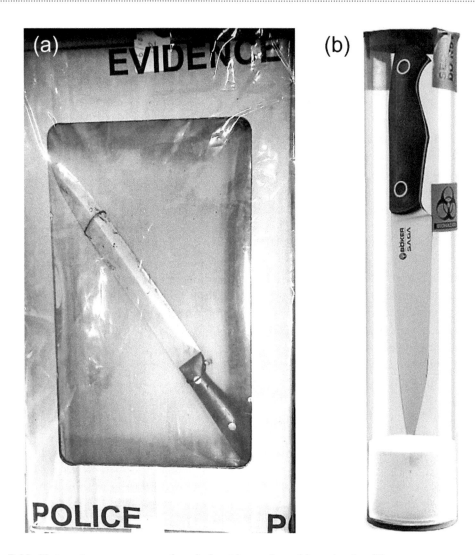

▲ **Figure 5.11** Knives in tamper-proof sealed evidence box (a) and tube (b).

(see below), in addition to the main report detailing the autopsy findings and opinion, statements may be required to clarify any further questions that might arise from the investigation. It is essential that in preparing statements for use in court, the pathologist must have access to all findings relating to the examination such as toxicology, imaging report from the radiologist, and the results of all relevant ancillary investigations.

## Further Examination of the Deceased

The pathologist may well find it beneficial to re-examine the deceased in the mortuary after several days have passed. Skin marks such as bruises may develop and become darker and more diffuse. Patterned injury in particular may be more pronounced in some cases. Furthermore, in relation to stab wounds, bruising around a wound on the skin may become visible if not previously seen, and possibly indicate a hilt mark of a knife. Such an observation will give the examiner some guidance as to whether the full length of the blade had impacted on to the body surface.

Where death is the subject of a criminal investigation, the victim may also require to be re-examined by another pathologist who has been appointed by advocates representing a person charged in relation to the death. This is carried out usually within a week or two after the pathologist has been engaged, although this may vary widely according to a number of practical issues.

The second examination will always be much more challenging to assess accurately the findings at the first autopsy because of the necessary dissection at the first examination, with all that entails. On occasions, when the period between the first and second examination is prolonged, the effect of intervening post-mortem changes may also modify the appearance of injuries. It is therefore essential that the second pathologist should have access to all images taken in relation to the first examination and results of further investigations made available to him/her

in a timely manner. In many cases, it is beneficial for the first pathologist to be present at the second autopsy to confirm the initial findings. In stabbing cases this is particularly important as it is difficult, if not impossible, in most cases to carry out any accurate assessment of the direction and length of wound tracks and other essential findings, for example the presence and quantity of blood in body cavities.

# References

Bajanowski T, West A, Brinkmann B. (1998). Proof of fatal air embolism. *Int J Legal Med* 111, 208–211.

Bolliger SA, Ruder TD, Ketterer T, Gläser N, Thali MJ, Ampanozi G. (2014). Comparison of stab wound probing versus radiological stab wound channel depiction with contrast medium. *Forensic Sci Int* 234, 45–49.

Burton J, Rutty R. (2010). *The hospital autopsy: a manual of fundamental autopsy practice.* Chapter 10 pp 119-121. 3rd Edition. CRC Press, Boca Raton.

Crown Office, Procurator Fiscal Service. (2015). The role of the procurator fiscal in the investigation of deaths. Information for bereaved relatives. https://www.copfs.gov.uk/Death/ (accessed October 2019).

Evans S, Baylis S, Carabott R, Jones M, Kelson Z, Marsh N, Payne-James J, Ramadani J, Vanezis P, Kemp A. (2014). Guidelines for photography of cutaneous marks and injuries: a multi-professional perspective. *J Vis Commun Med* 37, 3–12.

Fais P, Cecchetto G, BoscoloBerto R, Toniolo M, Viel G, Miotto D, Montisci M, Tagliaro F, Giraudo C. (2016). Morphometric analysis of stab wounds by MSCT and MRI after the instillation of contrast medium. *Radiol Med* 121, 494–501.

Kawasumi Y, Hosokai Y, Usui A, Saito H, Ishibashi T, Funayama M. (2012). Postmortem computed tomography images of a broken piece of a weapon in the skull. *Jpn J Radiol* 30, 167–170.

Richter M. (1905). *Gerichtsarztliche Diagnostik und Technik.* Hirzel, Leipzig.

Ruder TD, Ketterer T, Preiss U, Bolliger M, Ross S, Gotsmy WF, Ampanozi, G Germerott T, Thali MJ, Hatch GM. (2011). Suicidal knife wound to the heart: challenges in reconstructing wound channels with post mortem CT and CT-angiography. *Leg Med (Tokyo)* 132, 91–94.

Saukko P, Knight B. (2015). *Knight's forensic pathology.* 4th Edition. CRC Press, Boca Raton.

Schnider J, Thali MJ, Ross S, Oesterhelweg L, Spendlowe D, Bolliger SA. (2009). Injuries due to sharp trauma detected by post-mortem multislcice computed tomography (MSCT): a feasibility study. *Leg Med* 11, 4–9.

Spitz WU, Spitz DJ. (2006). *Spitz and Fisher's medicolegal investigation of death: guidelines for the application of pathology to crime investigation.* 4th Edition. Charles C Thomas Publisher, Springfield.

Thali MJ, Schwab CM, Tairi K, Dirnhofer R, Vock P. (2002). Forensic radiology with cross-section modalities: spiral CT evaluation of a knife wound to the aorta. *J Forensic Sci* 47, 1041–1045.

Thomsen AH, Jurik AG, Uhrenholt L, Vesterby A. (2009). An alternative approach to Computerized Tomography (CT) in forensic pathology. *Forensic Sci Int* 183, 87–90.

Waters BL. (2006) *Handbook of autopsy practice.* 4th Edition. Humana Press, Ottowa.

Winskog C. (2012). Precise wound track measurement requires CAT scan with object in situ: how accurate is post-mortem dissection and evaluation. *Forensic Sci Med Pathol* 1, 76–77.

# Further Reading

Pomara C, Karch SB, Fineschi V. (eds). (2010). *Forensic autopsy a handbook and atlas.* 1st Edition, CRC Press.

Royal College of Pathologists. (2019). Autopsy guideline series. https://www.rcpath.org/profession/guidelines/autopsy-guidelines-series.html (accessed March 2020).

Sheaff MT, Hopster DJ. (2005). *Post mortem technique handbook.* 2nd Edition. Springer Science and Business Media.

■ Chapter 6

# Patterns of Wounding and Demographic Factors in Homicidal and Other Sharp Force Assaults

## Introduction

This chapter discusses principally the various patterns of injuries and demographic factors seen in homicidal sharp force trauma and their interpretation in different scenarios. Such patterns are closely interrelated with other aspects of wounding including the dynamics, epidemiology and morphological appearance. Comparison with other manners of injury – suicidal and accidental – are also alluded to, although details of these will be found in their respective chapters. For the sake of clarity, I have described the regional distribution of injuries and defensive injuries in Chapters 8 and 9, respectively.

From careful analysis of the pattern of injury that is seen, the pathologist may be able to draw a number of conclusions regarding the dynamics (movements) between the assailant and victim, length of the assault, whether there was more than one assailant and whether the wounds were self-inflicted or accidental. Of course, the assessment of how the deceased met their death and its reconstruction cannot be made without consideration of all other factors such as the appearance of the scene and trace evidence collected, as well as all other evidence relevant to the case.

There are many publications which survey series of sharp force trauma, particularly from the use of knives. Such studies include the number of injuries on each victim, whether stab or incised, their location, gender, age, defence injuries and comparison between self-inflicted or accidental injury.

In this section I will deal in the main with injuries from knives although I will also refer to sharp force trauma patterns from other implements such as glass and chopping wounds from heavier implements such as axes.

## Number of Wounds

The number of wounds inflicted in homicide cases, frequently allows the investigator to have a clearer understanding of the circumstances of the assault, which might include length of time of the attack, motive, relationship between the victim and the offender, psychological factors involved and the use of drugs and alcohol and so on.

### Victim–Offender Relationship

The majority of homicidal fatal stabbings and related sharp force trauma fatalities occur in altercations between males and most of the victims know their attacker. Karlsson (1998) found that 63% of 130 homicides were as a result of males killing males and 25% were males killing females. Rodge et al.'s (2000) series found that from 121 homicides 21 were committed by women (15%) and in 19 cases their victims were male. The study by Au and Beh (2011) found that the number, severity and regional distribution correlated with victim–offender relationships which they categorised into three groups: spouse/intimate partner; acquaintance; stranger. They found that intimate partners as the offenders inflicted the highest number of injuries with greater severity, and on the victims' head, face and neck, whereas victims killed by strangers had the lowest number of injuries over the head, neck and face and elsewhere on the body. Karlsson's (1998) Swedish series found that the infliction of more than ten wounds gave a statistically lower probability that the perpetrator and the victim were strangers to each other, supporting the findings of Au and Beh's (2011) study.

## Single-Stab Wounds

The medico-legal investigation of fatal stabbings involving a single stab injury from a knife, may be potentially more problematic than dealing with deaths where more than one stab wound is present. Single stab wounds in homicide cases account for around a third to two-thirds of all stabbing cases (Rouse 1994; Hunt and Cowling 1991; Murray and Green 1987; Levy and Rao 1988; Thoresen and Rognum 1986; Ormstad et al. 1986). When a single stab wound is found to the body, it is most commonly seen on the chest or neck. The heart is the most commonly involved organ either solely or together with injuries to the lungs (Rouse 1994).

Its singular nature lends itself to the possibility of being considered by an advocate representing a defendant accused of murder as being accidental, i.e. the deceased ran onto a knife while it was being held firmly in the assailant's hand, or at least came towards the implement thus contributing to its speed of impact against the body (see Chapter 14).

Burke et al. (2018) reviewed single stab injuries in order to identify features which may aid in the differentiation between cases of homicide, suicide and accidental death. The single stab injuries were to the left chest in the majority of deaths from homicide and from suicide. The victim was nearly always stabbed through clothing in cases of homicide, but was also seen in some cases of suicide. The knife was found in situ in 9 of the 11 cases of suicide involving a chest injury, but was not seen in any of the cases of homicide.

Gill and Catanese (2002) reviewed the case records of all fatalities due to sharp injuries in New York City in 1999 and found that deaths due to a single stab wound occurred in 34% (34/101) of the homicides

and 24% (4/17) of the suicides. Of these, 38 deaths (58%) of the wounds were at the front of the chest and 71% injured the heart and/or great vessels. The remaining deaths with single stab wounds involved the femoral artery, abdominal organs or head.

## Multiple Wounds

Whilst one or two wounds are most commonly seen in victims – 58% in Ormstad et al.'s series (1986) – it is of interest to note that both the latter authors and Hunt and Cowling (1991) found that female assailants tended to cause fewer wounds than their male counterparts.

On the other hand, in respect of the number of wounds sustained, Thomsen et al. (2019) found no significant difference in the presence of multiple stab wounds between male and female victims.

Rouse (1994) found that following single stab wounds, there was a steep fall in the number of wounds seen. Most series have grouped together the stab wounds and, in many cases, included the incised wounds, so that the overall range for single wounds from four large series (Rouse 1994; Karlsson 1998; Katkici et al. 1994; Hunt and Cowling 1991) is 31%–45%, from two to nine wounds 31%–49%, and over nine wounds 20%–25% (Table 6.1).

Solarino et al. (2019) examined cases where there had been a large number of wounds which they described as "overkill" and examined the reasons for such an excessive number of injuries. In particular, there was in many cases an intimate relationship between assailant and victim. The weapons used (including scissors and screwdriver) were mostly brought by the perpetrator, suggesting premeditation; sometimes they found their "weapon" on site. Seventy-eight per cent of the victims (11 cases) were killed with stab wounds to the chest. Defence incised wounds in seven cases were detected on the hands and forearms.

Table 6.1 Number of stab wounds in homicide cases from a number of authors' series

| Author | Number of wounds | | | | | |
| --- | --- | --- | --- | --- | --- | --- |
| | 1 | 2–5 | 6–9 | 10–20 | 21+ | Total |
| Rouse (1994) | 67 | 41 | 24 | 8 | 8 | 148 |
| Hunt and Cowling (1991) | 39 | 36 | | 11 | 14 | 100 |
| Katkici et al. (1994) | 60 | 33 | 63 | 39 | - | 195 |
| Karlsson (1998) | 59 | 74 | | 41 | | 174 |

The author of this text has encountered a number of cases in which there have been multiple wounds in the so-called overkill scenario. In the two cases presented here (Figures 6.1 and 6.2) there did not appear to be any sexual motive or close relationship between the killer and the victim. Both appeared to be random homicides following break-in into their homes.

It has been stated by many forensic pathologists anecdotally that homosexual victims are subjected in many instances to much more severe and greater number of injuries than victims killed in other circumstances where sexual orientation and motivation do not play a part. Bell and Vila (1996), in their study to assess the extent of sharp force trauma in homosexual victims (in addition to examining other modes of trauma: gunshot wound; blunt trauma; multiple injuries), compared injuries in a homosexual and a control heterosexual group. Unfortunately, although they found some statistical significance between the two groups, their study for a number of reasons was methodologically flawed. As stated by Solarino et al. (2019) there are many other reasons for the infliction of severe and, as they describe, "overkill" injuries, with the release of rage in high emotional circumstances which do not include a sexual motive, as I have shown in the two case studies above. It should be appreciated that perpetrators who overkill may be psychotic individuals or have other mental issues; or indeed are individuals under the influence of drugs or very occasional serial and/or ritualistic killers.

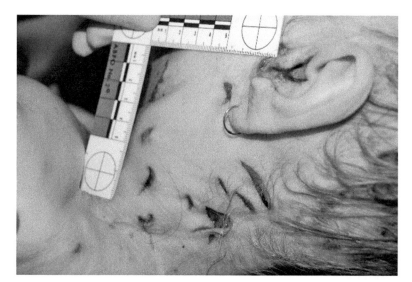

◀ **Figure 6.1a** Multiple stab wounds to the head and neck in an elderly woman living alone.

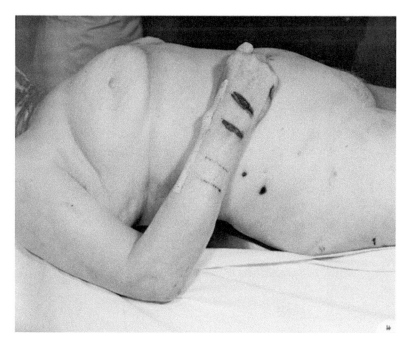

◀ **Figure 6.1b** The injuries on the right forearm and wrist were inflicted by the killer, possibly considering removing the hands. They appear to have been caused peri or post mortem by a serrated implement.

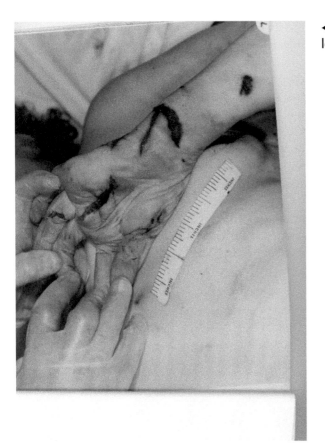

◄ **Figure 6.1c** Defence wounds are seen on the left hand and forearm.

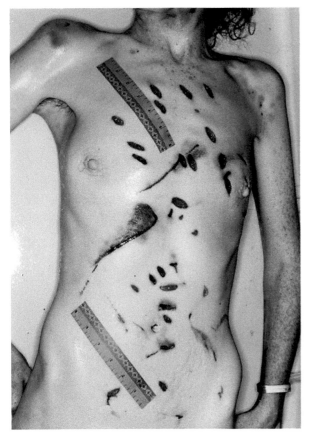

◄ **Figure 6.2a** This middle-aged female was found with multiple stab wounds distributed over her trunk.

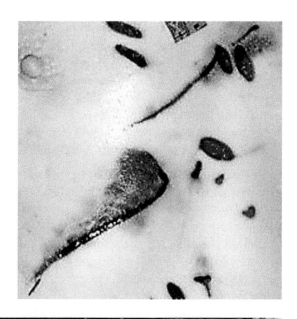

◀ **Figure 6.2b** Of note are the wounds which have not penetrated the skin but appear as linear abrasions. These injuries had been caused after the knife blade had become deformed and bent backwards near the tip during the assault.

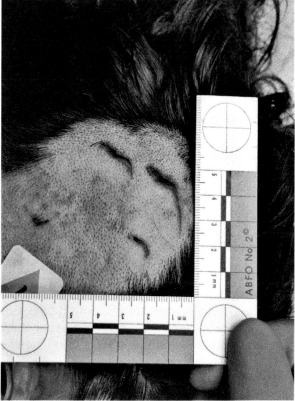

◀ **Figure 6.2c** In addition, she also suffered repetitive injuries to her head. Three curved stab wounds (due to the curved shape of the head) are seen in alignment on the shaved scalp. They appear to have been inflicted from the same direction in a repetitive manner.

# Physical Activity and Survival Time After Fatal Sharp Force Trauma

A victim's survival time and physical activity following a fatal injury from a sharp weapon is a frequently raised issue for forensic pathologists at trial. Most pathologists have dealt with cases where there has been significant activity after stabbing, including running, fighting back vigorously, and in some cases not even being aware that they had been stabbed until they collapse after engaging in a certain amount of physical activity. The extent and duration of physical activity is expected to vary in different fatal stab wound cases, depending on the severity and extent of the internal injuries, which should be taken into account when they are assessed by the pathologist. In the autopsy study carried out by Thoresen and Rognum (1986) on 109 victims with sharp force trauma, they found that the survival time was the least with those with multiple injuries, particularly to the heart and great vessels. Karger et al. (1999) analysed the physical activity of 12 cases of suicide resulting from sharp-pointed weapons and witnessed by one or more persons. In cases with heart wounds they found that in one group of four cases, physical activity was between 2 and 10 minutes. In a shorter-term group of two cases it was approximately 10 seconds and in one case there was immediate incapacitation. In the longer-term group, the size of the myocardial perforation was 7–10 mm in length compared to 1.4–2 cm in the short-term group. The authors concluded that small perforations of the heart offer a potential for considerable physical activity. Significant physical activity after injuries to the vital organs and large vessels were also observed by Levy and Rao (1988). Of 22 stab wounds in their series, they found that 16 (71%) survived longer than 5 minutes after they were stabbed. They found that in some cases victims with injuries to vital organs of large vessels were quite physically active before collapsing.

Cros et al. (2013) carried out a retrospective study on homicide cases to assess whether one could associate the extent of injury using an Injury Severity Score (ISS) with survival time. In their series, there was no association of survival time with ISS in stab wounds, which were the most common cause of death. On the other hand, blunt trauma and firearm injury fatalities did show a significant association.

A not-uncommon example of the type of activity that might occur in someone who has been fatally stabbed is described by Franchi et al. (2016). They report the case of a 15-year-old boy who was stabbed with a knife on the left chest. Closed circuit television showed the victim holding his chest and beginning to chase the perpetrator. The victim was active for exactly 38 seconds before collapsing and was still moving on the ground for a further minute. Despite prompt medical assistance, the victim died. At his autopsy, it was found that he had a stab wound of the left lung, the lower left part of the pericardium, a 2 cm stab wound of the left ventricle at the apex of the heart and a haemothorax measuring 660 ml. Savageau et al. (2006) proposed the following five factors as outcome predictors of sharp instrument injuries with regard to post-injury physical activity and survival length: site of injury; wound size; number of lesions; amount of blood loss; cardiac tamponade.

## Wound Orientation and Manner of Death

It has been reported by Karlsson (1998) that the orientation of an entrance stab wound may be another variable which should be considered in the classification of the manner of death, i.e. whether due to homicide, suicide or accident. In his comparative study of 174 homicidal and 105 suicidal sharp force deaths in the Stockholm area, he found a significantly higher number of vertical stab wounds located on the chest in the homicide cases. The suicides comprised more horizontal wounds. When counting the injured areas, irrespective of the number of injuries, abdominal wounds and horizontal chest stab wounds were also significantly found more often in victims of homicide. These findings were also observed by others including Brunel et al. (2010) who found a highly significant association between the longitudinal (vertical) axis of wounds and homicide, comparing 45 homicides with 21 suicides and by Krywanczyk and Shapiro (2015). The latter in their series of 21 homicides and 25 suicides involving blade wounds found vertical stab wounds of the chest in 5 homicides but none in suicides.

## Homicide, Suicide or Accident?

Differences between the various findings seen between the homicidal and suicidal sharp force trauma are alluded to throughout this chapter and in chapters 9 and 10. In addition, I have summarised below the typical different findings/indicators of each manner of death, including those related to accidental trauma (Table 6.2).

**Table 6.2** Comparison of typical findings/indicators seen between homicidal, suicidal and accidental deaths from sharp force trauma

| Homicide | Suicide | Accident |
| --- | --- | --- |
| No tentative cuts | Tentative cuts common | No tentative wounds |
| Any number of wounds frequently seen | Single or very few deep wounds | Usually single |
| Wounds not regularly placed unless victim immobilised | Regularly placed wounds are common | Usually single wound |
| Target vital areas | Sites of election | Random location |
| Often repetition in "frenzied attack" | Often repetition (each wound close to each other) | Usually single |
| May be injured anywhere | Accessible parts of the body | Random location |
| Deep | Deep | Variable depth |
| Defensive injuries | Self-mutilation | Absent |
| N/A | Usually in private | Either private or in presence of others |
| Stab through clothing | Usually clothing lifted | Stab through clothing |
| Usually scene disturbance | No scene disturbance | May be scene disturbance |
| Weapon usually removed from scene | Weapon usually still at scene near deceased | May be at scene depending on type of incident |

*Source:* Vanezis 2020

# Age

Most victims of stabbing are young and the number of cases decrease as middle age is approached. Age range depends very much on the population make-up, social attitudes and behaviour in different regions and communities. In the Scandinavian series by Rogde et al. (2000) the age range was between 20 and 50 years. Gill et al. (2002), found in their series from New York City that the age range was 5–84 years with a mean age of 34 years. The average age of homicide victims in another series from Bexar County Texas was very close at 35 years (Kemal et al. 2013). The gender and age in their homicide and suicide victims' population were comparable to those described in other similar investigations with a relative predominance of younger male victims in homicides than in suicides (Rouse 1994; Rogde et al. 2000; Fukube et al. 2008).

# Gender and Location of Assault

Males far outnumber female victims in deaths from homicide including sharp force trauma. All large series show that between a fifth to a third of victims are female and more likely to die within a domestic environment whereas males are more likely to be involved in assaults outside their residence, many of them in places such as pubs or other establishments where alcohol is sold (Rogde et al. 2000; Gill and Catanese 2002, Vassalini et al. 2014).

# Motive/Circumstances

In the majority of cases involving a male perpetrator with a male victim the stabbing results from a fight, in many cases with the assailant and victim under the influence of alcohol and or drugs. Thomsen et al. (op cit) commented in their paper that many male homicides in their series occurred following a

**Table 6.3** Motives/circumstances in sex-related multiple stabbing homicides

| | Number | Percentage |
|---|---|---|
| Jealousy | 27 | 45 |
| Other marriage and relationship issues | 10 | 16.66 |
| Cheating | 7 | 11.66 |
| Rape | 6 | 10.00 |
| Sexual deviant psychiatric patients | 5 | 8.33 |
| Homosexual related | 3 | 5.00 |
| Paedophile related | 2 | 3.33 |
| Total | 60 | 100 |

Adapted from Radojević et al. 2013

trivial event such as spilling beer or giving the wrong glance to someone or appearing threatening, with a large proportion of the victims suffering single stab wounds.

Male to female confrontations may be either in a domestic environment or associated with a sexual motive. Radojević et al. (2013) found that among the 110 victims of multiple stabbing homicides, the percentage of sex-related homicides for the female group was 68.18% (30 out of 44 cases), while it was 45.45% (30 out of 66 cases) for the male group. The same authors also found that jealousy was the most common motive in sex-related multiple stabbings (Table 6.3).

In terms of the regional distribution of wounds, Stermac et al. (2001) suggested that victims sexually assaulted by intimate partners tended to sustain more injuries to the head, face, neck, and groin area when compared to victims assaulted by an acquaintance.

The author investigated a case of a male in his late 50s who gave a lift in his car to a 20-year-old male. The young man said to the older man that he had nowhere to sleep that night as he was travelling from the South East of England to the North where his parents lived. The older man offered to put him up for one night at his home since it was near night fall. He lived alone and made it plain that he would be happy for the company. As the evening progressed within the host's house all seemed well, and following dinner and a number of drinks they prepared to retire. At this point the older man apparently made unsolicited advances towards his guest. It appears that the latter was so horrified with this and with the continued persistence of the older man, that he "snapped" and assaulted him with a broken glass bottle, whilst in a highly emotional state causing him multiple incised wounds to his throat (Figure 6.3). He confessed to the police the following day.

One of the more common motives for knife crime in particular, and which can be seen in a number of countries including the United Kingdom, involves the use of these weapons by street gangs, resulting in an alarming recent increase in both morbidity and mortality (see chapter 2).

Other less common circumstances in which sharp weapons are used include robbery, terrorism, racism and honour killings (Ozdemir et al. 2013). The latter authors carried out a retrospective survey between 2000 and 2010 of cut-throat deaths in Turkey from Sanliurfa and Malatya which are two major provinces in south-eastern and eastern part of that country. In terms of motive, they found homicide honour killings to be the second most common reason in their series – 3 cases (1 male and 2 females) from 14 homicides (20%); only mental illness was more common at 26.7%. They also found in the honour killing cases that the mean number of wounds was 34.3 per case compared to 7.4 per case for other homicides and 2.0 per case for suicides. They explained that the larger number of wounds seen in honour killings was an expression of the extreme anger felt by the offender towards the victim.

# Terrorist-Related Stabbings

There has recently been a spate of terrorist-related stabbings in a number of countries including the United Kingdom. The use of knives is inexpensive and much easier to obtain than firearms or explosives. A recent attack in the United Kingdom was in Fishmonger's Hall on London Bridge, during a conference dealing with offender rehabilitation. Two people were killed and a number of others injured. The killer was a convicted terrorist released on licence to attend the conference (Culbertson and Sephton 2019). He was tackled by a number of others who attended the meeting, including by a person

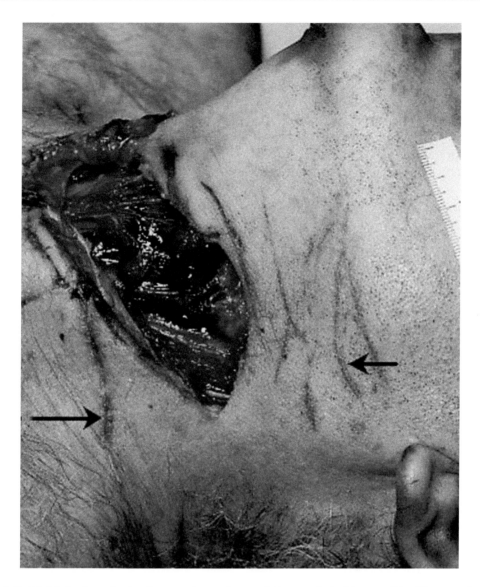

▲ **Figure 6.3** Multiple deep incised wounds to the neck in a male in his late 50s. The assailant was in a highly charged emotional state when carrying out the attack. Note the occasional double linear wounds seen (arrows), due to the impact of both parallel sharp edges of the broken bottle glass (see also Figure 7.46 Chapter 7).

85

brandishing a narwhal tusk from the conference hall. The killer, who was thought to be wearing a suicide belt (which in fact was a hoax device), was shot and fatally wounded by the police.

A number of studies have examined the differences between terrorist and non-terrorist attacks with sharp implements (Merin et al. 2017; Rozenfeld et al. 2018). The latter authors carried out a retrospective study of 1615 patients who had been intentionally stabbed in Israel during the period they describe as the "Knife Intifada" from January 2013 to March 2016. They divided these cases into two categories: terrorist related and due to interpersonal stabbing. They found that the terrorist-related stabbings comprised older patients, more females and more of a similar ethnicity. The time of day on which each type was more likely to occur, differed. Non-terrorist cases were more likely to occur throughout the week and at night time whereas terrorist-related cases occurred during the morning and afternoon, peaking around midweek. In relation to the injuries, the terrorist-related cases were more to the head and neck, whereas non-terrorist stabbings were more to the abdomen. Generally speaking, the terrorist-related cases displayed more severe injuries.

# Involvement of Alcohol and/or Drugs

A substantial proportion of incidents resulting in sharp force injury from brawls are associated with the victim and perpetrator being under the influence of alcohol, drugs or both. In a review of cases in Glasgow between 1998 and 1999, the author (Vanezis 2003) found that in 72 victims tested, there was a positive blood alcohol in 50 (69.4%). Other series demonstrated similar findings Karlsson (1998), 62% from 174 victims; Rogde et al. (2000), 65% of males and 35% females had no post-mortem alcohol. From a South African series of 173 cases, (Mitton and du Toit-Prinsloo 2016), a positive alcohol concentration in the blood was reported in 109 (66%) cases (a range of 0.01 g/100ml to 0.35 g/100ml). Exsanguination was the leading mechanism of death in 85% of cases.

Cocaine or its metabolites were also detected. Fifteen males and seven females were not tested for drugs – the remainder of the cases were negative with regard to drugs. In the Karlsson study (1998), drugs were detected in 27 (22%) of 112 victims where analysis of narcotic compounds had been carried out; amphetamine was found in nine, tetrahydrocannabinol in six, opiates in four, benzoylecgonine in one, and combinations of these in seven cases. Rodge et al. (2000) found that thirteen males and eight females tested positive for drugs in post-mortem blood. In seven of the males and seven of the females a benzodiazepine was found. Other drugs included amphetamine, methadone, morphine and tetrahydrocannabinol. In no instances were cocaine or its metabolites detected.

# Implement Used in Assault

The vast majority of sharp force injuries caused intentionally, either by assault or self-infliction, are by knives most of which have a single sharp side and commonly found in the kitchen. Rodge op. cit. from 141 homicides by sharp force trauma homicides, found only 19 male and 13 female victims where it was known that the weapon was a kitchen utility knife. A further five males were killed with a dagger and one female with a bayonet. Other weapons included broken glass, scissors, axe and screwdriver. The one female with head injury had been struck with an axe. In most of the cases, however, the weapon was registered as a knife without any further description.

# Additional Violence

Victims of sharp force trauma, frequently have evidence of additional violence caused by another type of injury, and which may, on occasions, contribute substantially to the cause of death. In 19 female victims (39%) of Rodge et al.'s cases (op. cit.), there were signs of additional violence, even though death was caused by sharp force trauma. In 13 cases the additional violence resulted from the use of blunt force injury. Strangulation was additionally seen in one further case and in the other five cases both sharp and blunt injury were found in combination with a third type of injury. Among the males, additional violence was found in 31 victims (34%); blunt force injuries in 29 cases and a gunshot injury in one case and one victim had been dismembered. A larger study by Behera and Sikary (2019) in New Delhi during the 20-year period from January 1996 to December 2015 of 187 autopsied cases where multiple methods were used (13.6% of all homicides), found that the combination of methods commonly involved were sharp trauma, blunt trauma and strangulation. Although in total, a larger number of combined trauma types was in males (112 males compared to 75 females), from all homicides during the study period comprising 1,048 males and 323 females, the combined method was shown to be more common amongst the female deaths at 23.2% compared to males at 10.7%. In male victims, the most common combination was blunt impact head injury and stabbing in the chest or abdomen (Figure 6.4); in female victims, it was ligature strangulation and smothering. Fischer et al. (1994) also found a predominance of female victims in combined trauma and explained it on the basis that conflicts in relationships can cause extreme emotional outbursts, leading to the use of multiple aggressive injuries.

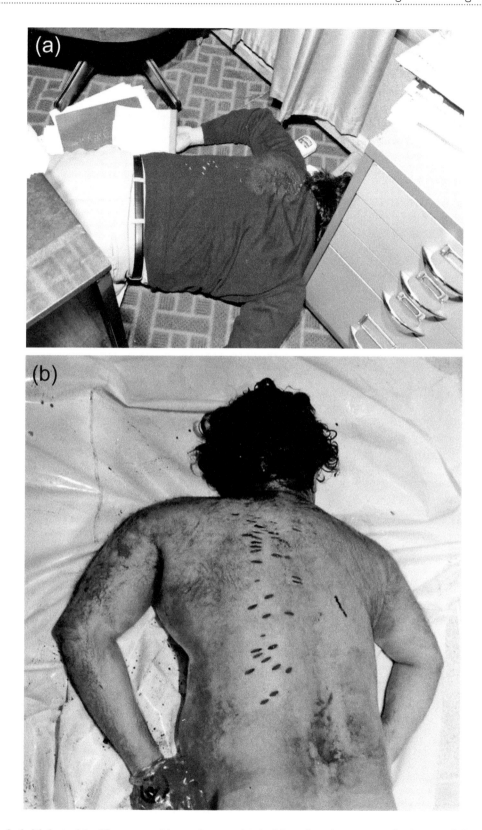

▲ **Figure 6.4** Male in his 40s was subjected to multiple blunt head trauma which immobilised him and then stabbed multiple times in his back whilst laying prone. (a) At the scene; (b) multiple stab wounds to the back.

A further related issue which needs to be considered when different types of violence are found in combination, is the number of perpetrators that may have been involved in each homicide and whether more than one type of weapon was used by one or more perpetrators. Behara and Sikary (2019) found that only one perpetrator was responsible in 70.6 % of homicide cases: males: 72.3% (81 from 112 cases) and females, 68.0% (51 females from 75 cases). Two perpetrators were involved in attacks against 31 males (27.7%) and 24 females (32%). With two perpetrators they observed that knives or other sharp instruments were mostly used either for stabbing or for producing cutthroat injuries predominantly in males. The second method used in addition to sharp weapon injury mostly involved blunt head trauma. The authors found that there were no cases where more than two perpetrators were involved.

## Injuries to Perpetrators

Examination of perpetrators shortly after the homicide may reveal injuries which have been accidentally inflicted as a result of the blade of the instrument used, slipping back into the hand during the assault. Karlsson (1998) found that of 113 perpetrators physically examined shortly after the homicide, 30 (27%) had evidence of sharp force injuries on their hands and four had self-harm injuries. They also found in two further cases where the perpetrator had hurt himself in an effort to prove that he himself had been attacked.

## Homicide Followed by Suicide (Dyadic Death)

Dyadic death, the phenomenon where an assailant kills a person or persons, (the victim or victims being mostly either family members or close acquaintances), is followed by the killer then committing suicide. Alternatively, the circumstances could also be an agreed suicide pact. Most

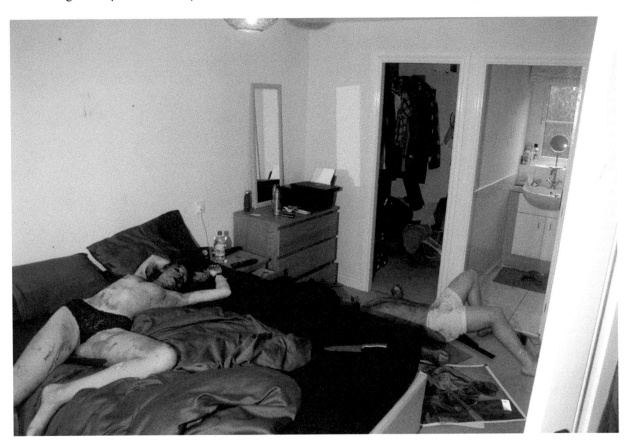

▲ **Figure 6.5a** Female lying on bed with knife close by. Male perpetrator is on the floor near to the bed.

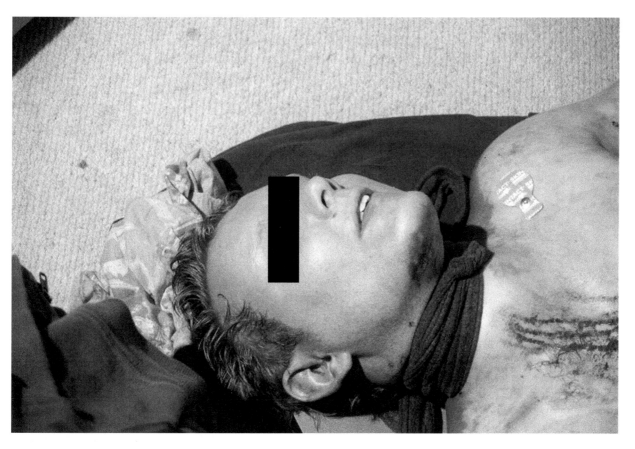

▲ **Figure 6.5b** Close up of deceased male with clothing used as a ligature seen tied around his neck.

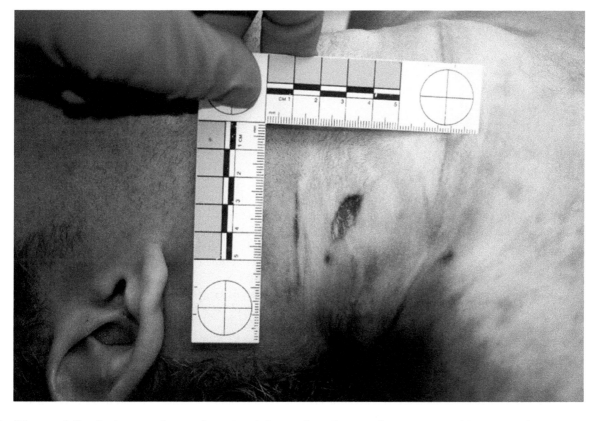

▲ **Figure 6.5c** Stab wound on right side of the neck with a small puncture and linear marks nearby.

homicide victims in published series (Copeland 1985; Milroy 1993, 1995; Betz and Eisenmenger 1997) have been described as suffering gunshot wounds with a much fewer number sustaining fatal sharp force or blunt force trauma. An example of a dyadic death involving sharp force trauma is given below.

A 23-year-old male manually strangled his 19-year-old girlfriend during an altercation following attending a night club and while he was under the influence of cocaine. Immediately afterwards, he stabbed himself in the neck and before collapsing was also able to tie a ligature around his neck. The ligature material covered the stab wound and the knife used was found nearby (Figure 6.5).

# References

Au KI, Beh SL. (2011). Injury patterns of sharp instrument homicides in Hong Kong. *Forensic Sci Int* 204, 201–204.

Behera C, Sikary AK. (2019). Homicide by multiple fatal methods: a study from South Delhi, India. J Interpers Violence, March 28, 1–11. Epub.

Bell MD, Vila RI. (1996). Homicide in homosexual victims: a study of 67 cases from the Broward County, Florida, Medical Examiner's Office (1982–1992), with special emphasis on "overkill" *Am J Forensic Med Pathol* 17, 65–69.

Betz P, Eisenmenger W. (1997). Comparison of wound patterns in homicide and dyadic death. *Med Sci Law* 37, 19–22.

Burke, M. P., Baber, Y., Cheung, Z., & Fitzgerald, M. (2018). Single stab injuries. *Forensic Science, Medicine, and Pathology, 14*, 295–300.

Brunel C, Fermanian C, Durigon M, de la Grandmaison GL. (2010). Homicidal and suicidal sharp force fatalities: autopsy parameters in relation to the manner of death. *Forensic Sci Int* 198, 150–154.

Copeland AR. (1985). Dyadic death-revisited. *J Forensic Sci Soc* 25, 181–188.

Cros J, Alvarez JC, Sbidian E, Charlier P, de la Grandmaison GL. (2013). Survival time estimation using Injury Severity Score (ISS) in homicide cases. *Forensic Sci Int* 233, 99–103.

Culbertson A, Sephton C. (2019). https://news.sky.com/story/police-dealing-with-incident-on-london-bridge-amid-reports-of-shots-fired-11873505. (accessed 30 November 2019).

Fischer J, Kleemann WJ, Tröger HD. (1994). Types of trauma in cases of homicide. *Forensic Sci Int* 68, 161–167.

Franchi A, Kolopp M, Coudane H, Martrille L. (2016) Precise survival time and physical activity after fatal left ventricle injury from sharp pointed weapon: a case report and a review of the literature. *Int J Legal Med* 130, 1299–1301.

Fukube S, Hayashi T, Ishida Y, Kamon H, Kawaguchi M, Kimura A, Kondo T. (2008). Retrospective study on suicidal cases by sharp force injuries. *J Forensic Leg Med* 15, 163–167.

Gill, JR, Catanese, C. (2002). Sharp injury fatalities in New York City. *J Forensic Sci* 47, 554–557.

Hunt AC, Cowling RJ (1991). Murder by stabbing. *Forensic Sci Int* 52, 107–112.

Karger B, Niemeyer J, Brinkmann B. (1999). Physical activity following fatal injury from sharp pointed weapons. *Int J Leg Med* 112, 188–191.

Karlsson T. (1998). Sharp force homicides in the Stockholm area, 1983–1992. *Forensic Sci Int* 94, 129–139.

Katkici U, Ozkok MS, Orsal M. (1994). An autopsy evaluation of defence wounds in 195 homicidal deaths due to stabbing. *J Forensic Sci Soc* 34, 237–240.

Kemal CJ, Patterson T, Molina DK. (2013). Deaths due to sharp force injuries in Bexar County, Texas, with respect to manner of death. *Am J Forensic Med Pathol* 34, 253–259.

Krywanczyk A, Shapiro S. (2015). A retrospective study of blade wound characteristics in suicide and homicide. *Am J Forensic Med Pathol* 36, 305–310.

Levy VI, Rao VJ. (1988). Survival time in gunshot and stab wound victims. *Am J Forensic Med Pathol* 9, 215–217.

Merin O, Sonkin R, Yitzhak A, Frenkel H, Leiba A, Schwarz AD, Jaffe E. (2017). Terrorist stabbings-distinctive characteristics and how to prepare for them. *J Emerg Med* 53, 451–457.

Milroy CM. (1995). The epidemiology of homicide-suicide (dyadic death). *Forensic Sci Int* 30, 117–122.

Milroy CM. (1993). Homicide followed by suicide (dyadic death) in Yorkdhire and Humberside. *Med Sci Law* 33, 167–171.

Mitton L, du Toit-Prinsloo L. (2016). Sharp force fatalities at the Pretoria Medico-Legal Laboratory, 2012–2013. *S Afr J Surg* 54, 21–26.

Murray LA, Green MA. (1987). Hilts and knives: a survey of 10 years of fatal stabbings. *Med Sci Law* 27, 182–184.

Ormstad K, Karlsson T, Enkler L, Law B, Rajs J. (1986). Patterns in sharp force fatalities—a comprehensive forensic medical study. *J Forensic Sci* 31, 529–542.

Ozdemir B, Celbis O, Kaya A. (2013). Cut throat injuries and honor killings: review of 15 cases in eastern Turkey. *J Forensic Leg Med* 20, 198–203.

Radojević N, Radnić B, Petković S, Miljen M, Curović I, Cukić D, Soć M, Savić S. (2013). Multiple stabbing in sex-related homicides. *J Forensic Leg Med* 20, 502–507.

Rogde S, Hougen HP, Poulsen K. (2000), Homicide by sharp force in two Scandinavian capitals. *Forensic Sci Int* 109, 135–145.

Rouse DA. (1994). Patterns of stab wounds: a six year study. *Med Sci Law* 34, 67–71.

Rozenfeld M, Givon A, Peleg K. (2018). Violence-related versus terror-related stabbings. *Ann Surg* 267, 965–970.

Sauvageau, A., Trépanier, J. S., & Racette, S. (2006). Delayed deaths after vascular traumatism: two cases. *Journal of clinical forensic medicine, 13,* 344–348.

Solarino B, Punzi G, Di Vella G, Carabellese F, Catanesi R. (2019). A multidisciplinary approach in overkill: analysis of 13 cases and review of the literature. *Forensic Sci Int* 298, 402–407.

Stermac L, Bove GD, Addison M. (2001). Violence, injury, and presentation patterns in spousal sexual assaults. *Violence against Women* 7, 1218–1233.

Thomsen AH, Hougen HP, Villesen P, Brink O, Leth PM. (2019). Sharp force homicide in Denmark 1992–2016. *J Forensic Sci.* doi: 10.1111/1556-4029.14244. [Epub ahead of print].

Thoresen SO, Rognum TO. (1986). Survival time and acting capability after fatal injury by sharp weapons. *Forensic Sci Int* 31, 181–187.

Vanezis P. (2003). Sharp force trauma, in *Forensic medicine, clinical and pathological aspects*, Eds., Payne-James J., Busuttil A., Smock W. Greenwich Medical Media Ltd, London, Chapter 22, 307–320.

Vanezis P. (2020). Sharp force trauma, in *Essential forensic medicine*, Ed Vanezis P. Chapter 8, 111–127. Wiley & Sons, Chichester, West Sussex.

Vassalini M, Verzeletti A, De Ferrari F. (2014). Sharp force injury fatalities: a retrospective study (1982–2012) in Brescia (Italy). *J Forensic Sci* 59, 1568–1574.

# Chapter 7

# Morphology of Sharp Force Injuries and Type of Implements Responsible for Causing Them

## Introduction

Although the vast majority of wounds are from knives, the morphology of injuries from other sharp and/or pointed implements will also be discussed, describing the individual variations that one would expect to see from different types of sharp edges (not exhaustive) and will include broken glass or sharp-edged broken fragments from ceramic objects, axes, machetes, cleavers, scissors, screw drivers (Philips and flat head screw drivers being the most common), razors, arrows, crossbow bolts and any object capable of penetrating the body that has a reasonably long cylindrical or elongated component and is pointed to a greater or lesser extent.

The pathologist, by describing in detail the appearance of injuries produced aims to assist in the identification of the nature and size of the implement (weapon) used and advise on the force, as well as angle of impact including the reaction and movement of the victim during the time the injury or injuries are sustained.

It is appropriate at this stage to emphasise the need to use appropriate and consistent terminology when measuring wounds both on the skin surface and their tracks inside the body. From time to time in post-mortem reports, one sees the longer distance (longitudinal axis) on the skin surface of a stab wound referred to as the width of the wound. The reason is, that it is associated with the width of the blade or other similar surface, to contrast with the distance the weapon has entered the body (length of the track of the wound). The degree to which the wound gapes on the surface is the width or gape of the wound (Figure 7.1). When the wound edges (syn. margins) are carefully apposed using clear adhesive tape it allows the pathologist to make a more accurate assessment of the wound shape in relation to the blade characteristics and particularly in cases where the wound is notched because of change of direction between its entry and exit (see Chapter 5).

An important point that should immediately be appreciated about tracks of wounds into the body, is the difference between the depth of a wound track and its length. Length is the distance travelled inwards from the skin and can be shallow or deep, depending on the angle of entry. On the other hand, depth refers to the perpendicular distance from the entry point (90° from where the measurement is taken).

93

## Factors Relating to the Appearance of Wounds

The appearance of any cutting injuries, whether, stab, incised (slash), chopping or perforating (aside from firearms), requires a thorough appraisal of their appearance to assist the investigation of a case. The following are important considerations in any case of sharp force trauma since they will determine, to a greater or lesser extent, the appearance of the inflicted wound and may assist in the identification of the injuring agent.

The shape of wounds on the surface and underlying tissue, for example from the use of a knife, may vary significantly when there are a number of wounds depending on how the weapon is used and the dynamics involved during the assault. It is also possible that different morphological features may indicate the use of more than one knife. One also needs to consider the effect that intervening layers of clothing may have on the appearance of any wound.

The angle of impact and direction into body of a knife or other sharp-edged instrument is an essential consideration in every case. Assessment by the

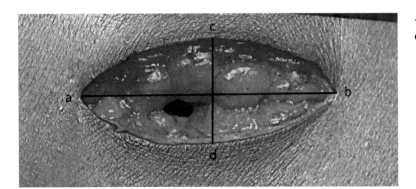

◀ **Figure 7.1** Stab wound length on skin surface a-b; width (gape) c-d.

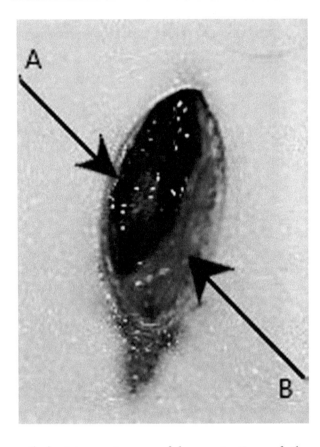

◀ **Figure 7.2** Stab wound showing undercutting edge (A), and shelved edge together with the direction of the track of the wound (B). The graze which appears as a short tail at the lower end of the wound indicates the direction of exit of the knife.

pathologist requires careful examination of the wound on the skin surface as well as the direction of the track. When the blade of a knife enters the body at a non-perpendicular angle to the body, its direction is indicated by the way subcutaneous tissue has been cut, with one side being shelved and the corresponding opposite surface being undercut (Figure 7.2).

The extent of underlying trauma to soft tissue and organ damage, including markings or fractures on bone or cartilage, will also be directly relevant to the dynamics of the assault, which includes a number of important factors related to the ease with which the implement may have penetrated the body, how it is used by the assailant and by the resistance offered by movement of the victim and by their clothes, skin and internal tissues (see chapter 3.)

# Demographic Factors

One should not lose sight of the fact that there are frequently many demographic factors, including the effect of wound numeracy, assailant/victim relationship, gender, age, location (environment), number of assailants or more than one weapon, motive, pattern of injury and other evidence which will complement

the physical appearance of wounds. Such issues are discussed in detail in chapter 6.

# The Effect of Sharp Force Impact on Clothing

The pathologist should be aware of the effect of sharp force trauma on the clothing of a dressed victim, particularly from knives which can add further information to the wounds seen on the body and inform us of the dynamics during an assault between one or more individuals. Items of clothing may be creased or folded over, and damage from one stabbing action may be seen on the same item of clothing more than once, giving the false impression of more than one deliberate blow. The situation becomes even more complicated when there are different layers of garments showing defects in different positions, due to movement of clothing such as by pulling, during an altercation. One should always bear in mind, the type and number of layers of clothing, how loosely or tightly worn and the variables which determine its resistance to penetration.

It is particularly important, not just for the fabric analyst to assess marks on clothing in a thorough and cautious manner, but also for the pathologist not to misinterpret such findings, particularly in situations where the deceased is skeletonised, badly decomposed, mutilated in some way, including from animal predation, or when only clothing is found without the corresponding body.

The variable factors which affect the type of damage seen on the body will also, to a greater or lesser extent, be applicable to the marks and defects seen on clothing. One must bear in mind however, that different types of fabrics may be damaged in slightly different ways. This has to be taken into account by the fabric analyst when testing the material in question.

Examples of defects (cuts and tears) made in clothing from cases encountered by the author are shown in Figure 7.3 . It is not unusual that in some, the marks on the clothing may not match underlying injuries for the reasons just given (Figure 7.4).

The effect of stabbing through up to three layers of clothing was studied by Sarkisian and Fedorov (2014). They considered the direction of

stabbing through clothing. The injuries had all been inflicted by kitchen knives having the blades of practically identical length and width but differently shaped tips. A total of 480 skin wounds and 720 damaged clothing specimens were available for the examination. They found that injuries to the skin unprotected by clothing had a different shape and length of the edge and end portions, depending on the shape of the blade tip and the direction of the stab. With regard to the effect of layers of clothing, they observed that the length of all wounds inflicted through clothing decreased as the number of layers increased. The wounds had their linear shape, contusion collar and flattened area become narrower and the shape of the back edges of the wounds altered when inflicted through a three-layer barrier.

Assessment of fabric severance morphology, which is common practice in forensic science, was studied by Cowper et al. (2015) on similar fabrics (not laundered and laundered). They were evaluated after impact with kitchen knives. They found knife-withdrawal technique to be an important variable when evaluating severance appearance but that, depending on the scenario, controlled laboratory simulation test methods were likely to be of limited use to recreate fabric severances for comparison to a crime.

Kemp et al. (2009) found from their research that they were able to differentiate between different types of blades and could estimate the direction of impact by examining the shape and size of the severance in the fabric and the appearance of its constituents. The above authors point out that the results of fabric damage assessment typically at varying levels is at least partly subjective. On the other hand, examination at the fabric level concentrates on the degree of distortion in the fabric surrounding the severance changes to the "normal" yarn (thread) spacing, the direction of the severance line relative to the yarn direction and the relative position of severed yarn ends, depending on the fibre type and the weapon used.

95

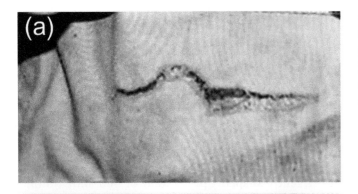

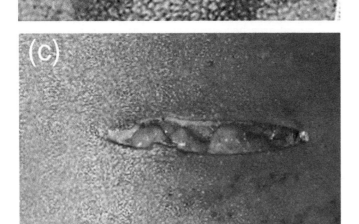

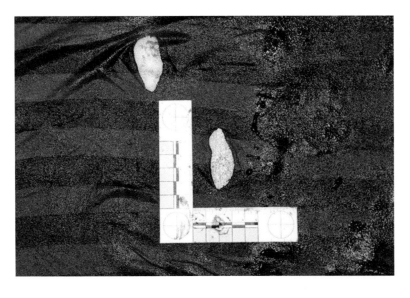

◀ **Figure 7.3** Two layers of clothing (a) outer and (b) inner, showing cuts from the use of a kitchen knife. The notch in both layers indicates the change of direction of the knife on withdrawal. (c) Corresponding wound on the skin.

◀ **Figure 7.4a** Large cuts in thin T shirt from two stab wounds. Shirt is soaked with blood.

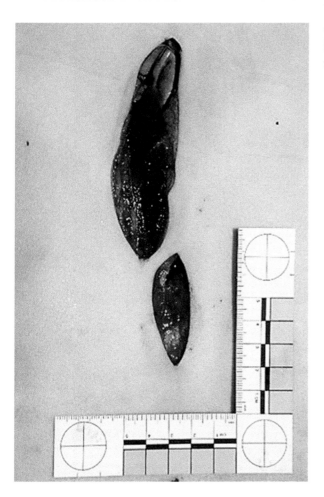

◀ **Figure 7.4b** Corresponding stab wounds on lower thorax in slightly different orientation due to creasing of shirt during the stabbing action.

## Case of Azaria Chamberlain

A high profile case in point in Australia, where reliance had to be placed on marks on clothing, is the disappearance of nine-week-old Azaria Chamberlain in 1980 at Ayres Rock. Lindy Chamberlain, her mother, was convicted of her murder and given a life sentence. Her husband Michael was convicted as an accessory after the fact and given a suspended sentence. Their baby daughter Azaria went missing on 17 August 1980 from the family tent at the base of Uluru (Ayres Rock) where Lindy Chamberlain, her husband, Michael, and their three children were camping. Lindy said she saw a dingo leave the tent with the baby. Police and Aboriginal trackers instituted a massive search but only found a blood stained jumpsuit (Figure 7.5), singlet and nappy near a dingo's lair. A coroner's inquest accepted the account given by the parents but was quashed, and in 1982 Lindy was charged with murder and Michael with accessory after the fact. At their trial evidence was heard that Lindy Chamberlain had cut Azaria's throat with a pair of scissors in the family car and deposited the jumpsuit in a place where it

would be found so as to simulate an attack by a dingo. They did not believe her story that the baby was wearing a matinee jacket at the time.

There has been much controversy over how death was caused; whether the baby had been taken by a dingo or whether it had had its throat cut with a pair of scissors (Tullet 1986). In January 1986, Mr David Brett died after he lost his footing and fell whilst climbing Uluru. His body was found eight days later in an area where there were dingo lairs. In addition they also found a white matinee jacket as described by Azaria's mother (Figure 7.6). Lindy Chamberlain was released from prison and The NT Supreme Court acquitted the Chamberlains in 1988. The independent findings of a Royal Commission of Inquiry (1987) were adopted at a fourth inquest in 2012 (NTMC 20 (2012)) as well as further evidence given about the finding of the further clothing near a dingo lair and the fact that dingoes had been observed attacking young children. Azaria's mother Lindy Chamberlain, was exonerated on the basis of the civil level of proof, i.e. the balance of probability.

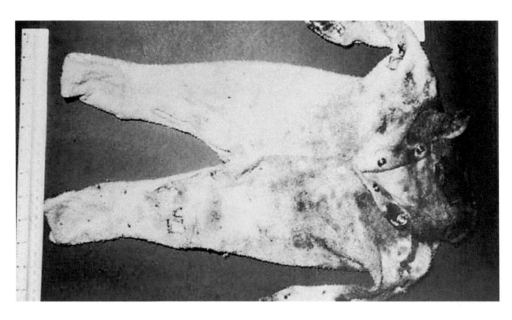

▲ **Figure 7.5** Azaria Chamberlain's torn and bloodied jumpsuit (NT PoliceSource: News Limited).

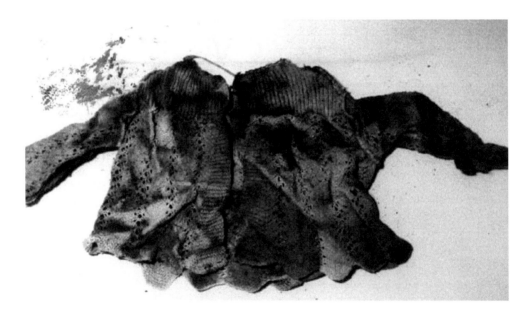

▲ **Figure 7.6** Matinee jacket: Police searching for a fallen hiker found Azaria's matinee jacket near a dingo's lair on Uluru. (NT Police Source: News Corp Australia)

# Morphological Appearance of Wounds on the Skin and Factors Affecting their Shape and Size

## Wound Shape and Dynamics

Assessment of the morphology of wounds is essential in order to reconstruct how they were caused in relation to the type, shape and size of the implement used and the dynamics which affect their appearance, including force, direction and the relative movements between the assailant and victim during their infliction.

The shape of a wound, its length and width (gape) on the skin surface as shown in Figure 7.1; whether

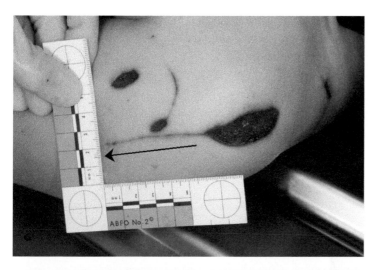

◀ **Figure 7.7a** Stab wounds impacting on the shoulder region, producing a tail from one end of two of the wounds due to the rounded nature of location caused from partial tangential contact with the skin. The tail ends are caused as the knife is withdrawn from the body with most probably the victim moving (direction of withdrawal shown by arrow).

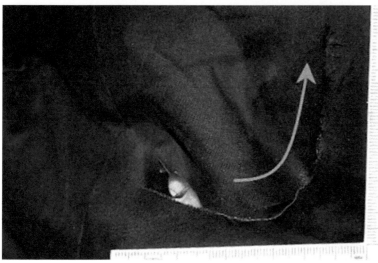

◀ **Figure 7.7b** Garment showing a corresponding defect and tail (arrow shows direction of withdrawal).

99

the wound appears regular or irregular, may well be altered with differing angles of impact and the location on the body, for example curvature of the skin and/or whether over bone, may produce a stab wound with a tail as the knife is retracted from the body, particularly when the victim is also moving (Figure 7.7).

## Laceration or Incised Wound?

Lacerations when sustained over bone, particularly to the head, may resemble incised wounds and require careful assessment to determine their true nature. In such circumstances the skin may split neatly leaving a wound which is almost indistinguishable from an incision. It is especially important to examine the underlying bone, such as the skull, to look for scored marks or chips from which may have been caused by a knife and distinguish from fractures typical of blunt impact (Figures 7.8 and 7.9).

Further difficulties may arise when the weapon used has a sharp and blunt component as with an axe or a machete. With such implements, there is a combination of crushing injury, showing both features of incisions and lacerations. Such injuries are referred to as chopping wounds.

Further confusion may arise when misleading terminology is used amongst medical professionals (see chapter 1) where the term laceration is used for a cutting injury and vice versa (Milroy and Rutty 1997). A typical linear laceration which is sometimes erroneously referred to as a "cut" is shown in Figure 7.10 and shows typical subcutaneous bridging tissue between the two split edges.

The angle of impact will influence whether shelving with undercutting is present and thus give some guidance as to the direction of the impact (Figure 7.2.). If the knife blade enters perpendicular to the plane of the body, the wound defect will not show evidence of

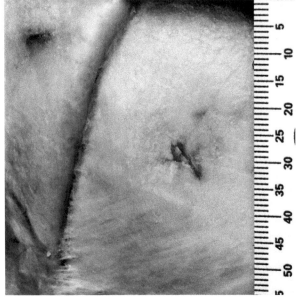

**◄ Figure 7.8a** Stab wound in the left frontal region of the skull.

**◄ Figure 7.8b** The scalp has been reflected to reveal the skull periosteum to show chipped bone with a linear component. The subcutaneous aspect of the stab wound which has caused this injury is seen at the bottom left hand corner.

shelving or undercutting on the opposite side. With shelving, the angle made between the skin and the underlying soft tissue and skin surface on one side of the wound is obtuse. With undercutting, the same interface angle with the other side of the wound is acute. If the knife blade enters at an upward, downward or sideways (e.g. from left to right) angle at the point of entry then these features are commonly seen and can be used as a guide as to the angle of entry into the body rather than directly into the body at 90 degrees.

However, one should appreciate that side to side movement of the body and weapon are a common feature of stabbing in a dynamic situation, and thus will need to be considered in the overall assessment of the direction of the impact and wound track. In the vast majority of cases the pathologist will find and describe a wound track as a combination of upward or downward tilting of the knife track from the point of entry as well as movement with sideways direction from left or right. Occasionally when examining a single

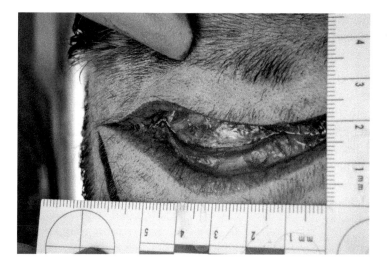

◄ **Figure 7.9a** Tangential incised wound to the crown of the head.

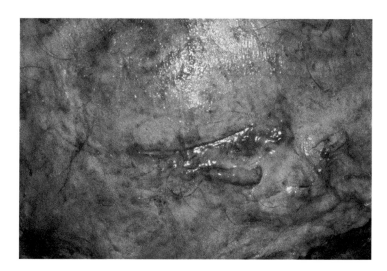

◄ **Figure 7.9b** The linear score mark on the underlying skull assists in differentiating between a linear laceration and a cutting injury.

101

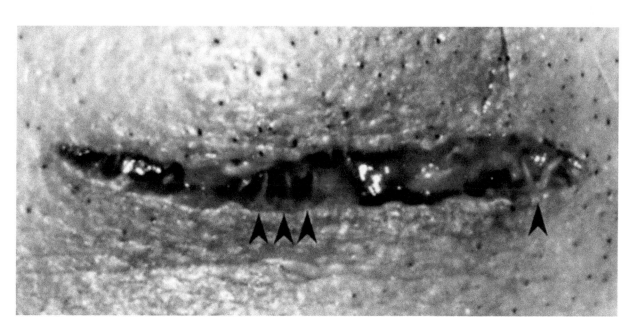

▲ **Figure 7.10** Linear laceration on chin. Bridging strands of tissue (arrows) are seen in the wound.

wound, there may be more than one wound in the heart for example, close to each other. Such further wounds occur as a result of movement of the knife and /or victim as well as the heart itself during the stabbing action.

The angle of impact will also affect the depth of penetration into the body as opposed to the length of the track of the wound. When there is movement between the assailant and the victim it may sometimes be difficult to assess which impacts were intended stabs or slash wounds; and frequently, where there are multiple sharp trauma wounds, a combination of both is seen (Figure 7.11).

The ubiquity of security cameras is an accepted part of everyday life and not infrequently one is able to capture and watch the assault, slow down the speed and confirm the direction of impact from an assailant or assailants and therefore have a much clearer understanding of the size of weapon, type of thrust (whether overarm, underarm, from a sideways position, from behind), length of the attack, as well as the relative positions of the victim and attacker at the time. All this information can then be correlated with the post-mortem findings.

## Wound Shape and Knife Shape

The shape of the knife (its blade and hilt) frequently broadly correlates with certain characteristics which are found on a wound that it causes. Such marks may vary as described above according to the variable factors involved in its production.

One of the features of most knives is some form of hilt (guard). Murray and Green (1987) in their series of 74 fatal stabbings providing 143 stab wounds found only five wounds with a mark made by the hilt of a knife. They concluded that hilt marks were more related to the site of injury rather than force of impact. In addition, it should be appreciated that it is not only the site of injury, but also the position at the wound, whether uniform around the wound, or at one side or the other, will depend on the angle of impact of the knife to the skin and whether at that point the blade length has entered its full length into the tissue (Figure 7.12).

In relation to the cutting edge of a blade, most stab wound injuries seen are caused by blades with a single straight (as opposed to serrated) cutting edge, and this is reflected in the characteristic shape of the wounds, showing a pointed end with the other end

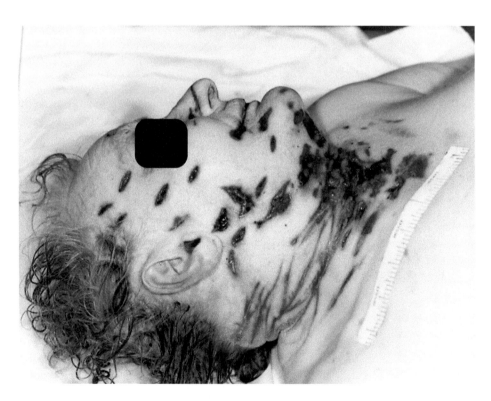

▲ **Figure 7.11** Combination of stab and incised wounds.

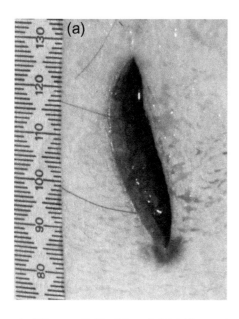 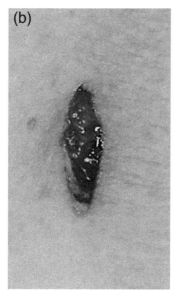 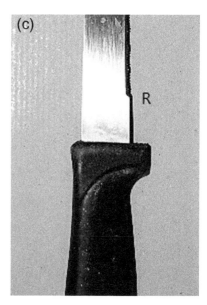

▲ **Figure 7.12** (a) and (b) Hilt marks at the lower end of both stab wounds. (c) The knife detail shows a pronounced hilt which surrounds the end of the blade beyond the ricasso (R) and incorporates the rest of the black handle.

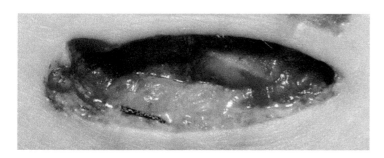

◄ **Figure 7.13** Stab wound caused by knife with single sharp edge and the other side showing a "fish tail."

103

having a squared off, ragged or "fishtail" appearance (Figure 7.13).

Serrated knives may also produce a clean sharp-ended wound with clean cut sides, resembling a smooth cutting surface, when the knife impacts the body such as to enter and be withdrawn rapidly out of the body. In single stab cases it may be impossible to differentiate between the two types of cutting edge. However, in many cases there may be superficial or angular (non-perpendicular) wounds which demonstrate interrupted linear abrasions caused by serrations, as shown in Figures 7.14 and 7.15.

Occasionally, it is possible to carry out superimposition of the image of a suspected knife with superficial wounds with a serrated pattern (Figure 7.16). The pathologist will not be able to positively identify a particular knife from having caused such injuries but may be able to state whether the injuries were consistent with being caused by such a weapon or one of a similar type. Direct comparison of a suspected

knife with wounds over the body is entirely inappropriate so as not to cause any contamination and affect the integrity of the evidence in the case.

Kaliszan et al. (2011) encountered a homicide case where doubt arose as to whether a knife thought to have caused the wound had a smooth cutting edge or was serrated. The knife that was involved was smooth bladed but had a serrated pattern to its hilt adjacent to the blade (Figure 7.17). They carried out an experiment on a human cadaver (Figure 7.18) and were able to demonstrate a striated pattern similar to the wound in their homicide case

A good example of a knife with a serrated edge is the survival knife (Figure 7.19). This weapon has a serrated surface on the back of the blade as well as a non-serrated smooth cutting edge on the other side. A case is presented by Ciallella et al. (2002) demonstrating the appearance of the injuries produced by stabbing and sawing across the skin to produce the interrupted marks seen (Figure 7.20).

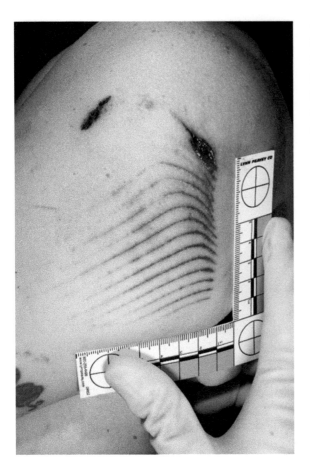

◀ **Figure 7.14a** Forearm of stabbed victim indicating the dynamic nature between the assailant and victim resulting in an angular thrust with the serrated edge of the blade dragging across the skin before entering the skin in a stabbing action and exiting on the other side, where a short tail is seen.

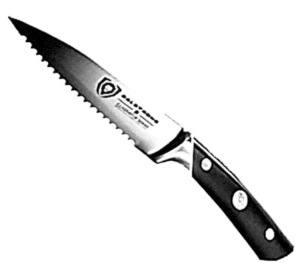

◀ **Figure 7.14b** Typical serrated kitchen knife.

The degree of tapering of a knife and whether pointed, will also influence the appearance of the injury. A bruised area (collar) may be present if the knife has a prominent hilt, assuming that the full length of the knife blade had entered into the body. It is also necessary to take into account the elasticity of the skin and its location when assessing blade width.

It should also be appreciated that the tip of the knife affects the force required to penetrate the body and to a great extent determines whether the wound produced will be clean cut or ragged and the degree of surrounding bruising frequently seen. A number of experiments to demonstrate the effect of blade tip, its radius and cutting angle were carried out by Ní Annaidh et al. (2013) (see chapter 3).

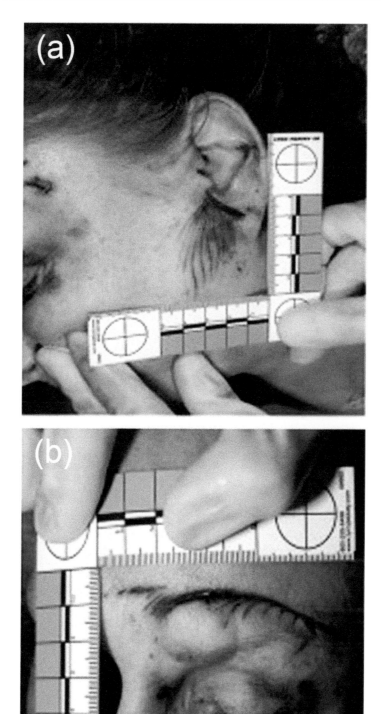

▲ **Figure 7.15** Same victim as in Figure 7.14 showing a variety of wounds caused by the same knife.

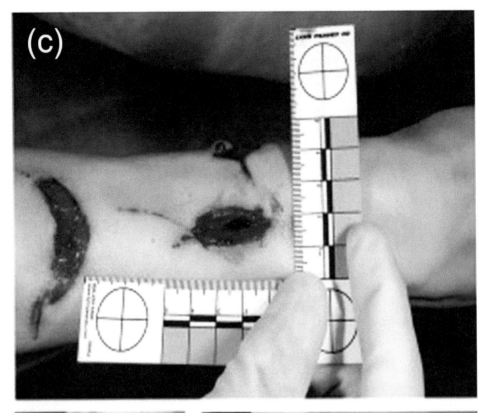

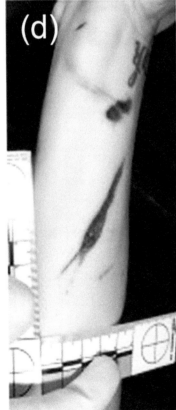

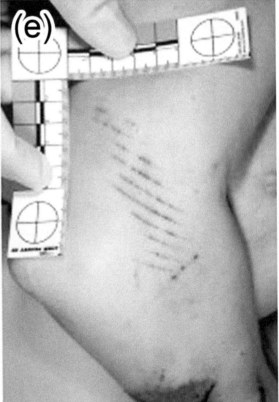

▲ **Figure 7.15** (Continued)

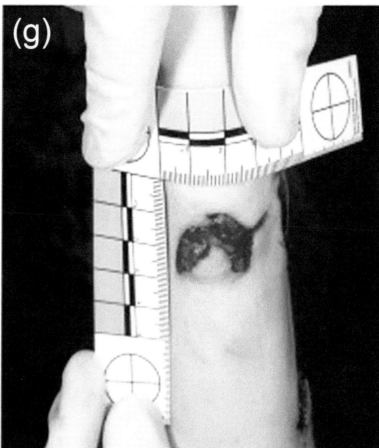

▲ **Figure 7.15** (Continued)

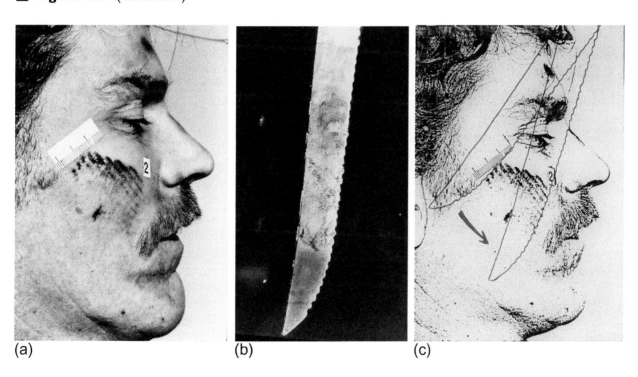

(a)  (b)  (c)

▲ **Figure 7.16** (a) Linear facial wounds. (b)Serrated knife blade. (c) Overlay of outline of knife blade with wounds to assess consistency in matching them with the serrated teeth of the knife.

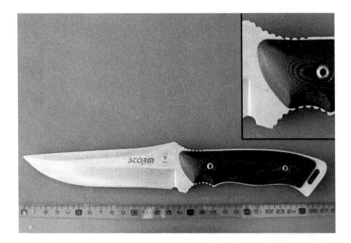

◀ **Figure 7.17** Striated pattern adjacent to hilt and back of knife. Source: (Courtesy, Kaliszan et al. 2011).

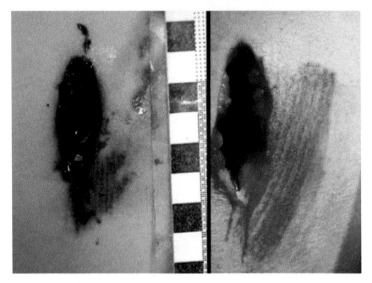

◀ **Figure 7.18** Homicide wound (left); Experimental wound (right). Source: (Courtesy, Kaliszan et al. 2011).

108

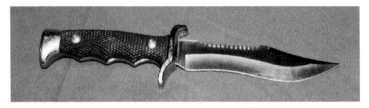

◀ **Figure 7.19** An example of a survival knife. Source: (Courtesy, Ciallella et al, 2002).

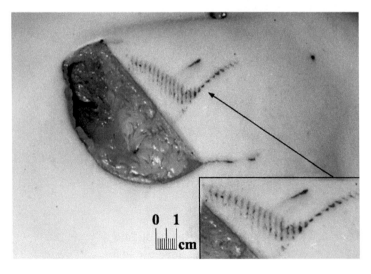

◀ **Figure 7.20** The patterned appearance of the wound on the skin with the particular feature showing the edges of the wound changing from linear to V-shape, almost reproducing in the skin the mechanism of stabbing then withdrawing of the weapon. Source: (Courtesy, Ciallella et al, 2002).

## Notched Wounds

Frequently, wounds show a notch or change of direction along their margin on the skin (Figures 7.21, 7.22 and 7.23). This is caused by relative movement of the knife and the body during the stabbing action thus causing the exit track of the wound to be slightly modified. In the case reported by Menon and colleagues (2008), the external wound had an extension described by them as "swan tail" with two wounds to the heart and lungs, indicative of movement of the internal organs from change in position during movement.

The shape of a wound may sometimes be distorted giving a rectangular or cigar-shaped appearance.

This pattern may arise from an angled impact as well as in some cases, from notching of the wounds, a product of the dynamics of the stabbing (Figure 7.24).

## Identification of Weapon Used from Wound Morphology

Pathologists are frequently requested to give an opinion on the type of weapon that caused injury to the victim. The features which will be considered in assisting the type of weapon, will be the proportion and dimensions of the anatomical parts, particularly of a knife, which is by far the most significant weapon used in sharp force trauma.

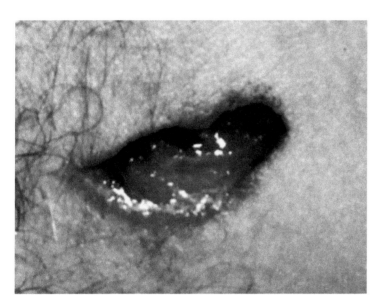

◀ **Figure 7.21** Stab wound showing a slight central notch on its upper margin. The lower margin shows "shelving", with underlying tissue visible. (This refers to an angled penetration of the skin in a stab wound. The undercut is the half of the skin that is angled out over the cut, while the shelf is the other half of the skin that is under the angled entry of the stab.) Such wounds give the investigator an indication of the direction of their track on entry and exit.

109

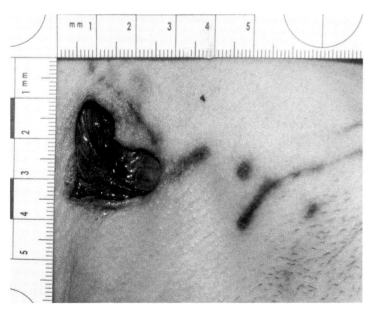

◀ **Figure 7.22** Stab wound with central notch giving the appearance of a "V" shape indicating the blade direction had changed appreciably through the knife turning or from the movement of the victim.

(a) (b)

▲ **Figure 7.23** Extension of wound indicating that the direction of the track on exit had altered slightly. The upper wound (a) appears slightly shorter than when the edges of the same wound (b) have been apposed.

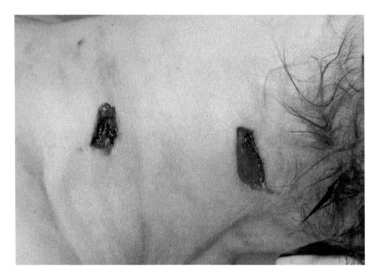

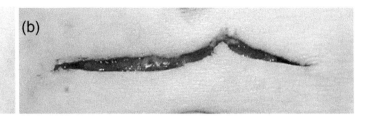

◀ **Figure 7.24** Two stab wounds on the neck with a rectangular appearance from a large single sharp-edged kitchen knife.

In terms of the anatomy of a knife, the following features will require consideration together with wounds on the body (see also chapter 3):

- overall weight
- design
- handle, including hilt
- blade: width, length, pointedness, sharp surfaces
- any deformity of knife

*Wound Size and Blade Width*

Blade width from the examination of stab wounds can only approximately be assessed. The blade width frequently tapers from a maximum width near the hilt to a point. Furthermore, if the full length of the blade has not come into contact with the body, the length of the wound on the skin surface may only be compared with the length of the blade that had entered the body. Having stated the above, wounds that have been caused by penetration at or near an angle of 90 degrees are the most likely to be closely related to the blade width.

Barber (2009) carried out stabbing experiments on pig skin using four kitchen knives of differing sizes and ensuring that the blade of each knife penetrated to the hilt and impact being at 90 degrees. The skin wounds were measured by opposing the cut edges and comparing with the maximum width of each blade. It was observed that the wounds were either the same size as the blade width or narrower. The author also analysed retrospective autopsy data from 40 homicide cases where the cause of death was given as single or multiple stab wounds. The knives causing the injuries were known. The results in almost all cases demonstrated similar results to the pig skin data with wound lengths which were equal to or smaller in size when compared with the width of the knife blade.

Estimation of blade width is certainly not an exact science in case work and is further complicated by distortion of a wound which can occur for a number of reasons, including the angle of impact on the body which is related to the direction of the impact as well as the curvature of the location. The "superficial" stab wound which impacts at a very shallow angle to the body and does not enter a body cavity, may be useful for considering and identifying the stabbing weapon which created the wounds. It has been suggested that a superficial stab wound has a shallow wound cavity which runs almost parallel to the surface of the body and additionally its wound cavity shape may reflect the original profile of the weapon (Ohshima 2005).

In addition, wounds from the same knife which are produced on the body from the same direction onto a broadly similar region on the body, may appear different due to the direction of the lines of cleavage (Langer's lines) as reported by Byard et al. (2005) (Figure 7.25 and 7.26).

Stabbing experiments that were carried out by Pollak and Fischer (1991) using a single-edged blade on skin preparations taken from three regions of the body (anterior chest wall, abdominal wall, lumbar region), showed that the most gaping stab wounds were found, as anticipated, if the blade was stabbed perpendicular to Langer's lines. If the blade entered parallel to these lines, which depend on the pattern of cutaneous fibres, narrow slit-like wounds were produced; the dimensions of wounds from stabs

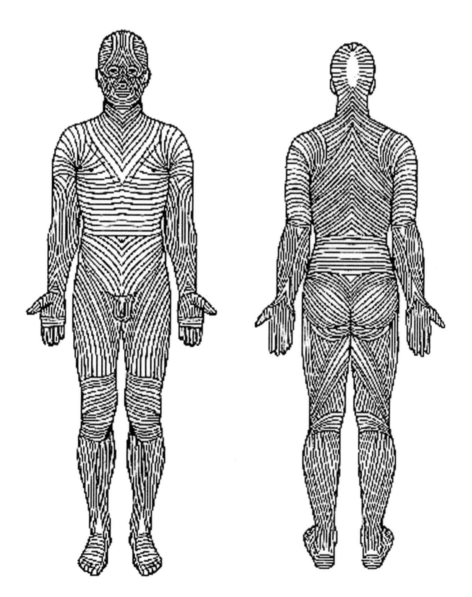

▲ **Figure 7.25** Langer's lines, sometimes called cleavage lines, are topological lines drawn on a map of the human body.

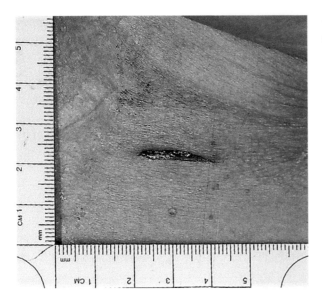

◀ **Figure 7.26a** Linear slit-shaped stab wound on left side of neck aligned with Langer's lines.

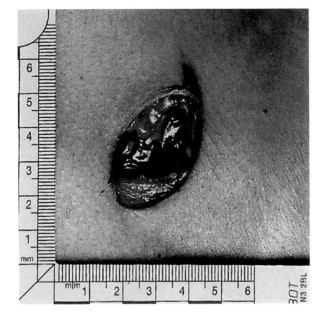

◀ **Figure 7.26b** Gaping stab wound on right side of neck cutting across Langer's lines.

at an angle of 45 degrees to Langer's lines, were between the two extreme patterns.

They also found that the length of the skin wounds in stabbing (without lateral cutting movement) was greater in the abdominal region than in the chest and lumbar regions, but never reached the full width of the penetrated blade, even after approximating the edges of a gaping wound.

As stated by Ohshima (2005), superficial wounds may assist in the identification of the knife or other weapon used for stabbing. They discuss the appearance of the cavities formed by shallow stab wounds

and discuss two cases where the profile of the blade could be assessed from such injuries.

Finally dealing with examination of skin surface wounds, it should always be borne in mind that where there are multiple wounds on the body, there is a greater possibility of damaging the knife in some way. This generally occurs from repeated impact against hard tissue such as bone particularly during a prolonged attack. In such circumstances the knife tip may be broken off or the blade twisted, bowed or bent in some way during an attack and produce wounds which may mirror the damage seen on a knife, thus aiding its identification as the weapon used (Figure 7.27).

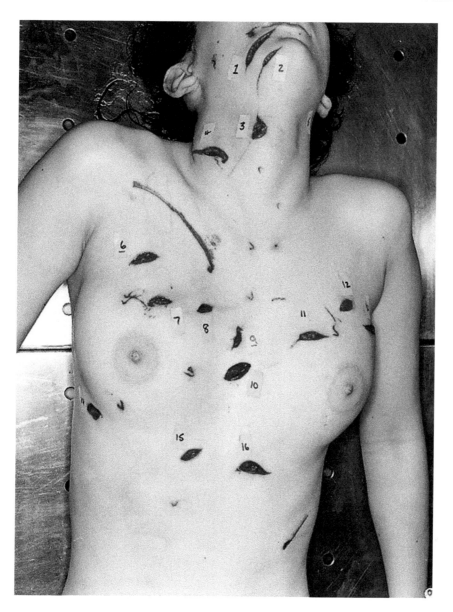

▲ **Figure 7.27a** Young woman with multiple stab wounds.

# Appearance Inside the Body and Factors Affecting Shape, Size and Length of Track

It is important to appreciate that the tracks of wounds can provide a wealth of information which will assist the pathologist to determine the dynamics of the stabbing and the injuries caused internally.

The methods of inflicting a stab wound which indicate the direction of movement before impact on the body (taking also into account the movements of the victim) include the following:

- overarm movement

- thrust towards the victim which may be horizontal forward or from the side of the assailant, towards the victim

- upper cut motion towards the body

See also chapter 3.

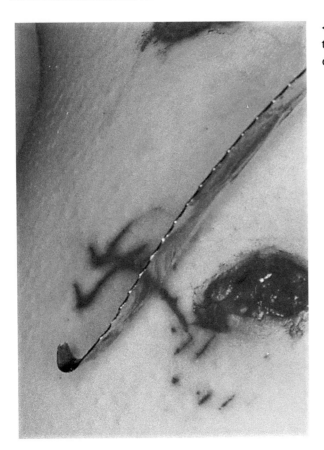

◀ **Figure 7.27b** The knife had become bent at the tip, causing the later injuries to conform to the damage seen to the implement.

114

# Direction of the Track of a Stab Wound

The direction of the track within the body, from the direction of impact, is generally predictable but may vary significantly from what is expected, due to the extent and type of movement between the assailant and victim.

Assessing the direction of the track within the body will assist in reconstructing the positions of the assailant and victim, how the knife was held by the assailant and the method of delivery of the stab. It should be understood that the track direction may be significantly affected by the stance of the victim. The position of the victim may vary when multiple wounds have been sustained from standing to lying flat, and any position in between rendering reconstruction of events very difficult.

Beillas et al. (2009) demonstrated that that there is marked change in organ position between being upright and supine. Their work was in relation to human modelling for car crash research. They imaged the thorax and the abdomen of nine subjects in four postures using a positional MRI scanner. The four postures were seated, standing, forward-flexed and supine. They were selected to represent car occupants, pedestrians, cyclists and a typical position for medical imaging, respectively. They found that only the supine posture was affected by changes to organ volumes and their positions in the spinal frame, but the other postures were mostly unaffected. The supine posture was associated with a motion of all solid organs of up to 39 mm and a reduction of the thoracic cavity volume of up to 1300 cm³. Subject-to-subject variations were especially large for the volume of the spleen and the position of the kidneys.

The situation in a mortuary, where the deceased is supine on a table, will alter the position of the thoraco-abdominal organs from being in their upright position governed by the effects of gravity, to a horizontal position in which gravity is spread evenly throughout the truncal organs to an extent which may have a significant effect on the true direction of the wound track within the body.

Surgeons operating on such injuries in hospital are well aware how damage to vessels or other organs can be overlooked unless it is appreciated that the direction of a wound track or tracks may appear different in theatre, because of the change of position of the victim from the position in which they were injured.

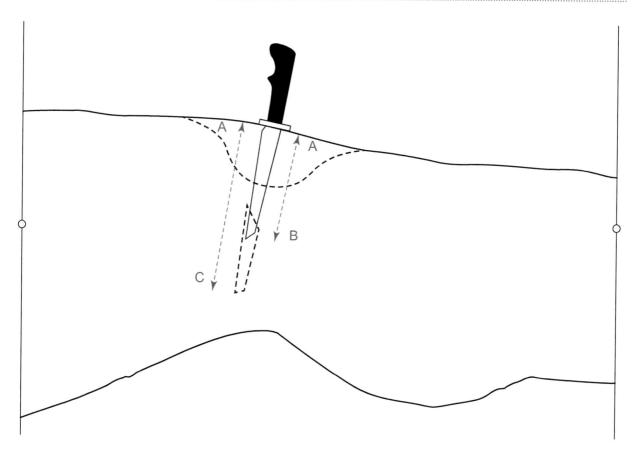

▲ **Figure 7.28** Knife penetrated to the hilt showing the position before abdominal compression and then as a result of compression by the instrument being pushed into the abdominal cavity. The length of the blade of the knife (A-B) will therefore be shorter than the estimated length of the track (A-C).

115

The length of a stab wound track (which is not the same as the depth into the body) can be difficult to assess with accuracy unless there is a known end point where the knife has terminated, such as a mark or chip in bone, particularly the spine or ribs. One of the main reasons for estimating the length of a wound track is to assess the length of the blade of a knife, assuming the full length of the blade has entered the body. However, making such an assessment as blade length can only be an approximation. The reason for this is that the skin particularly over the abdomen is very yielding to an impact by a knife before it is breached, thus giving the impression when the track is measured at the autopsy, that a longer blade was used, than may have actually been the case (Figure 7.28). This to a lesser extent can also occur in the thorax which is compressible to an extent on impact, particularly in younger persons.

Fais et al. (2016) and Bolliger et al. (2014) used imaging (MSCT and MRI) with contrast medium to attempt to demonstrate tracts of wounds. This was generally successful insofar as compact tissue was concerned but not superior to layer-by-layer dissection or even probing. Probing should, however, be used with caution as there is a danger of producing false tracts or distorting already existing ones. Tracts in body cavities may be unpredictable and imaging in any event is difficult, limited and may be misleading. The gold standard remains careful layer-by-layer dissection.

Track assessment may be an especially inaccurate estimation, where the wound terminates at a non-fixed point in the chest or abdominal cavity. The reason may well be due to the difference of the position of the victim when they are being stabbed compared to when they are lying supine on a mortuary table.

The pathologist will assess the direction of impact of a knife on to the body and orientation of the wound, its location and track length, with reference to distance from anatomical landmarks and planes on the body. The purpose of this is to obtain as full a picture as possible of how the assault occurred, including the relative position of the assailant and victim.

Where there are multiple stab wounds, particularly if they are grouped together and sometimes overlapping, it may be difficult if not impossible, to be precisely sure which wound on the skin was responsible for which internal wound/s.

The size and shape of injuries seen on internal softer organs such as the lungs, heart, liver and so on, should be interpreted with caution, bearing in mind that movement of a knife may cause it to change direction from being a single straight entry and exit thrust to the body. Such movement of the weapon may distort wounds as it is withdrawn in a slightly different direction from the entry tract. This occurs as a result of movement between the assailant and the victim and on rare occasions, as a result of the assailant deliberately twisting the knife within the victim's body. A detailed description of internal injuries in different regions is found in chapter 8.

## Analysis of Marks on Bone and Cartilage Caused by Sharp Force Trauma

Further investigation of the characteristic of a knife or other sharp implement, may involve close examination of damage to bone, cartilage and soft tissue in addition to the surface characteristics of wounds as well as marks on clothing, at both a macroscopical and microscopical level by a number of different forensic specialists. Mark analysis in skin and cartilage has been described by (Sitiene et al 2006); saw mark and dismemberment analysis by Symes et al (2010), Saville et al (2006), and weapon identification from mark analysis in bone by Bartelink et al (2001), Humphrey and Hutchinson (2001), Tucker et al (2001), Alunni-Perret et al (2005).

More recently Love et al (2019) reviewed the research on the effect of sharp force trauma on cartilage and bone by carrying out an extensive review of the literature. They concluded that although saw and cut mark analyses are based on a strong scientific foundation, there is still much work to do. They stress the need for uniformity on error rates of matches which currently are only specific to individual studies. Large databases of cut and saw mark features are required to be collected from test marks made with a large variety of known tools to allow more accurate assessment with less intra-individual variability of marks made with the same tool and inter-individual variability of marks made from different tools. They also state the need for statistical models (such as classification tree) to define the potential error associated with cut and saw marks.

It should be appreciated, however, particularly when the knife or other sharp implement is not available for comparison with the findings on the deceased, that identification can only be made in terms of the type of weapon that is involved. In that way, at least a large number of possible agents causing injury can be eliminated from an investigation.

## Scars from Previous Trauma

The documentation of the presence of previous injuries from sharp force trauma is essential in assessing the overall injury profile of the victim and whether or not he/she had been involved in previous such assaults (Figure 7.29). Self-inflicted scars are described in Chapter 10.

## Chopping Wounds

### Axe or Hatchet (Type of Hand Axe)

Chop or incised wounds (usually deep) are produced by sharp-edged tools such as an axe or a machete. The weight of the implement, together with the sharp chopping surface, leads to the production of injuries with both blunt and sharp features (Figure 7.30).

Wounds to the head frequently carry a high mortality rate, producing severe fragmented skull fractures and extensive cerebral contusions (Figure 7.31). Handlos et al. (2019) present a case of a violent death of a 57-year-old-man. The autopsy revealed deformation of the right side of the head. A total of 23 slash, stab and cut wounds as well as contused lacerations were identified on the scalp as well as the face and the neck.

In situations where the victim is alive, the use of CT scanning with 3-D reconstruction may be

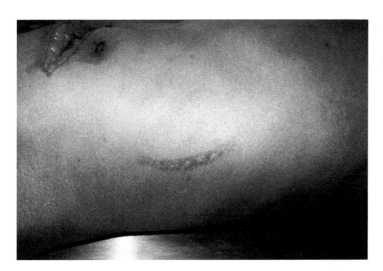

◀ **Figure 7.29** Stab wound victim. Previous scar from assault with a knife is shown in the right axillary line.

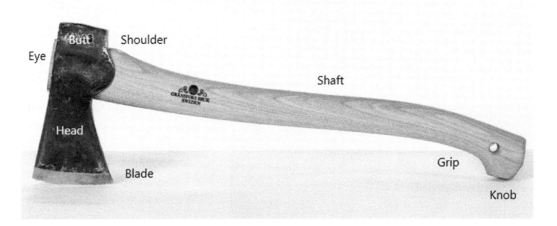

▲ **Figure 7.30** Main components of a typical axe.

117

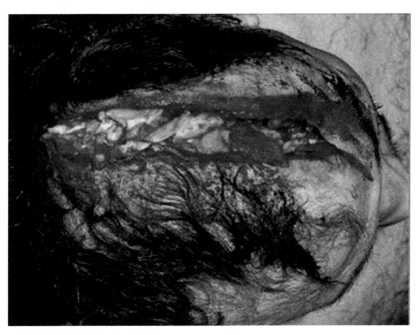

▲ **Figure 7.31** Fatal axe chopping wound. Open fatal injury, showing underlying soft tissue, comminuted fractures and lacerated cerebral tissue.

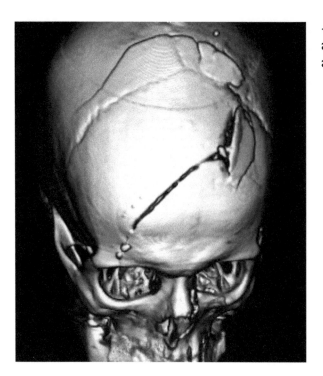

◀ **Figure 7.32a** 3-D CT reconstruction of the anterior skull showing chop wounds with associated fragmented and linear fractures.

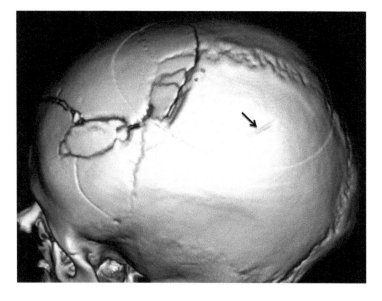

◀ **Figure 7.32b** View from the left side and top of skull vault. Two chop fracture sites are seen with lifted external components and separate short linear bone groove on the left side of the vault (arrowed) (Courtesy Johnson et al 2014).

particularly useful in demonstrating underlying fractures. Johnson et al (2014) demonstrated this very elegantly in the case they reported of an adult male with axe injuries to the head. They point out that for forensic investigative purposes in living patients, because no autopsy is available, a 3D reconstruction of the skull clearly demonstrates the pattern of typical chopping injury. This can be carried out after treatment in life-threatening situations and after the patient has stabilised (Figure 7.32).

## Meat Cleaver Injuries

The meat cleaver is designed to cut through meat and bone with a less sharpened cutting edge than a knife in order thus crushing as well as an incising through tissue. In addition to the heavy rectangular blade, many have a hand protector with a sturdy handle (Figure 7.33). There are many varieties of cleaver, but the injuries they produce are typical chopping type (Figure 7.34), also seen with axes and hatchets.

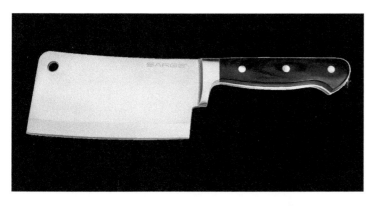

◀ **Figure 7.33** Meat cleaver.

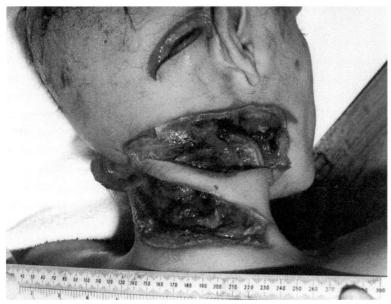

◀ **Figure 7.34a** Meat cleaver incised wounds to the back of the head and neck.

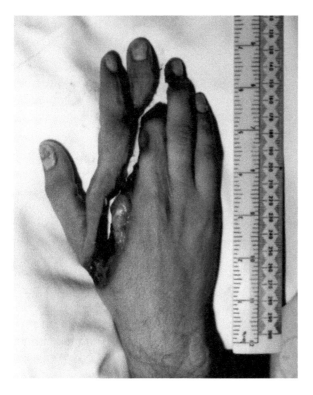

◀ **Figure 7.34b** Deep and mutilating defence wound of the right hand. The wounds have dried and abraded margins.

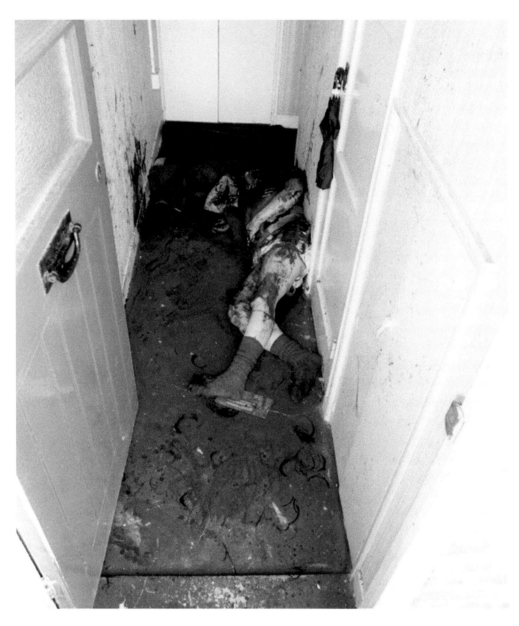

▲ **Figure 7.35a** Homicide scene. The deceased is seen in the passage way of his apartment with extensive bloodstaining on and around him. He was attacked just inside his front door.

The author investigated the case of a Vietnamese male in his late 30s who was found deceased at home in the passage to the front door. He used a type of cleaver used by Asian chefs called a Chinese cleaver (also called a Chinese chef's knife) which is a sharper and lighter implement than a butcher's cleaver and can slice vegetables, meat as well as well as chop bone. The perpetrator confessed to the police saying that he killed the deceased because he had threatened him and his family if he did not give him a large amount of money (Figures 7.35, 7.36, 7.37 and 7.38).

## Machete Injuries

Machete injuries are unusual in an urban environment (Donnally et al 2017). These authors examined the spectrum of upper extremity injuries sustained accidentally and from assaults in 48 patients (96% males of which 81% were assaulted). They noted that such injuries are much more frequently seen in rural settings where machetes are very common hand tools and particularly in developing countries in Africa and Asia where they are traditional and cheap agricultural tools.

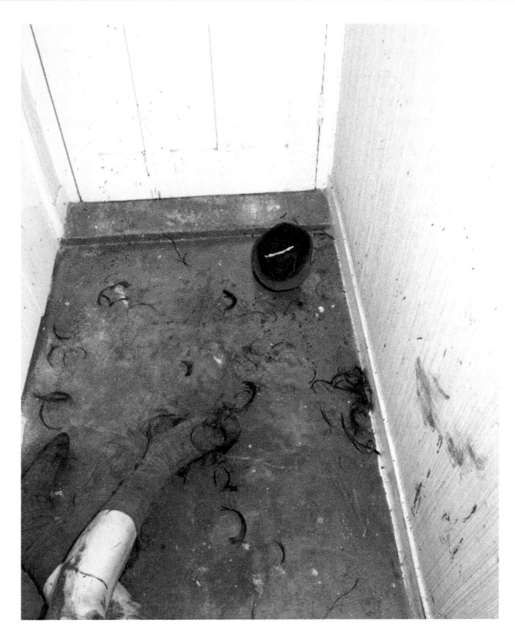

▲ **Figure 7.35b** View from the other end showing his lower legs and a large amount of cut head hair on the floor. The hair had been cut from his head during the attack with the cleaver which had a very sharp edge, using a quick repeated action. The perpetrator's cap can be seen near the door which he inadvertently left behind at the scene.

The author of this text, was personally involved with a number of other colleagues in the pathological investigation of victims from one of the most brutal massacres that occurred in Rwanda in 1994 in which the vast majority of victims died from assaults with agricultural implements, in particular machetes. I have given a brief review of the events below.

*Background of Rwanda Genocide*

In Rwanda there are two main tribal groups, the majority Hutu and minority Tutsi.

The Tutsi had dominated the political landscape during the colonial period when administered by Belgium and thus became the ruling class ruling through monarchy. Independence in 1961 changed

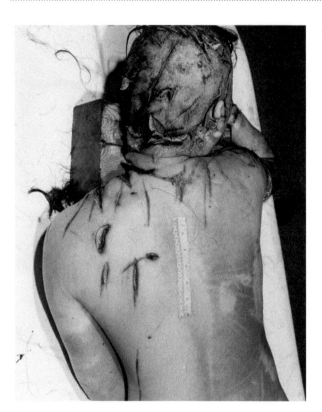

◄ **Figure 7.36a** Wounds to back and head.

◄ **Figure 7.36b** Defensive injuries to right hand and forearm.

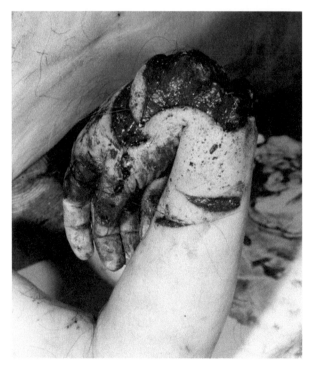

the position when Hutu, who were the majority, became the ruling class.

The killings began on 6 April 1994 when an airplane carrying President Juvénal Habyarimana along with the Burundian Cyprien Ntaryamira was shot down over Kigale, the capital city. Habyarimana was a Hutu and was the President of the Republic of Rwanda from 1973 until his assassination. During his 20-year leadership, he favoured his own ethnic group, the Hutus, against the Tutsi. His assassination

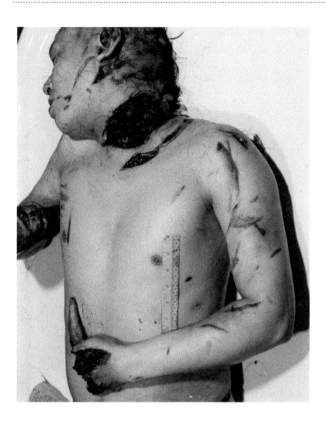

◀ **Figure 7.36c** Injuries to the front with a substantial incised area of wounding to the neck and defensive injuries to the left hand.

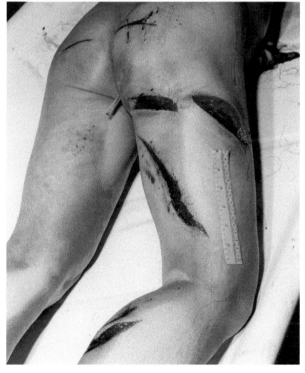

◀ **Figure 7.36d** Deep incised wounds to the back of the right thigh and calf area.

123

ignited ethnic tensions in the region and helped spark the Rwandan Genocide.

From April to July 1994, members of the Hutu ethnic majority murdered, by some estimates, as many as 800 000 people, mostly of the Tutsi minority.

The killing spree, which began in the capital Kigali, and spread throughout the country with staggering speed by local officials and the Hutu government who encouraged their fellow citizens to take up arms against their neighbours. The killings finally ended

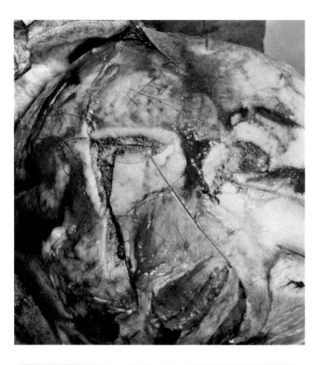

◀ **Figures 7.37a** Multiple skull fractures caused by a Chinese meat cleaver. Appearance of skull before removal of soft tissue.

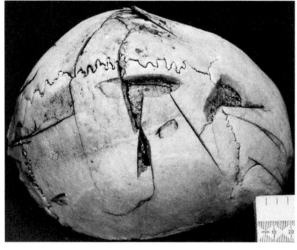

◀ **Figures 7.37b** Defleshed skull vault. Note wide chipped areas of the outer table and linear cuts and fractures.

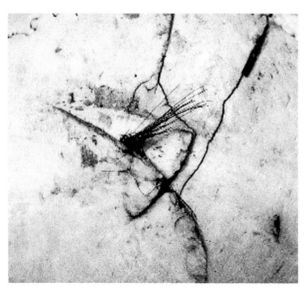

◀ **Figures 7.37c** Cut hair is shown trapped in one of the linear fractures.

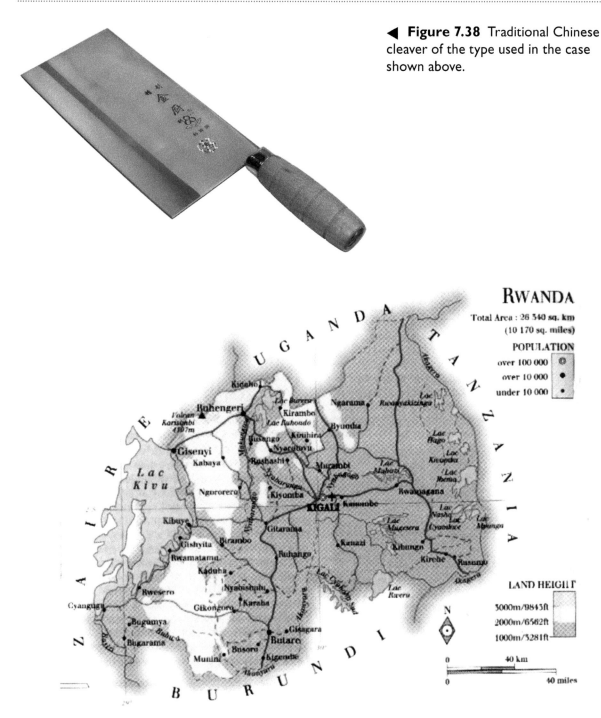

◀ **Figure 7.38** Traditional Chinese cleaver of the type used in the case shown above.

▲ **Figure 7.39a** Map of Rwanda.

when Tutsi-led Rwandese Patriotic Front gained control of the country through a military offensive in early July 1994.

Pre-exhumation assessment of the genocide by our forensic team identified hundreds of potential sites and graves to investigate in Rwanda. Our attention was directed to a mass grave near the Roman

Catholic church and Home St. Jean in the parish of Kibuye, above Lake Kivu in the northwest of the country (Figures 7.39, 7.40, 7.41 and 7.42). The killings here were instigated by the parish's former prefect, Clément Kayishema. From April 8–17, 1994, Hutu officials throughout the parish of Kibuye directed Tutsi civilians to aggregate in Roman Catholic churches, which they dubbed as "safe

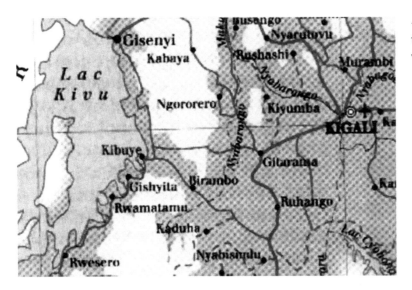

**◀ Figure 7.39b** Detail of parish town of Kibuye where mass graves were located.

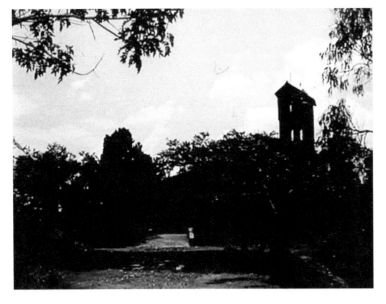

**◀ Figure 7.40** View of Catholic church.

126

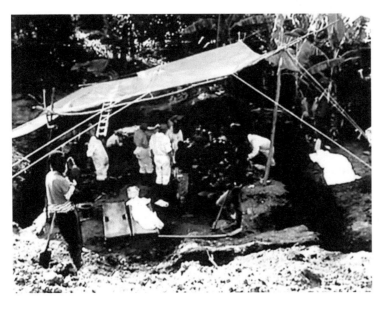

**◀ Figure 7.41** Mass grave site.

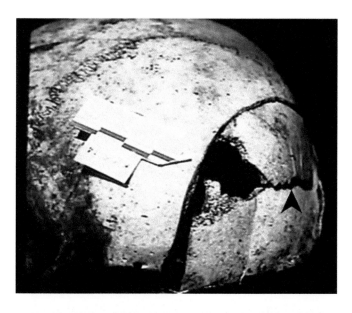

◀ **Figure 7.42a** Skeletonised victim from Rwanda mass grave showing a curved cut through the occipital bone. Below it is a crush fracture produced during the process of internment (black arrow).

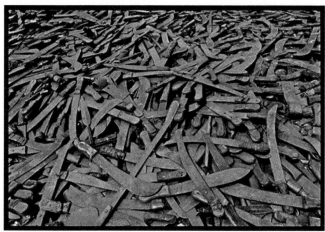

◀ **Figure 7.42b** Machetes, found in the homes of many farming families in Rwanda, were widely used in the 1994 genocide. This iconic photograph by Jim Nachtwey (photojournalist Time Magazine) was taken in 1994, towards the end of the genocide.

**127**

havens." On April 17 and 18 1994, the complex was surrounded by Hutu extremists and Interahamwe, a paramilitary organisation which enjoyed backing of the Hutu-led government in Rwanda leading up to and during the genocide, and the Tutsi who had gathered in this "safe haven" were brutally attacked. In the mayhem that followed, the Tutsi were clubbed and chopped to death. The killings in the parish of Kibuye were investigated in connection with the indictment of the parish's former prefect, Clément Kayishema, a trained medical doctor whom the Trial Chamber II of the International Criminal Tribunal for Rwanda established by the UN Security Council eventually sentenced to life in prison for the crime of genocide on 21 May 1999 (Peerwani 2017).

## Spade Injuries

Occasionally, spade injuries are seen; the vast majority are accidental and reported in agricultural regions of the world. As with other heavy hand tools with a sharp edge, they can produce both sharp and blunt wounds. Das (2014) reported on agricultural accidents in West Bengal, India, and found that the most frequently involved tools in hand injuries were the spade and the sickle. In particular, injuries were observed to the fingers and toes of the limbs followed by other parts of the extremities including ankles, hands, feet and wrists. Das and Gangopadhyay (2018) surveyed working preadolescents in the agricultural sector and concluded that repetitive work caused fatigue with an increased likelihood of the tool slipping in the hand causing injuries to fingers and toes.

# Glass Injuries

The edges and points of glass are usually extremely sharp and readily cause cuts of varying dimensions, as well as small linear and superficial punctate lesions, but deep puncture wounds are far less common. Most wounds are the result of household accidents, frequently from falling against glass door panels, and cases of suicide or homicide involving broken glass are rare. Rothschild et al (2001) reported three cases which presented with wounds similar to stab wounds caused by a single-edged knife and were initially suspected of being homicides. Thorough autopsy examination revealed that they had all been caused by impact against glass.

Injury from glass may occur during the course of a fight on the ground where there are numerous broken glass fragments as shown in Figure 7.43.

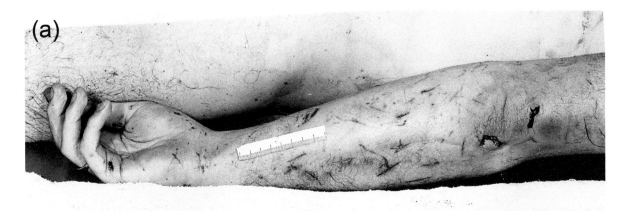

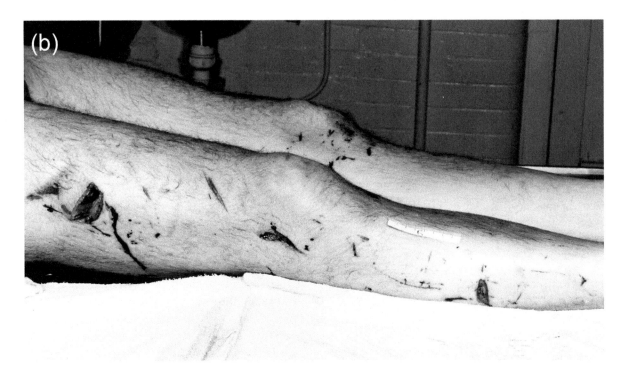

▲ **Figure 7.43** Multiple glass injuries on the upper (a) and (b) lower limbs, caused during a fight when the deceased was on the ground with broken glass scattered around him. Note double edged parallel linear components of a number of the wounds, particularly on the lower limbs, as well as the varying depth, size and direction of the wounds. Significant blood loss occurred from the large puncture wound on the right thigh.

Homicide from stabbing using a glass fragment is rare. Fracasso and Karger (2009) report a case of a woman who was killed by her boyfriend using a dagger-like fragment of a broken window glass to cause ten atypical stab wounds to the neck and face as well as several wounds elsewhere. The authors also point out that the risk of self-injury to the perpetrator's own hand is high from holding broken glass.

Sterzik et al. (2008) carried out tests with drinking glasses thrown at a skull–neck model to see whether when striking the model, the glasses would remain intact or splinter. They concluded that the glasses remain intact if they hit the object with the bottom or the lower part of the cylindrical glass body. In about half such cases, they observed a fractured skull. If the glass impacted with the rim or the upper part of the body, the glasses splintered producing superficial skin lesions, but no larger glass fragments penetrated into the depth of the skin. Adamec et al. (2019) also carried out tests on 1 litre beer steins which are used during the autumn festivals and beer halls in Southern Germany and Austria. They observed many serious and potentially life-threatening injuries from blows from these glasses. They found a discrepancy between the mechanical stability of brand new and used steins and the corresponding injuries, which they explained was due to a decrease in impact tolerance of the steins with their use. There was in most cases a combination of blunt and sharp force trauma; with the bottom of the glass being responsible for the more severe blunt head injuries, including skull fractures.

*Glassing* is a colloquial term used to describe the act of injuring someone with a glass object such as a drinking glass or a bottle. It is frequently seen at home as well as in pubs and other public places and in many cases accompanied by the use of alcohol. In a study of alcohol-related violence from Queensland Australia involving 4629 patients seen in an Emergency Department, 72% of which were men, and of these, 36% were aged 18 to 24 years; the authors found that 9% of alcohol-related assault injuries were as a result of glassing (Laing et el 2013). The home was the most common location for alcohol-related violence (33% were glassings). Overall, at home the most common glass object used was a bottle (75%); however, in pubs and clubs the numbers between bottles and drinking glasses were of similar proportions.

The exposed parts of the body, particularly the face and neck are targeted and the resulting wounds can be deep and disfiguring. The incised wounds, particularly when the rounded end of a bottle or glassware is thrust into the face or elsewhere, frequently have a curved linear shape with varying depth (Figure 7.44). Where the glass is drawn across the body then wounds tend to be long, although relatively more superficial (Figure 7.45).

Glass injuries may have the appearance of superficial tram-line incisions which are part of the broken surface of the glass edges. An example of such a broken piece of glass from a bottle (prepared by the author and not related to any cases in this book) is shown in Figure 7.46 (see also Chapter 6).

129

# Other Instruments Causing Sharp Force Trauma

## Scissors

Occasionally, injuries from scissors are seen in different authors' series. In the series reported by Rogde et al (2000), scissors amongst other objects were also used; although the number was not specified. In Karlsson's (1998) study of 174 cases, objects including scissors, broken glass, and razor blades were used in six cases (4%). One victim from a series of 13 from Solarino et al's study (2019) was stabbed simultaneously in the chest and head region with scissors and a screwdriver. Zhang and Yang (2016) reported a spinal cord injury from scissors stab wounds causing craniocervical junction in an eight-year-old boy who developed Brown Séquard-plus syndrome. Karadag et al's (2004) case was of a five-year-old girl who injured herself with scissors while trying to cut her hair. The scissors, with the blades open, had penetrated between C3 and C4 vertebrae and injured the ipsilateral vertebral artery (Figure 7.47).

The morphology of wounds caused by scissors will depend on a number of factors including most obviously whether the tool was used with open points or closed as well as the structure of the blades and shape of the scissors in general.

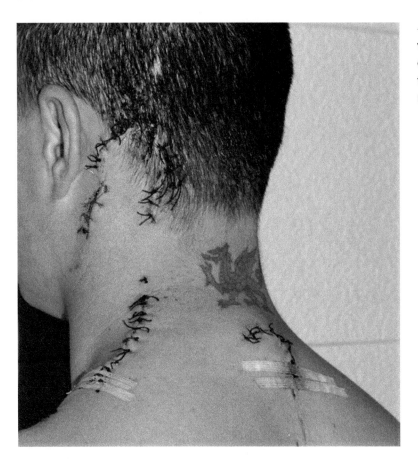

◀ **Figure 7.44a** Curvilinear wounds from a broken bottle produced by smashing an empty bottle twice on the back of the head and neck.

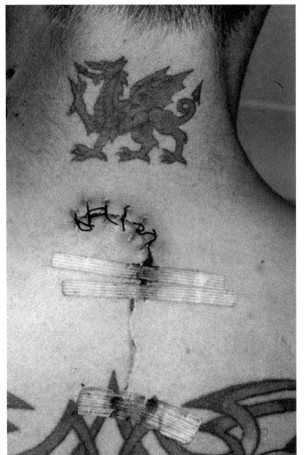

◀ **Figure 7.44b** Close up of one of the curved wounds.

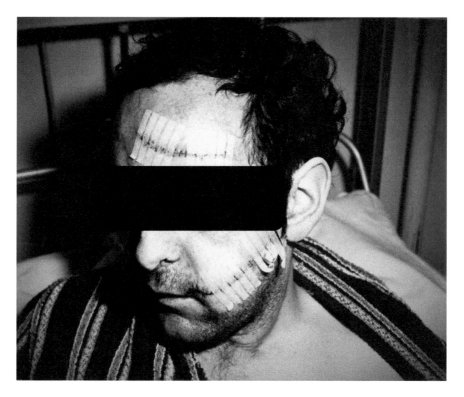

▲ **Figure 7.45** Slash wounds across the face caused by an assault with broken glassware.

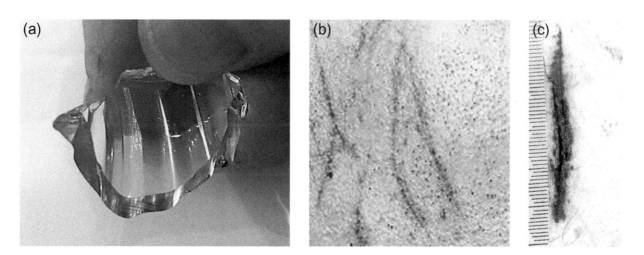

▲ **Figure 7.46** (a) View of broken edge of glass from a bottle showing double sharp edges which have a tendency for causing linear tramline appearance in some wounds, depending on the angle of impact. (b) and (c) Detail of superficial incised wounds showing a tramline appearance.

## Saws

There are a large variety of different types of saws which include both manual non-powered and powered (mechanised) saws. Injuries from these frequently show a characteristic teeth pattern in soft tissue, bone and cartilage (description of the marks produced is described elsewhere).

The most severe injuries are caused by powered saws and there have been many publications describing injuries from different types such as band saws, chain saws, circular saws, etc. (Rubin et al 2007; Sritharen et al 2018; Frank et al 2010). Mostly such injuries are caused as a result of accidents in an occupational setting, or occasionally as a method of suicide or rarely, homicide. Manual hand and powered saws are also

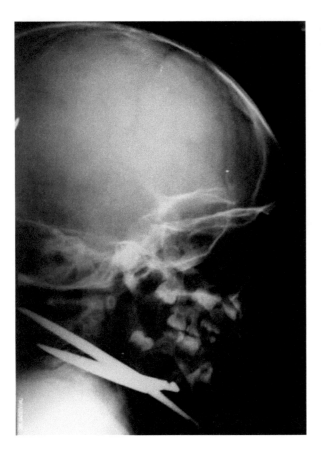

◀ **Figure 7.47a** Lateral radiograph of the cervical spine showing the scissors passing between the C3 and C4 cervical vertebrae without any obvious bone fracture.

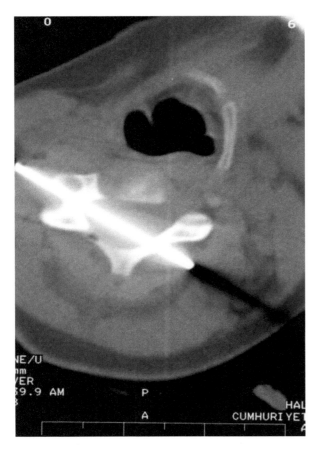

◀ **Figure 7.47b** CT scan of the cervical spine demonstrating the metal blade traversing the spinal canal at C3–C4 junction (British journal of neurosurgery, 18, 545–547 (Source figures 1 and 2); Used with permission courtesy Taylor & Francis).

frequently used to dismember a body usually to facilitate disposal. A more detailed description of saw fatalities as well as their use in dismemberment is to be found in chapters 11 and 12.

## Crossbow, Bow and Arrow and Other Pointed Objects with a Shaft or Rod-Shape Causing Penetrating Trauma

The crossbow was the most important weapon of foot soldiers during the Middle Ages. This weapon is now mainly used for sport or hunting purposes. Traumatic crossbow injuries, whether self-inflicted or otherwise, are very seldom encountered these days in forensic medicine or in hospitals. Closely related to crossbow injuries and nowadays even more unusual are long bow injuries caused by longbows or compound bows. Grellner et al (2004) encountered four fatalities (two homicides and two suicides) and two non-fatal injuries (grievous bodily harm and an accident). All the victims were male, between 31 and 54 years. The weapons used were described as high performance precision crossbows with telescopic sights and hunting bolts. The parts of the body that were injured involved the head or the thorax with the bolt remaining in the wound in four out of six cases. With regard to the morphology of the wounds produced, this will depend on whether the tip has multi-cut sides, producing incised wounds or whether the arrow tip is conical, producing a circular or slit mark (see also chapters 1 and 10).

## Screwdrivers

Screwdriver injuries are regularly reported and serious injuries in particular have involved either the spine or head and neck regions (Bhutta et al 2008; Faller-Marquardt and Pollak 1996). The morphology of different types of screwdriver have been examined by Kieser et al (2008) who carried out experiments on the cranial head of the pig. Their study demonstrated clearly that wounds inflicted by different types of screwdriver may be grouped into three categories. Firstly, the straight-head screwdriver produces a wound that is characteristic and clearly identifiable from all the others. The second grouping consists of wounds inflicted by square- (Robertson) and star-head screwdrivers, and the third group consists of the Posidriv and Phillips screwdrivers.

The author of this text has seen a number of cases where screwdrivers have been used as single weapon or in combination with another sharp implement or blunt trauma. The following two cases demonstrate examples of such injuries.

Elderly male who was the victim of a robbery, sustained multiple injuries with a straight head screwdriver to the chest and face as well as blunt impact injury to the head (Figure 7.48).

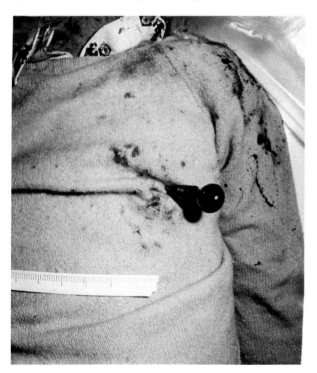

◀ **Figure 7.48a** Screwdriver embedded in the left chest through clothing. A number of defects produced by the implement are seen.

133

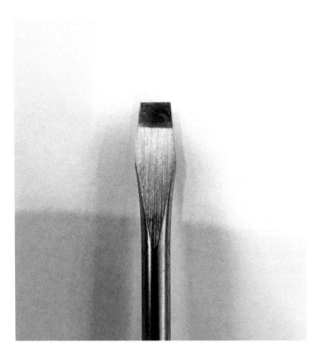

◀ **Figure 7.48b** Tip of straight head screwdriver.

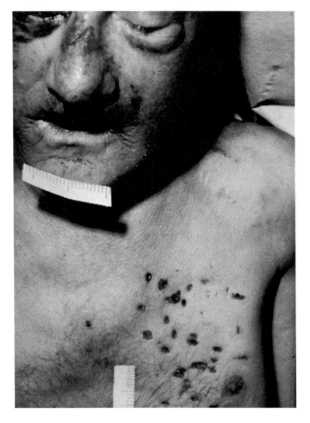

◀ **Figure 7.48c** Injuries to the chest, nose and right eye.

The other case involved a middle-aged male attacked by two men with a variety of weapons including a Phillips screwdriver as well as a small ornamental sword. In addition, he sustained stab wounds to the chest with a knife. He was then wrapped in plastic sheeting and thrown into a river, to be discovered four days later (Figure 7.49).

## Knife Sharpener

A unique case was seen by the author in which a rod-shaped knife sharpener was used to produce stabbing injuries (Vanezis 1989). The type of sharpener in question is heavy with a pointed end and contains longitudinal ridges along the steel rod. The deceased

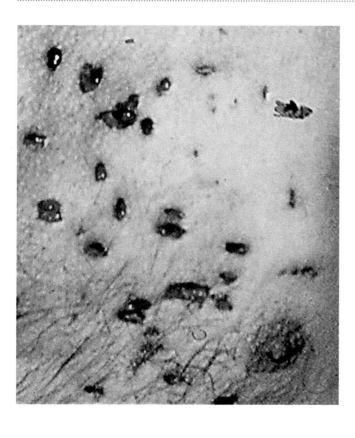

◀ **Figure 7.48d** Close up of chest injuries showing rectangular wounds.

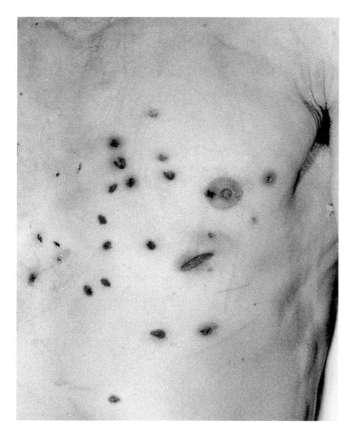

◀ **Figure 7.49a** Chest stab wounds.

135

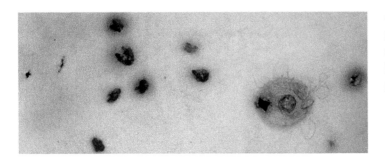

**Figure 7.49b** Close up views showing "puckered" wounds giving the appearance in some of a cross shape. Most have been caused by a small ornamental sword.

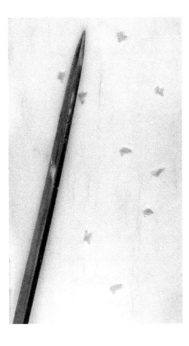

**Figure 7.49c** Cadaver skin tests with an ornamental sword showing similar wounds as in (b). The sword has four sides to the blade which then tapers to a point.

136

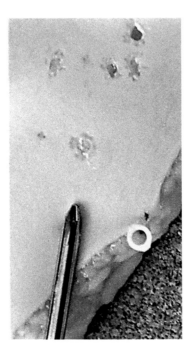

**Figure 7.49d** Skin test with a Philips screwdriver showing dissimilar wounds comprising a central round component with small satellite abrasions.

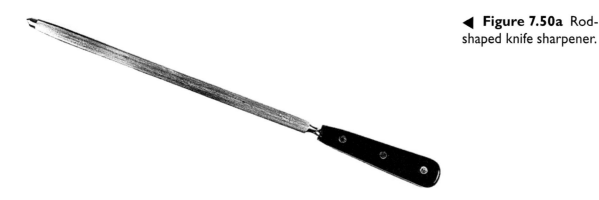

◀ **Figure 7.50a** Rod-shaped knife sharpener.

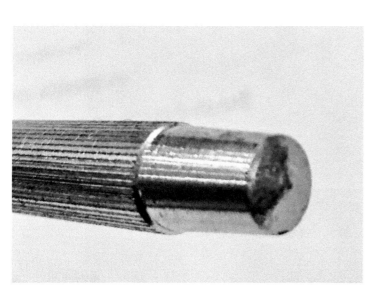

◀ **Figure 7.50b** The implement is pointed but the tip is blunter than most knives. The sides of the rod are fashioned into fine vertical ridges composed of hardened carbon steel.

was an elderly woman who lived alone. Her nephew who suffered from schizophrenia visited her on a regular basis. For no apparent reason he attacked her with a knife sharpener which from its size and shape required a substantial amount of force to produce the injuries seen to the head, neck and chest (Figure 7.50).

## Propellers from Watercraft

Semeraro et al (2012) described patterns of propeller injuries in soft tissue and bone, in their description of three cases. They are of the view that such injuries are examples of blunt force rather than sharp force trauma based on the fracture patterns in bone and the squared propeller edge rather than the bevelled edge seen in knives, axes, hatchets, saws etc. (Figures 7.51 and 7.52). They point out that objects without a sharp edge tend to cause, scoring, grazing or splintering of bone, compared to scoring across the bone surface or chipping as seen in stabs. With soft tissues, when a squared-off edge such as a propeller impacts the skin with speed, a clean wound resembling a cut is produced rather than one similar to a typical laceration.

Injuries from other sharp-edged objects including saws, razors and various pointed objects as well as injuries from animals are described principally in Chapters 10, 11 and 12.

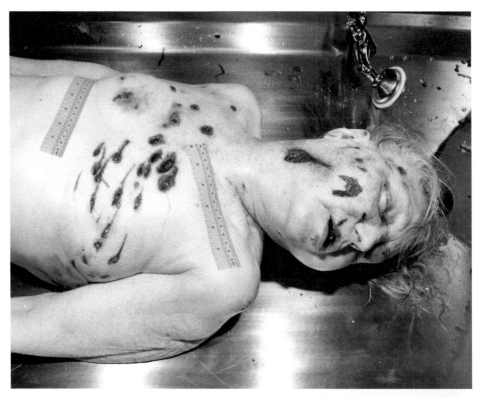

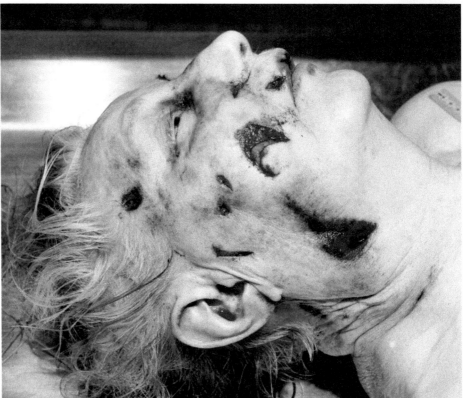

▲ **Figure 7.50c and d** Show multiple wounds to the face, neck and chest with abraded collars caused by the ridged edges of the sharpener.

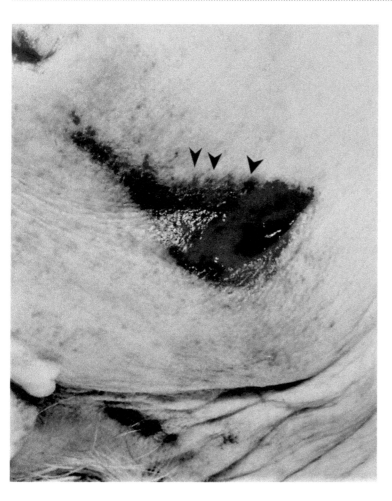

◀ **Figure 7.50e** Detail of one of the wounds showing a pattern of teeth marks caused by the ridges, trailing from the upper end of the wound (arrows).

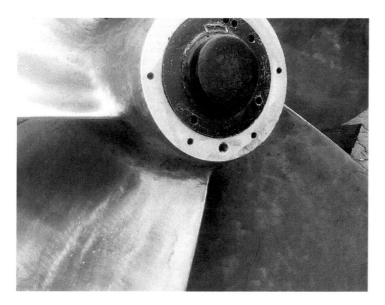

◀ **Figure 7.51a** Close view of a large propeller.

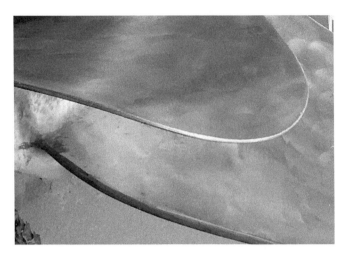

◀ **Figure 7.51b** Squared-off edge (unlike bevelled edge of knives etc.).

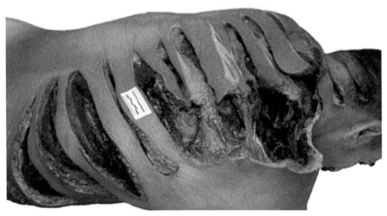

◀ **Figure 7.52** Wounds from a motor boat propeller (Semeraro DI, Passalacqua NV, Symes S, Gilson T. (2012). Patterns of trauma induced by motorboat and ferry propellers as illustrated by three known cases from Rhode Island. *J Forensic Sci* 57, 1625–1629 (Source figure 3); Used with permission and courtesy of the authors)

# References

Adamec J, Dorfner P, Graw M, Lochner S, Kunz SN. (2019). Injury potential of one-litre beer steins. *Int J Leg Med* 133, 1075–1081.

Alunni-Perret V, Muller-Bolla M, Laugier J, Lupi-Peégurier L, Bertrand M, Staccini P, Bolla M, Quatrehomme G. (2005). Scanning electron microscopy analysis of experimental bone hacking trauma, *J. Forensic Sci.* 50, 213–216.

Barber LR. (2009). Matching the wound to the weapon: the correlation between the size of stab wounds on the skin and the size of weapon in homicide victims. MSc Dissertation, Queen Mary, University of London.

Bartelink EJ, Wiersema JM, Demaree RS. (2001), Quantitative analysis of sharp-force trauma: an application of scanning electron microscopy in forensic anthropology, *J. Forensic Sci.* 46, 1288–1293.

Beillas P, Lafon Y, Smith FW. (2009). The effects of posture and subject-to-subject variations on the position, shape and volume of abdominal and thoracic organs. *Stapp Car Crash J* 53, 127–154.

Bhutta MA, Dunkow PD, Lang DM. (2008). A stab in the back with a screwdriver: a case report. *Cases J* 1, 305.

Bolliger SA, Ruder TD, Ketterer T, Gläser N, Thali MJ, Ampanozi G. (2014). Comparison of stab wound probing versus radiological stab wound channel depiction with contrast medium. *Forensic Sci Int* 234, 45–49.

Byard RW, Gehl A, Tsokos M. (2005). Skin tension and cleavage lines (Langer's lines) causing distortion of ante- and postmortem wound morphology. *Int J Legal Med* 119, 226–230.

Ciallella C, Caringi C, Aromatario M. (2002). Case report: wounds inflicted by survival-knives *Forensic Sci Int* 126, 82–87.

Cowper EJ, Carr DJ, Horsfall J, Fergusson SM. (2015).The effect of fabric and stabbing variables on severance appearance. *Forensic Sci Int* 249, 214–224.

Das B. (2014). Agricultural work related injuries among the farmers of West Bengal, India. *Int J Inj Contr Saf Promot* 21, 205–215.

Das B, Gangopadhyay S. (2018). Occupational agricultural injuries among the preadolescent workers of West Bengal, India. *Int J Adolesc Med Health* [published online ahead of print, Dec 10 2018].

Donnally CJ III, Hannay W, Rapp DA, Lekic N, Dodds SD. (2017). Machete injuries to the upper extremity. *Arch Orthop Trauma Surg* 137, 1615–1621.

Faller-Marquardt M, Pollak S. (1996). Homicide with a screwdriver and simulation of a similar offence by self-infliction of injuries. *J Clin Forensic Med* 3, 141–147.

Fais P, Cecchetto G, BoscoloBerto R, Toniolo M, Viel G, Miotto D, Montisci M, Tagliaro F, Giraudo C. (2016). Morphometric analysis of stab wounds by MSCT and MRI after the instillation of contrast medium. *Radiol Med* 121, 494–501.

Fracasso T, Karger B. (2009). A glass fragment for a dagger—Never mind your own hand. *Forensic Sci Int* 188, e15–e16.

Frank M, Lange J, Napp M, Hecht J, Ekkernkamp A, Hinz P. (2010). Accidental circular saw hand injuries: trauma mechanisms, injury patterns, and accident insurance. *Forensic Sci Int* 198, 74–78.

Grellner W, Buhmann D, Giese A, Gehrke G, Koops E, Püschel K. (2004). Fatal and non-fatal injuries caused by crossbows. *Forensic Sci Int* 142, 17–23.

Handlos P, Uvíra M, Dokoupil M, Marecová K. (2019). Axe injury pattern in homicide. *Forensic Sci Med Pathol* 15, 516–518.

Humphrey, J. H., & Hutchinson, D. L. (2001). Macroscopic characteristics of hacking trauma. *Journal of forensic sciences*, 46, 228–233.

Inquest into the death of Azaria Chantel Loren Chamberlain [2012] NTMC 20 (12 June 2012).

Johnson CP, Melmore SA, Johnson O, Campbell RS, Dunn A. (2014). Life threatening chop injuries to the head: optimising injury interpretation using three dimensional computerised tomography (3DCT) reconstruction of pre-treatment imaging. *J Forensic Leg Med* 2, 1–4.

Kaliszan M, Karnecki K, Akçan R, Jankowski Z. (2011). Striated abrasions from a knife with non-serrated blade—identification of the instrument of crime on the basis of an experiment with material evidence. *Int J Legal Med* 125, 745–748.

Karadağ O, Gürelik M, Berkan O, Kars HZ. (2004). Stab wound of the cervical spinal cord and ipsilateral vertebral artery injury. *Br J Neurosurg* 18, 545–547.

Karlsson T. (1998). Sharp force homicides in the Stockholm area, 1983–1992. *Forensic Sci Int* 94, 129–139.

Kemp SE, Carr DJ, Kieser J, Niven BE, Taylor MC. (2009). Forensic evidence in apparel fabrics due to stab events. *Forensic Sci Int* 191, 86–96.

Kieser J, Bernal V, Gonzalez P, Birch W, Turmaine M, Ichim I. (2008). Analysis of experimental cranial skin wounding from screwdriver trauma. *Int J Legal Med* 122, 179–187.

Laing AJ, Sendall MC, Barker R. (2013). Alcohol-related violence presenting to the emergency department: is 'glassing' the big issue?. *Emerg Med Australas* 25, 550–557.

Love JC. (2019). Sharp force trauma analysis in bone and cartilage: a literature review. *Forensic Sci Int* 299, 119–127.

Menon A, Kanchan T, Monteiro FNP, Rao NG. (2008). Atypical wound of entry and unusual presentation in a fatal stab injury. *J Forensic Leg Med* 15, 524–526.

Milroy CM, Rutty GN. (1997). If a wound is "neatly incised" it is not a laceration. *BMJ* 315, 1312.

Murray L. A., & Green, M. A. (1987). Hilts and knives: a survey of ten years of fatal stabbings. *Medicine, Science, and the Law, 27*, 182–184.

Nı´ Annaidh A, Cassidy M, Curtis M, Destrade M, Gilchrist MD. (2013). A combined experimental and numerical study of stab-penetration forces. *Forensic Sci Int* 233, 7–13.

Ohshima T. (2005). Diagnostic value of "superficial" stab wounds in forensic practice. *J Clin Forensic Med* 12, 32–35.

Peerwani N. (2017). The role of a forensic pathologist in armed conflict. *Acad Forensic Pathol* 7, 370–389. Academic Forensic Pathology: Invited Review. Official publication of The National Association of Medical Examiners.

Pollak S, Fischer A. (1991). Morphometric findings of stab wounds. *Beitr Gerichtl Med* 49, 219–25.

Rogde S, Hougen HP, Poulsen K. (2000). Homicide by sharp force in two Scandinavian capitals. *Forensic Sci Int* 109, 135–145.

Rothschild MA, Karger B, Schneider V. (2001). Puncture wounds caused by glass mistaken for stab wounds with a knife. *Forensic Sci Int* 121, 161–165.

Royal Commission of Inquiry into Chamberlain Convictions, Report, Commonwealth Parliamentary Papers (1987), volume 15, paper 192.

Rubin, L. E., Miki, R. A., Taksali, S., & Bernstein, R. A. (2007). Band saw injury in a butcher. *Occupational medicine (Oxford, England)*, 57, 383–385.

Sarkisian BA, Fedorov S. (2014). The morphological features of stab-and-slash skin wounds inflicted by the blades with differently shaped tips through the multilayer barrier. [Article in Russian]. *Sud Med Ekspert* 57, 28–31.

Saville PA, Hainsworth SV, Rutty GN. (2007), Cutting crime: the analysis of the "uniqueness" of saw marks on bone, *Int. J. Leg. Med.* 121, 349–357.

Semeraro DL, Passalacqua NV, Symes S, Gilson T. (2012). Patterns of trauma induced by motorboat and ferry propellers as illustrated by three known cases from Rhode Island. *J Forensic Sci* 57, 1625–1629.

Sitiene, R., Zakaras, A., Pauliukevicius, A., & Kisielius, G. (2007). Morphologic, experimental-comparative investigation as an identification of the injuring instrument method. *Forensic science international*, 167, 255–260.

Solarino B, Punzi G, Di Vella G, Carabellese F, Catanesi R. (2019). A multidisciplinary approach in overkill: Analysis of 13 cases and review of the literature. *Forensic Sci Int* 298, 402–407.

Sritharen Y, Hernandez MC, Zielinski MD, Aho JM. (2018). Weekend woodsmen: overview and comparison of injury patterns associated with power saw and axe utilization in the United States. *Am J Emerg Med* 36, 846–850.

Sterzik V, Kneubuehl BP, Ropohl D, Michael Bohnert M. (2008). Injuring potential of drinking glasses. *Forensic Sci Int* 179, e19–e23.

Symes SA, Chapman EN, Rainwater CW, Cabo LL, Myster MT. (2010), Knife and Saw Toolmark Analysis in Bone: a Manual Designed for the Examination of Criminal Mutilation and Dismemberment. National Institute of Justice Technical Report, National Institute of Justice, Washington, DC, 2010 Report no. 2005-IJ-CX-K016 2010.

Tucker B, Hutchinson D, Gilliland M, Charles T, Daniel H, Wolfe L (2001). Microscopic characteristics of hacking trauma, *J. Forensic Sci.* 46, 234–240.

Tullet T. (1986). The dingo baby case pp 190–211, in *Clues to murder*, The Bodley Head Ltd, London.

Vanezis P. (1989). Chapter 4. Penetrating injuries pp 29–30, in *Pathology of neck injury*. Butterworths, London.

Zhang XY, Yang YM. (2016). Scissors stab wound to the cervical spinal cord at the craniocervical junction. *Spine J* 16, e403–e406.

# Chapter 8
# Sharp Force Trauma – Regional Location and Consequences of Injury

## Introduction

Although sharp force injury is frequently found in more than one region of the body on the same person, it is useful to describe the particular injuries that might be seen in each location, how they are inflicted and the effects they have on morbidity and mortality, taking into account the structures seen in each region. It should always be borne in mind that the extent and severity of the overall impact of inflicted trauma, depends on many factors which include not just location, but the number of wounds, other types of trauma (e.g. the presence of blunt impact) prior state of health of the victim, force used and mode of death. The incidence and distribution of injury to different regions, and their location within each region, also depends on whether the wounds were inflicted by another person or persons, or were self-inflicted or produced accidentally.

In this chapter, injuries will be described from different body regions; broadly these will comprise head, neck, trunk and extremities. In addition, the effects that injuries in each region have on the victim will be described both as general consequences that one might find, irrespective of the region injured, as well as effects pertaining to more specific regional trauma.

The pathologist is required to take into account the various possible effects of sharp force trauma, including the impact of medical intervention on the overall outcome and possible contribution to morbidity and mortality. The chapter will deal with the issues that may be encountered by the forensic pathologist and includes the more recognised effects and complications of sharp force trauma at different stages after injury.

## Regional Distribution of Injuries and Manner of Causation

A retrospective study by Vassalini et al. (2014) demonstrated the differences in the regional infliction of sharp force trauma between homicide, suicide and accident. The above authors, from assessing all the injuries in their series of 92 homicide cases, including defence wounds, found the most common site injured was the left anterior chest (54.3%), followed by the neck (48.9%), the right anterior chest (35.9%), and the left posterior chest (30.4%). Their findings are supported by a number of other studies (Rouse 1994; Mitton and du Toit-Prinsloo 2016; Krywanczyk and Shapiro 2015) who found fatal injury or injuries in approximately the same order of regional distribution (Table 8.1.).

Concerning suicides, Vassalini and colleagues (op .cit.) found single sharp force injuries in 35.7% of fatalities (6 cases): single injuries were predominantly stab injuries located at the left chest. More than one injury was present in 64.3% of cases: only in one case, the wounds were more than 20. Analysis of all self-inflicted injuries, even nonlethal, showed that upper limbs were the anatomical sites most commonly involved: most injuries occurred on the left forearm (67.9%) and on the right forearm (50%). With regard to only fatal injuries, the upper limbs accounted for 39.3% of wounds (25% on the right and 14.3% on the left); the neck for 32% and the left anterior chest for 28.6%.

**Table 8.1** Percentage regional distribution of sharp force injuries by manner of death in four series

| Study/Series | Homicide | | | | Suicide | | | Accident |
|---|---|---|---|---|---|---|---|---|
| | 1* | 2* | 3* | 4* | 1* | 2* | 4* | 1* |
| **No. of cases** | **92** | **148** | **173** | **21** | **28** | **8** | **25** | **11** |
| Head and Neck | | 14.9 | | | 32 | 25 | | |
| Head | 3.3 | | 20.2 | 33.3 | | | | 18 |
| Neck | 35.9 | | 35.3 | 47.6 | 32 | | 32 | 27 |
| All Chest | | 75 | 64.7 | 70.9 | | 62.5 | 4 | |
| Left Chest | 44.6 | | | | 28.6 | | | |
| Mid-chest | | | | | | | | |
| Right Chest | 17.4 | | | | | | | 9 |
| All Abdomen | 7.6 | 6.1 | 13.3 | 9.5 | | 12.5 | 4 | 9 |
| Left Abdomen | 5.4 | | | | | | | |
| Mid-Abdomen | | | | | | | | 9 |
| Right Abdomen | 2.2 | | | | | | | |
| Upper limbs | | | 24.3 | 61.9 | 39.3 | | 48 | 18 |
| Crook of elbow | | | | | | | 12 | |
| Wrists | | | | | | | 40 | |
| Left Arm | | | | | 25 | | | 18 |
| Right Arm | | | | | 14.3 | | | |
| Lower limbs | 3.3 | 3.4 | 11 | 4.8 | 3.6 | | 8 | 18 |
| Left Leg | 3.3 | | | | 3.6 | | | 18 |
| Right Leg | | | | | | | | |
| All Back | 21.7 | | 26 | 14 | | | | |
| Left Back | 13 | | | | | | | |
| Right Back | 8.7 | | | | | | | |

1* Vassalini et al (2014); 2* Rouse (1994); 3* Mitton and du Toit-Prinsloo (2016)
4* Krywanczyk and Shapiro (2015)

Of the 11 accidental deaths seen in the Vassalini et al. (2014) study, six cases (54.5%) had a single sharp force injury. Where more than one injury was present these were mostly superficial and were caused by breaking glass producing fragments with sharp edges and pointed ends. Two fatal injuries were located on the head, three on the neck, one on the right anterior chest, one on the epigastrium, two on the left upper limb and two on the left lower limb.

It is hardly surprising that the data in large series in the literature from homicide cases reveal that the majority of wounds are found on the left side of the body in frontal confrontations, bearing in mind that most people are right handed and tend to hold the knife in the dominant hand. The location of wounds in homicides (including defence injuries) is confirmed from my own unpublished series of 87 stabbings in and around Glasgow (1998–99) (Table 8.2).

Most stab wounds, with a fatal outcome, as we can see from the above data, are to the trunk and less so the head and limbs. The mode of death may be straightforward or complex and depends also on the underlying organ damage. Frequently the injuries seen internally have damaged more than one organ, with rapid and devastating effect on the victim.

**Table 8.2** Location of stab wounds in 87 fatal stabbing homicides in Glasgow 1998–99

| Location | Left (%) | Right (%) | Midline (%) | Total (%) |
|---|---|---|---|---|
| Thorax front and back | 125 (51.2) | 96 (39.3) | 23 (9.4) | 244 (58) |
| Abdomen and lower back | 29 (72.5) | 10 (25) | 1 (2.5) | 40 (9.5) |
| Neck | 13 (48) | 11 (40) | 3 (11.1) | 27 (6.5) |
| Head | 24 (60) | - | 16 (40) | 4 0 (9.5) |
| Arms | 22 (56.4) | 17 (43.6) | - | 39 (9.4) |
| Legs | 19 (63.3) | 11 (36.7) | - | 30 (7.1) |
| **All regions** | **232 (55.2)** | **145 (34.5)** | **43 (10.2)** | **420 (100)** |

*Note:* Unpublished material

# Acute and Longer-term General Effects of Injury

Before a description of injuries, it is appropriate to describe some of the more general effects of trauma that may cause morbidity or mortality which are seen both in the acute phase after injury and the longer-term complications.

## Exsanguination – Hypovolaemic Shock

Blood loss leading to hypovolaemic shock is the primary outcome in most cases. In many victims the small amount of blood seen externally belies the extensive amount of internal haemorrhage from damaged vasculature one sees with chest wounds, and frequently accompanied by haemothorax and/or pneumothorax. Hypovolemia refers to a massive decrease in blood volume by excessive loss of blood, from damage to major organs and blood vessels causing death by exsanguination. It is the most common acute cause of death in fatal stabbing cases. Although some pathologists do not like to use the phrase "hypovolaemic shock" since it is essentially a clinical diagnosis, it seems to me to be perfectly acceptable terminology for a pathologist to conclude as the mode of death since it conveys exactly the outcome. The cause of death should, however, indicate the underlying trauma.

## Infection Following Trauma

The major problem, once the patient has been initially stabilised, is the risk of infection while they are recovering in hospital. Because of improvements in the control of haemorrhage after trauma, people who have survived injuries still face a number of obstacles before full recovery. Two-thirds of patients who die following major trauma now do so as a result of causes other than exsanguination (Lord et al. 2014). Trauma facilitates a systemic reaction that includes an acute, non-specific, immune response associated, paradoxically, with reduced resistance to infection. This results in damage to multiple organs caused by the initial cascade of inflammation aggravated by subsequent sepsis to which the body has become susceptible and which frequently leads to multi-organ failure. Furthermore, age has a profound influence on the chances of surviving trauma irrespective of the nature and severity of the injury. In this respect, elderly people have a significantly worse prognosis after trauma, independent of the nature or severity of their injury, and despite adjustment for comorbidities.

The author of this book dealt with a case of a 42-year-old male with HIV who cut his right index finger whilst opening a champagne bottle on his birthday whilst on holiday. Within 24 hours of the accident, his arm became swollen and dark in colour. When he arrived at the hospital he was found to have cellulitis and necrotising fasciitis (Staphylococcus aureus was cultured) and required an urgent operation for debridement (Figure 8.1). During surgery he suffered a cardiac arrest with a down time of two minutes before being resuscitated. Post operatively he developed multi-organ failure and was transferred to ITU. Two days later he was taken back to theatre for further debridement because of the aggressive

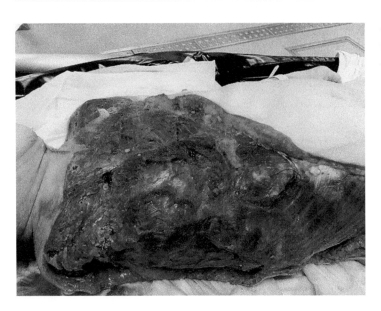

◀ **Figure 8.1** Wide area of debridement is shown incorporating amputation of the right arm.

progression of the necrotising fasciitis, but unfortunately died during surgery. He had developed septic shock and coagulopathy in addition to multi-organ failure.

## Loss or Diminished Function

Loss of or diminished function may occur, following direct damage or by diminished blood flow to organs and musculoskeletal system. Indeed, loss of blood supply to injured limb vasculature may result in ischaemia followed by amputation. Asirdizer et al. (2004) evaluated 372 cases of post-traumatic extremity vessel lesions, for which the Forensic Medicine Council, Istanbul, Turkey, prepared medico-legal evaluation reports between 1998 and 2000. There were 378 artery (74.5%) and 131 vein injuries (25.5%) out of a total of 509 limb vascular injuries. The most frequently injured arteries and veins were the femoral artery (n = 73), and the deep femoral vein (n = 41), respectively. Cutting and stabbing injuries accounted for 160 cases (43.0%); between a quarter and a third of these injuries were accompanied by local nerve and bone lesions. They showed that almost all the injuries were life threatening and many with a substantial loss of organ function.

## Formation of Pseudoaneurysms and Fistulae

Blood vessels may develop aneuryms. The walls are weakened and are liable to dissection and with the possibility of the development of arteriovenous

fistulae or fistulae between different organs. A pseudoaneurysm or false aneurysm, arises from a disruption in arterial wall continuity and is not an enlargement of any of the layers of the blood vessel wall. Sometimes a tear can occur on the inside layer of the vessel, resulting in blood filling in between the layers of the vessel to create a pseudoaneurysm. These lesions may result from inflammation, trauma or iatrogenic causes such as surgical procedures. Blood dissects into the tissues around the damaged artery and forms a sac that communicates with the arterial lumen.

Naouli et al (2015) reported two cases of pseudoaneurysm of the profunda femoris artery (deep femoral artery (DFA). One of their cases was of a 23-year-old man who sustained a stab wound in the middle of the posterior right thigh, which required suturing. Two months later, he was admitted with increasing pain and swelling in the right thigh and after investigation with Color Doppler and 64-slice multidetector CT aniography was found to have a pseudoaneurysm of the deep femoral artery from the second perforating branch of the DFA, and there was also a communication of approximately 2 cm visualised between the cystic lesion and the deep femoral vein with arterialization of the normal venous flow within the vein (Figure 8.2). Following surgical repair, the postoperative course was uncomplicated and the patient was discharged on the fifth postoperative day.

In addition to false aneurysms, acute arterial injuries can often be complicated by the development of an arteriovenous fistula (AVF). An AVF may present

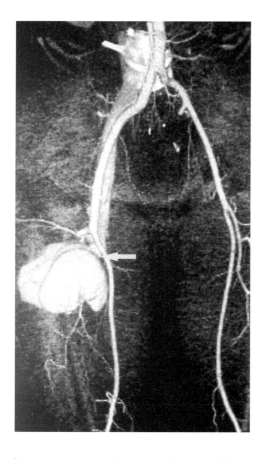

◀ **Figure 8.2** Computed tomography angiogram of the lower limbs showing a pseudoaneurysm of the second perforating branch of the DFA with femoro-femoral arteriovenous fistula (arrow) (Courtesy Naouli et al 2015).

acutely at the same time as the arterial injury. There may be signs of bleeding followed by the development of shock, an expanding pulsatile hematoma, absence of distal pulses and the onset of neurological deficiency. Early diagnosis and treatment is essential in order to avoid serious long-term complications. Robbs et al. (1994) in their large series of 202 cases of arteriovenous fistulae, found that 198 were caused by penetrating trauma. Knife stab wounds were found in 177 cases (63%) and 52 (26%) from gunshot wounds. There were four iatrogenic fistulas (2%) following transcutaneous arterial cannulation in one patient and operative injury in three. In terms of their anatomical distribution, over half (54%) involved vessels of the neck and mediastinum. The commonest single vessels involved were the common carotid artery in 42 and the internal jugular vein in 63. The upper limbs and lower limbs were injured in 22% and 20% of cases, respectively.

Elsewhere, they accounted for 4% of cases. Multiple fistulae were seen in eight patients. One of them had sustained multiple stab wounds in the neck and developed fistulae between the brachiocephalic and subclavian vessels.

In the case reported by Nagpal et al. (2008) of a 27-year-old man who had sustained a stab wound from a kitchen knife in his left thigh, prompt treatment ensured a favourable outcome. He had a 2 cm wound on the posterolateral aspect of his mid-thigh with no active bleeding and no distal neurovascular deficit. The following day, however, he developed disproportionate swelling to his thigh in relation to his injury and was referred to the vascular surgeons. Digital subtraction angiography confirmed an AVF between the superficial femoral artery and vein in the left distal thigh. The fistula was successfully repaired and he made a full recovery.

# Head

Although I have separated the description of head injuries from those seen to the neck, it should be appreciated that frequently and unsurprisingly, injuries are seen to both regions in individual victims. Fatal solitary wounds to the head are unusual, whereas they are frequently accompanied by wounds elsewhere on the body as well as on the neck. Although the skull appears to offer significant resistance to penetration by a manual assault from a sharp implement, there are a number of vulnerable areas of the cranium which can be penetrated by a sharp implement relatively easily. These include the squamous temporal region and the skull foramina, especially in the orbits. According to the literature most stab wounds of the brain occur through the orbits or the temporal region (DiMaio and DiMaio 2001). Although this seems plausible bearing in mind the thinness of the skull in these areas, the existing data suggest that there is a more even distribution. The sites of scalp and skull penetration appear to be more evenly distributed with a majority of wounds in the parietal (40%) and frontal (21%) regions in data from South Africa (Du Trevou and van Dellen 1992). Furthermore, Bauer and Patzelt (2002) found no significant regional preference in their cases. The latter authors concluded that a more even distribution of injuries supports the contention that difference in bone thickness is not the most important parameter for effective intracranial penetration in knife assaults and that under suitable conditions a knife attack to the head will penetrate the skull regardless of the site of injury.

De Villiers and Sevel (1975) in their series of ten cases of trans-orbital stabbing cases found that none of their patients was below the age of 20. Six of their ten patients were stabbed with a knife or a wire. One was stabbed with a sharpened stick, and the only female in their series was stabbed with a pointed pencil. In one case the object used by the assailant was not known but was probably a knife. The left eye was involved more frequently than the right side (6:4) possibly because the vast majority of people are right-handed. In six patients the globe of the eye was damaged (3 in the left eye and 3 in the right) and in four of these the intraocular contents were markedly disrupted; three of the four died.

The author of this textbook has seen a case in a 30-year-old man who accidentally sustained a penetrating injury with a pointed cane during horseplay with a friend. The cane was partly removed prior to death and the tip and part of the shaft were retained in the brain (Figure 8.3).

The thin calvarium in children is also a vulnerable structure to penetrating trauma. Bauer and Patzelt

(2002) from their series, found that penetrating cranio-cerebral knife injuries were rare and occurred almost exclusively in homicides. Over a period of 30 years from autopsies performed in their institute, they found only 13 cases with intracranial stab wounds. Of these, only four cases were found to be lethal injuries to the brain.

## General Features of Injury

As noted above, fatal cranio-cerebral stab wounds and other sharp trauma injuries are reported infrequently in forensic and emergency medical literature and most frequently they accompany fatal wounds which are in the neck chest or elsewhere. Most are of an accidental or suicidal nature (Chui et al. 2002; Hirt and Karger 1999; Iwakura et al. 2005; Mohan et al. 2005) but some are homicidal (Bhootra 2007; Cosan et al. 2001; Davis et al. 2004; Deb et al. 2000; Gluncic et al. 2001).

Often, the victim does not die at the scene but is admitted to hospital. The capacity to act is known to be present in many cases after stab wounds with penetration of the brain, and may lead to an incorrect assessment of the life-threatening nature of the sustained injury (Deb et al 2000). The prognosis of these victims depends on the cerebral regions affected and on the increasing intracranial pressure of the injured brain.

It appears that this is a male-specific type of violence which is assumed to be related to the need for a greater degree of force to penetrate the skull than elsewhere on the body. Penetration by a knife or a pointed implement such as a screwdriver, can be expected to occur if the blade is sharp and rigid (ridged shaft with the use of a screwdriver or other non-bladed pointed implement) and the force on impact created is high. The force necessary for skull penetration requires to impact onto a very small surface area. Any movement of the skull relative to the stab direction would probably prevent skull penetration and cause the knife to be deflected. However, it is not essential for the head to be fixed if the impact force is high enough.

As observed by Dempsey et al. (1977), a stab wound creates a narrow haemorrhagic infarction which is largely restricted to the wound tract. Concentric zones of coagulative necrosis do not result from stab wounds as they do from explosives or firearm

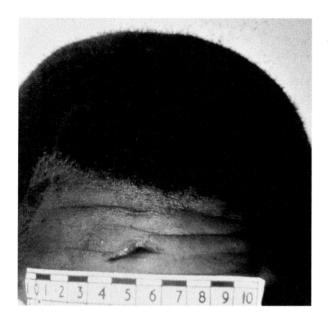

◄ **Figure 8.3a** Stab wound jut to the right of the midline on the forehead.

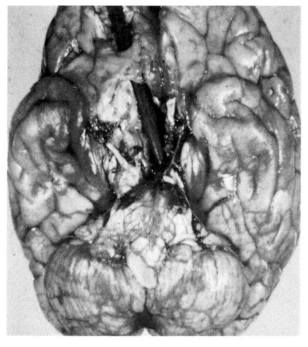

◄ **Figure 8.3b** The tip of the cane is at the base of the brain, having penetrated through the underside of the right frontal lobe and terminated at the Circle of Willis.

149

missiles. The lesion is focal and provided there is no injury to the brain stem or a major vessel, the prognosis may be good.

## Accidental Injury

Accidental penetrating sharp trauma injuries are exceedingly rare. Rothschild et al. (2001) describe the case of a very drunk 34-year-old man who had fallen into a window pane during an altercation and remained lying on the ground with a bleeding wound to his right eye. He was found to have a stab wound which extended deep into his skull. It was at first thought to be a homicide. The autopsy revealed a 15 cm wound channel, passing from the right eye socket, through the roof of the orbit and extending into the basal ganglia and ventricular system. The cerebral tissue contained a 4 cm glass fragment. Another had been removed at operation prior to death. The only issue remaining was whether the man had fallen against the glass or whether he had been deliberately pushed.

# Neck

The neck is second to the chest as the most common region to suffer fatal sharp force trauma. Injury may either be homicidal, suicidal or accidental. The author, in common with the study by Robbs et al. (1994), found that stabbings to neck structures varied in incidence from around a quarter to over a third of all cases (Table 8.2).

The neck which carries many vital structures within such a tight space and acts as a conduit between the brain and the rest of the body, when subjected to sharp force trauma, may result in devastating effects on the individual. The anterior neck structures which are not protected by the cervical spine, are particularly vulnerable to trauma.

The injuries seen are essentially penetrating, as in stab wounds or incised (slash) wounds which are longer rather than deeper and produced by impacting on the skin in a tangential manner. Furthermore, quite often multiple wounds are directed to both the head and neck, resulting in combination of wounds to both regions. In such circumstances the fatal injury or injuries are most commonly seen in the neck (Figures 8.4 and 8.5).

## Zonal Trauma Evaluation

Clinicians for the purposes of evaluation of trauma since the 1970s have divided the neck into three anatomical zones. Zone I (base of the neck) extends from the sternal notch to the cricoid cartilage, Zone II (mid-neck) from the cricoid to the mandibular angle and Zone III (upper neck) from the angle of the mandible to the base of the skull. However, the evaluation and management of hemodynamically stable patients with penetrating neck injury has evolved considerably over the previous four decades. During that time, mandatory endoscopy and angiography for Zone I and III penetrations, or mandatory neck exploration for Zone II injuries had become popular. Currently, modern sensitive imaging technology, including the use of multi-detector computed tomography angiography (CTA), is widely available and imaging triage can now accomplish what operative or selective evaluation could not, i.e. a safe and non-invasive evaluation of critical neck structures to identify or exclude injury. As a result of such developments in the evaluation of the injured patient, the use of anatomical zones has been recently re-evaluated in favour of an evidence-based strategy employing a non-zonal approach to management in such cases (Shiroff et al. 2013; Low et al. 2014).

## Type of Implement Used

On most occasions a knife is used although other pointed objects are seen from time to time such as a screwdriver (Patel 1998; Schulz et al 1995). The latter authors describe the case of a 50-year-old female victim who died of recurrent pulmonary embolism, three months after having received multiple screwdriver stab wounds in the neck and upper spine. Autopsy showed that one stab had penetrated the middle part of the cervical spinal cord and thus

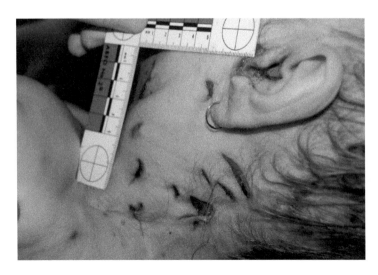

◀ **Figure 8.4** Multiple stab wounds on and behind and below the left ear. The fatal wounds were to the neck region.

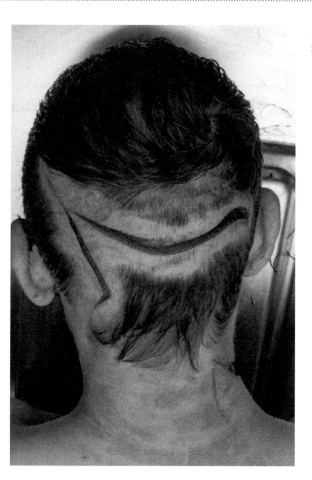

◄ **Figure 8.5a** Two incised (slashed) wounds across the back of the head.

151

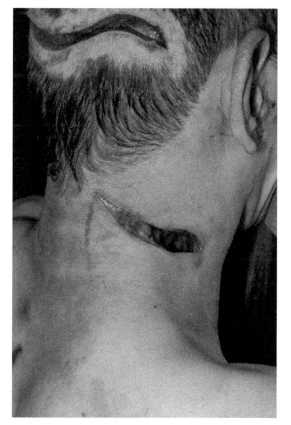

◄ **Figure 8.5b** View from right side shows accompanying elongated neck stab wound which proved to be the fatal injury.

caused an incomplete tetraplegia. In the region of the healed spinal cord and the affected meninges, a considerable amount of hair and textile fibres surrounded by foreign body giant cells and elastic fibres of spinal ligament were found, all of which had been carried into the stab canal by the blunt tip of the screwdriver. In addition to the primary clinical findings, this unusual transportation of matter into the depth of the stab canal allowed identification of the murder weapon. Hewett and Mellick (2012) further describe the case of a nine-year-old girl who, at school, fell on a sharpened pencil which penetrated the left side of her neck. Rothschild et al. (2001) reported the case of a 65-year-old male, who, during a fall down a staircase, knocked a picture from the wall breaking the glass frame which hit him in the neck and cut through his right vertebral artery. Glass fragments were noted within the track of the wound.

## Cervical Cord Injury

Stabbing injuries to the cervical cord are relatively rare. Burney et al. (1993) in the United States, found that spinal cord injury comprised 2.6% of all trauma cases, with approximately 1% of those attributed to stab wounds. Saeidiborojeni et al. (2013) found 40% cervical spinal cord injuries in their study of 57 patients with spinal cord stab wounds who attended an Iranian hospital emergency department between 1999 and 2011. The weapons used involved sharp

objects such as a knife, dagger, whittle and Bowie-knife. An earlier and larger study in South Africa in 1977 found that 450 of 1,600 patients admitted with stab wounds over a period of 13 years had sustained spinal cord injury, 30% of which were to the cervical region (Figure 8.6) (Peacock et al. 1977).

Most stab wounds to the neck, track in a downward or horizontal direction, whereas only around 10% travel upwards. Rubin et al. (2001) in relation to cervical spine injury, found that laterally directed horizontal stab wounds, were particularly dangerous because the blade could pass between two vertebrae to transect the cord resulting in irreversible injury. The more common stab wounds, inflicted from behind, usually produce incomplete cord damage. According to Peacock et al. (1977) this outcome is due to protection of the spinal cord by the spinal processes causing the blade to be deflected laterally.

Beer-Furlan et al (2014) report the case of a 34-year-old man brought into hospital with a single stab wound from an assault with a screwdriver. Neurological examination revealed an incomplete Brown-Sequard syndrome, with grade IV motor deficit on the left leg and contralateral hemihypoalgesia below T9 level. The screwdriver had been retained in the neck and was seen on radiological examination at T9 level. The authors were of the view that the incomplete deficit was as a result of the Phillips screwdriver dissecting, rather than cutting through tissue, thus minimising damage. It should also be

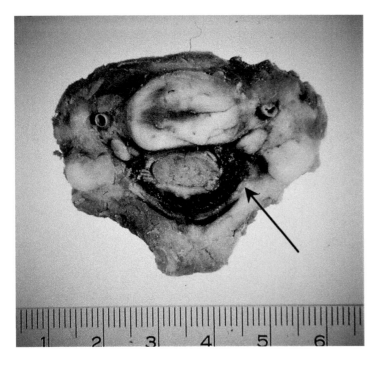

◄ **Figure 8.6** Transverse section of the cervical spine at C3 level showing spinal subarachnoid haemorrhage from stab wound to the back of the neck (arrow).

appreciated that a weapon such as a screwdriver with a rigid shaft will concentrate a large amount of force over a small area, allowing easier penetration of bone compared to a knife. Less damage will also occur when the knife blade is deflected laterally on the vertebrae as discussed above.

Occasionally the tip of the knife may break and be retained in the cervical spine, particularly if there is a turning motion of the victim or the knife whilst it is within the spine. Zaldivar-Jolissaint et al. (2015) describe a case where a broken knife blade was retained in the cervical spine when their patient sustained a stab wound to the supraclavicular triangle from a small pocket knife. It was initially managed in a local hospital by simple primary wound closure without any radiological examinations then discharged. He continued to have mild local persistent neck pain, and subsequent radiological investigations revealed a foreign body (the broken blade of a pocket knife) embedded in the left neural foramen between the C6 and C7 vertebrae penetrating the disc space. The blade was lying between the left C7 nerve root and the ipsilateral vertebral artery. Initially, he was neurologically normal but a few days later, he developed a delayed left C7 radicular deficit and following urgent exploration, the blade was successfully removed.

Occasionally stab wounds may also occur at the craniocervical junction. In such cases, the instrument used is deflected by the occipital squama into the atlanto-occipital or atlanto-axial interspace. The surface wound itself which is situated in the sub-occipital or retromastoid region may appear insignificant. De Villiers and Grant (1985) in a series covering a period of eight years, found 11 patients with stab wounds at this level, seven were on the left and four on the right. Penetration of the dura mater, with cerebrospinal fluid leakage, followed by meningitis, occurred in five patients and vertebral artery injuries were seen in four (Figure 8.7).

## Self-inflicted versus Homicidal Stabbing Of the Neck

Stabbing of the neck is from most authors' accounts, an unusual mode of suicide (Gee 1972; Vanezis and West 1983). Although most victims are adult males, Hasekura et al. (1985) reported such an injury in a ten-year-old child. Generally, differentiation between different categories of stabbing is not difficult. There are occasions, however, when the circumstances may not be straightforward and conclusions initially reached may be challenged later in court. The pathologist should be mindful of the scene findings (see Chapters 4 and 10).

In homicidal stabbing, wounds are frequently multiple and accompanied in many cases by wounds elsewhere on the body including defensive injuries. Self-inflicted wounds are frequently accompanied by tentative wounds (Vanezis and West, 1983).

153

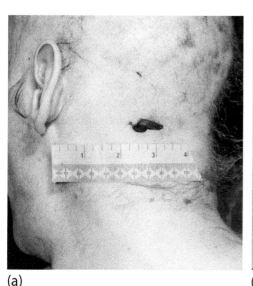
(a)

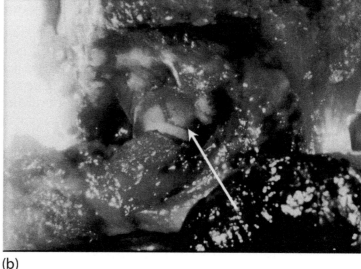
(b)

▲ **Figure 8.7** (a) The surface wound caused by a knife has deflected downwards after impacting against the left occipital condyle (arrow in (b)) resulting in severance of the vertebral artery.

## Accidental Neck Stabbing

Accidental stab wounds to the neck from knives are rare. King (1885) reported a case in which a knife became detached from a machine consisting of a large revolving wheel with a number of sharp knives at its circumference which was used for shaving down spokes of wheels. The unfortunate victim who was standing 10 feet (over 3 metres) away was struck and suffered a deep stab wound to his neck.

Road traffic injuries may occasionally include penetrating wounds to the neck due to splintered glass or indeed from sharp pieces of broken metal detached from a vehicle. Penetrating injuries may also occasionally be encountered in other accidents involving glass, such as falling on to or through plate glass or mirrors (Polson et al 1985). The latter authors describe the case of a five-year-old girl who fell while running with a sharpened pencil in her hand and stabbed herself through the jugular vein.

## Vascular Neck Injuries

Shirkey et al. (1963) from a series of 225 patients, found 350 separate injuries involving 52 different structures. Of the injuries in this series, 136 involved arteries or veins, the structure most often injured was the external jugular vein. In my own series of 49 cases of penetrating and incised neck wounds (Vanezis 1989), the common carotid artery and the internal jugular vein were the most commonly injured vessels (Table 8.3).

Indeed, the common carotid artery has been found in most series to be the most frequently injured part of the carotid arterial system, followed by the internal and then the external carotid. Associated venous injuries are frequently present and contribute significantly to the mortality in such cases (Figure 8.8).

### Ischaemic Changes to the Brain and Other Complications of Vascular Neck Trauma

There may be ischaemic brain changes due to diminished blood supply to a region from the effects of penetrating or blunt trauma. Karnecki et al. (2014) reported two cases of ischaemic stroke secondary to traumatic internal carotid artery thrombosis leading to middle cerebral artery thrombosis. One of the cases was of a 57-year-old man, a carpenter who sustained a penetrating injury to his neck from a fragment of wood. He was in his warehouse when he was struck very hard in the face, in the region of

**Table 8.3** Distribution of vascular injuries from 49 penetrating and incised wounds seen by the author during the period 1974–1986

| Vessel injured | Percentage Incidence (from 49 cases with 54 injuries) |
| --- | --- |
| Common carotid artery | 35 |
| Internal jugular vein | 33 |
| External jugular vein | 16 |
| Internal carotid artery | 10 |
| External carotid artery | 8 |
| Vertebral artery | 6 |
| Subclavian artery | 2 |

*Source:* Vanezis 1989

his left cheek by an irregularly shaped wood fragment which resembled a large splinter (measuring about 26 cm in length, and with the greatest cross-sectional dimensions of 3.5 × 1.5 cm) that broke off from the board being processed on his machine. The autopsy revealed a thrombus occluding the left internal carotid artery and the proximal segment of the left middle cerebral artery, a large area of infarction in the temporal lobe and adjacent parts of the frontal and occipital lobes of the left hemisphere of the brain, brain oedema with features of subfalcine and tentorial herniation, a comminuted fracture of the left maxilla and an occipital bone fracture in the region of the occipital condyle with the fragment impression. There were no atherosclerotic lesions in the carotid and basal cerebral arteries.

Penetrating neck trauma frequently leads to arterial wall injury in the form of contusion or vessel wall dissection with the formation of intramural haematoma, outer arterial layer damage (adventitia) and the formation of pseudoaneurysm or segmental vessel spasm. Suppurative inflammation may also develop in the periarterial space, should the patient survive long enough after the trauma. The above-mentioned primary vessel wall injuries, associated with an injury limited to at least endothelium and intima, predispose to the development of thrombosis with subsequent vessel occlusion and ischemic stroke.

### Vertebral Artery Injuries

Injuries to the vertebral arteries are uncommon because of their relatively well-protected position. Park et al. (2007) relate the case of cerebellar infarction in a 50-year-old woman caused by vertebral artery injury

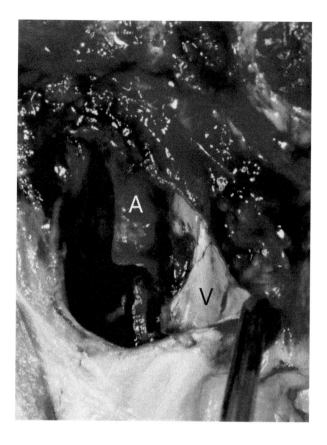

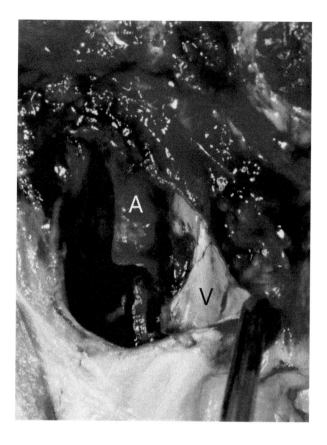◀ **Figure 8.8** The left common carotid artery (A) and the left internal jugular vein (V) are transected as result of a single stab wound.

from a stab wound that severed the vessel between the transverse processes of C3 and C4. She had a hypoplastic contralateral vertebral artery and as a result, she ultimately suffered infarction of the cerebellum due to the lack of preservation of the posterior inferior cerebellar artery blood flow. Shirkey et al. (1963) found three vertebral artery wounds caused by stabbing from a series of 136 vascular injuries. Nevertheless, vertebral artery trauma is probably still underdiagnosed, not only because of the relative inaccessibility of the vessels but also because of the lack of awareness of the possibility of such injury (Figure 8.9). Penetrating wounds of the neck region frequently injure a number of structures along their track and therefore it is not difficult to overlook wounding to the vertebral artery. Occasionally such injuries have been misdiagnosed as carotid artery injuries. Vertebral artery lesions not initially recognised may lead to complications including fistulae and/or aneurysm formation (see earlier in the chapter).

*Incidence of Different Types of Neck Trauma*
The incidence of different types of neck injuries and their effects is described by Demetriades et al. (1997). They demonstrated that 20% of stab wounds to the neck in a prospective study of 223 patients were associated with significant injuries to vital structures.

The incidence of types of structures injured is shown in Table 8.4.

*Asphyxia from Airway Obstruction*
*Following Sharp Force Injury*
Vanezis (1989) reported an unusual acute complication involving a young man who developed asphyxia from airway compression following a stab wound to the neck. He had a partial incision of the right common carotid artery as well as injury to other smaller vessels nearby. The blood had tracked through tissue planes of the neck and compressed his trachea, thus resulting in virtual closure of his airway (Figure 8.10). In one of the cases reported by Farley et al (1964) only a small haematoma was sufficient to cause airway obstruction.

Asphyxia is also a major mode of death in cases where blood has been inhaled and the larynx and trachea have been injured. Frequently, in such cases substantial haemorrhage is also present and the mode of death should be regarded as a combination of events.

Other anterior neck structures such as the laryngeal complex and tracheal airway, oesophagus and pharynx are seen in stabbings and they are commonly combined with major vascular injury (Figure 8.11).

155

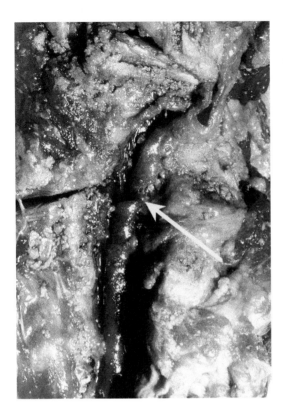

*Incised (slash) Wounds of the Neck*

**156**

Such wounds are characterised by greater length on the skin than depth of penetration. Most so called "cut throat wounds" are either self-inflicted or homicidal. Very occasionally they may be accidental in nature; they are seen particularly in road traffic collisions where such injuries may be caused by fragments of glass.

The distinction between self-inflicted and homicidal wounds may be a difficult if not impossible one to make on autopsy examination alone. The circumstances surrounding the death, including assessment of the scene where the body was discovered and antecedent history, are essential considerations in the examination of such cases.

A number of features in the character and distribution of such wounds, nevertheless, are frequently of value in making the distinction between self-infliction and homicide. Self-inflicted injuries when made by right-handed persons, normally begin high on the left side of the neck and pass downwards across the front to end on the right side. They are deeper at their origin and then tail off on the right. Such wounds may also be horizontal, lying across the front of the neck. They are usually linear and clean cut, since the skin is likely to have been held under tension. Separate shallow wounds (*tentative* or *hesitation* incisions) are strongly indicative

**Table 8.4** Incidence of type of injuries from neck stab wounds

| Injury | Stab wound (%) |
|---|---|
| Vascular | 14.6 |
| Aero-digestive | 3.4 |
| Spinal cord | 1.1 |
| Peripheral or cranial nerves or sympathetic | 4.5 |
| Haemo or pneumothorax | 13.5 |

*Source:* Demetriades et al. 1997

of self-infliction. There are often accompanying incised wounds to the wrists or occasionally tentative stab wounds, particularly on the chest. Some self-inflicted incised wounds may be extremely deep, leaving multiple pronounced score marks on the cervical spine. It is also not unheard of for a victim to excise his own larynx (Giles 1956). Indeed, in a case described by Schuessler (1944) the victim, using a single-edged razor, pulled out the hyoid bone, larynx, trachea and part of the anterior oesophagus. With prompt treatment he survived and his oesophagus was reconstructed.

Homicidal wounds as a rule do not have the regular planned appearance of those that are self-inflicted

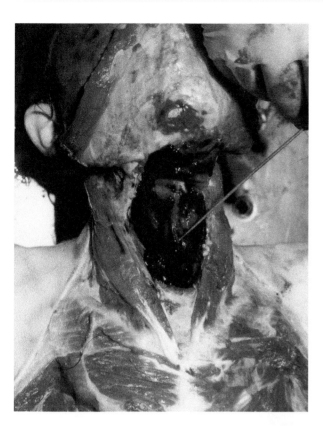

◀ **Figure 8.10** Young male stabbed in the neck. Blood has surrounded his larynx and compressed on his airway, causing asphyxia.

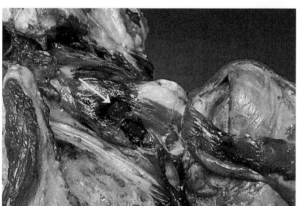

◀ **Figure 8.11a** Stab wound to left side of the neck with the track through the sternocleidomastoid muscle and cutting through the upper pole of the left thyroid gland and base of the thyrohyoid muscle then into the cricoid cartilage (arrow).

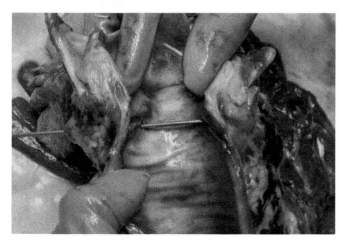

◀ **Figure 8.11b** Then exiting on the opposite side.

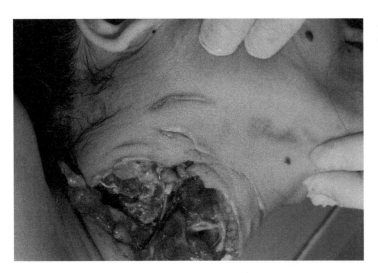

◀ **Figure 8.12a** Homicidal cut throat wounds.

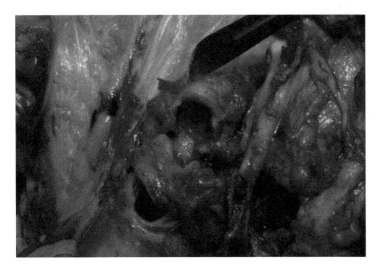

◀ **Figure 8.12b** Injured internal neck structures including the cricoid cartilage, trachea, left common carotid artery and internal jugular vein.

and they are unaccompanied by tentative wounds (Figure 8.12). Nevertheless, they are frequently accompanied by incised wounds which may be difficult to interpret without accompanying obvious self-inflicted injuries. As a rule, they are more haphazardly placed on the neck and in some cases have irregular edges. In addition, such wounds tend to be deeper, although this by no means is invariably so. Accompanying stab wounds may also be present on the neck and other parts of the body as well as defensive injuries to the upper limbs.

Accidental incised wounds may be caused by glass fragments from road traffic collisions and in such cases the cause is obvious. Such injuries may be accompanied by numerous small cuts caused by glass fragments. Small pieces of glass are also frequently found in wounds.

Cutting and tearing injuries can be produced by chainsaws (Pratt 1985). The classic injury incurred by contact between the neck and the moving chainsaw results from the motion of the saw blade. This is usually in a direction from below up, and produces multiple tears and cuts into the affected tissue. The wounds are relatively clean, in an approximately straight line and usually as multiple parallel cuts.

The internal structural injury caused by cut throat wounds was described by Rao (2015) in an autopsy study of 74 cases. He found that the external jugular veins were involved in all the cases. The larynx, trachea, carotid and internal jugular vessels were involved in 91.89% (68 of the cases) (Figure 8.13). The sternocleidomastoid in 56.76% (42 cases) and the oesophagus and thyroid cartilage in 18.92% (14) and 10.81% (8) of cases, respectively. The cervical vertebrae were least affected with injury being found in 8.12% (6 of the cases).

A 49-year-old female, seen by the author of this book, was the victim of attempted murder where she suffered severe incised neck wounds but fortunately survived. She sustained six separate cuts to her neck

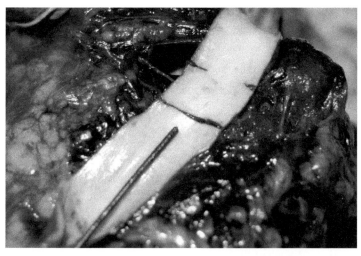

◀ **Figure 8.13** Two cuts across the right common carotid artery at the base of the neck which have been caused by a knife.

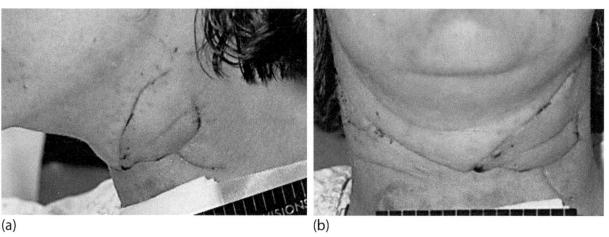

(a)                                            (b)

▲ **Figure 8.14** (a) Left side and (b) front of neck showing multiple healing scars from incised wounds.

(Figure 8.14). Her larynx and pharynx were incised at the level of the false vocal cords, through the pyriform fossa and into the prevertebral fascia. A large number of blood vessels were also cut. She required urgent medical intervention including blood transfusions and a tracheostomy to save her life and enable reconstruction of her larynx and pharynx. She made a full recovery.

# Thorax

The thorax is the most common area of injury in fatal sharp force trauma, in particular stabbing with the use of a knife. Neblett and Williams (2014) found in their series that the chest was the area most frequently stabbed at 42.1%. The heart was the most frequent sole organ injured (33.3%) in those with only chest wounds, and a haemothorax was present in 79.1% (Table 8.5.).

The predominance of left-sided chest wounds may principally be due to frontal assaults with most people being right-handed. It could also be due to awareness of the heart being on the left side of the chest. However, pathologists, in their assessment of the stab wound location should be cautious in reaching such conclusions, bearing in mind the various positions that the assailant and the victim may adopt in a confrontation.

The direction of the track from the external location of a stab wound to the thorax from a knife or from any other sharp implement needs to be carefully assessed since the internal structures damaged may well also involve injury to abdominal organs if the direction of the wound track is steeply downwards or it is situated in the lower thoracic region. Similarly, a steeply downward track in the lower part of the neck may enter into organs of the thoracic cavity.

**Table 8.5** Type of viscera injured and consequences in the victim with only chest wounds

| Viscera injured | | | Consequence | | |
|---|---|---|---|---|---|
| Type of organ involved | n | % | Pleural cavity | n | % |
| Lung alone | 3 | 12.5 | Normal | 1 | 4.2 |
| Heart alone | 8 | 33.3 | Haemothorax | 19 | 79.1 |
| Major blood vessel | 4 | 16.7 | Pneumothorax | 1 | 4.2 |
| Not documented | 2 | 8.3 | Not documented | 3 | 12.5 |
| Combined (more than one) | 7 | 29.2 | | | |
| **Total** | **24** | **100** | | **24** | **100** |

*Source:* After Neblett and Williams 2014

Mitton and du Toit-Prinsloo (2016) from their series of 173 fatalities found that more than one body region was injured in 79 cases (46%), and the same body region was injured in more than 96 cases (56%) once. Overall, the thoracic cage sustained the most injuries. Collectively, 112 wounds were recorded in the chest area, which indicates that sharp force injury to this region was documented in 65% of their cases. One hundred and twelve wounds were present in 93 cases. The cause of death in 79 of the latter was recorded as a stab wound to the chest, and as a stab wound to the heart in 14 cases. Only six of these patients were admitted to hospital. Ninety-four per cent of patients with the stab wounds in the chest died at the scene before the arrival of the emergency medical services.

## Cardiac Injuries

Penetrating cardiac injuries involve the right ventricle in around a third of cases due to its anterior left parasternal position and the left ventricle in around a quarter of cases, taking into account its more left lateral position (Karmy-Jones et al. 1997). The muscular left ventricle is the most likely to close over a small injury, followed to a lesser degree by the thin-walled right ventricle. The atria do not appear to have this ability.

It has been shown by Demetriades (1986) and Moreno et al. (1986) that 50–81% of patients with cardiac wounds succumb shortly after being injured, either from cardiac tamponade or bleeding. For patients who can be brought to the operating room with life signs and a recordable blood pressure, the survival rate should exceed 85% for stab wounds. Complex cardiac injuries that include injury to the left anterior descending artery are associated with a mortality rate of 64% for stab wounds.

In a study from Durban, South Africa, Campbell et al. (1997), examining cases seen between 1990 and 1992, found that 697 patients sustained cardiac stab wounds of which 66 reached hospital alive (just over 9%). When analysing the patients who did not reach hospital alive, 202 (18%) with tamponade due to an isolated stab wound were identified as a group who might have been saved with prompt treatment. The authors of the study concluded that delays in reaching hospital and in receiving treatment, accounted for such a high mortality rate. A case showing a cardiac tamponade from a single fatal stab wound to the left side of the chest is shown in Figure 8.15.

*Coronary Artery Injuries*

Injuries to the coronary arteries as a result of stabbing are rare, with the left anterior descending artery being the most frequently injured (Karin et al. 2001). Its anterior location renders it more vulnerable to injury than the other coronary arteries. A penetrating wound of a coronary artery may result in immediate, or rarely, delayed cardiac tamponade, intrathoracic bleeding or myocardial infarction. Later complications may develop such as a coronary artery aneurysm or fistula, either arteriovenous or with a cardiac chamber (arterio-cameral) (Rea et al 1969).

Bartoloni et al (2013) report the case of a previously healthy 29-year-old man who had sustained a single stab wound to the chest. He was admitted to hospital and following a chest radiograph and CT scanning, was found to have a left haemothorax which required draining. During the next 4 days, the patient only complained of mild chest discomfort and on the 5th day, he was discharged in a stable condition, only to be found dead at home four days later. At autopsy, he was found to have healing wounds to the

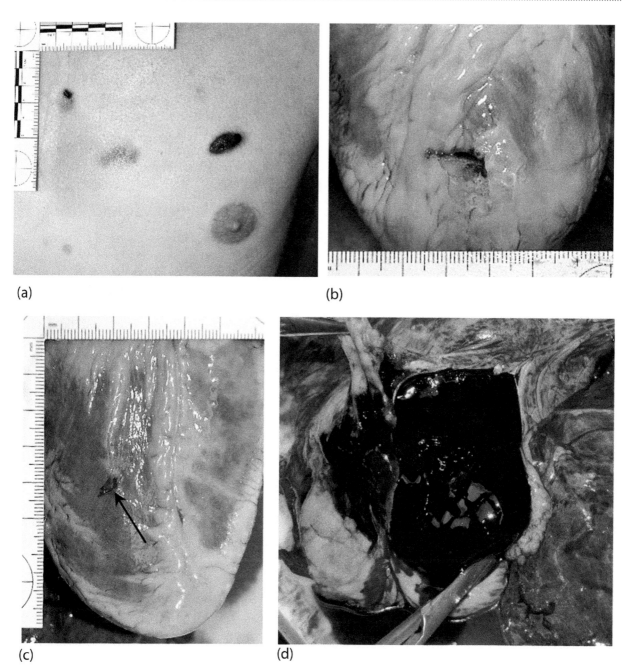

(a)

(b)

(c)

(d)

▲ **Figure 8.15** (a) Stab wound to left side of chest causing a perforating heart wound of the left ventricle and interventricular septum (b); (c) The exit wound is just visible at the posterior left ventricular wall (arrow). The victim succumbed from a fatal cardiac tamponade shown in (d).

left lung lingula and on the anterior surface of the pericardium. The pericardial cavity was filled with fluid blood and clots (400 c.c.). A round, fibrinoid-like excrescence was found on the antero-superior ventricular epicardial surface of the middle-third segment of the LAD coronary artery. Transverse sections showed that the LAD coronary artery segment had split longitudinally. There was also an occlusive thrombus and the coronary wall had ruptured,

resulting in a pseudo-aneurysm surrounding the artery as a hematoma adjacent to the epicardial surface. There was also an extensive, healing myocardial infarction involving the interventricular septum and the anterior free wall of the left ventricle.

Wall et al. (1997) in their series of 711 cases of penetrating cardiac injuries found that 384 (54%) were due to stab wounds. Traumatic coronary artery injuries due to penetrating cardiac stab wounds

161

**Table 8.6** Coronary artery injuries from stabbing

| Artery | Total | Died | Mortality |
|---|---|---|---|
| Left anterior descending | 14 | 9 | 64.3% |
| Right coronary | 5 | 2 | 40% |
| Left circumflex | 3 | 2 | 66% |
| Diagonal | 2 | 0 | 0% |
| All coronary arteries | 24 | 13 | 54% |

*Source:* After Wall et al. 1997

were uncommon and were found in 24 of the stabbing cases (6.25 %) with a high mortality from such injuries of 54% (Table 8.6.). Five of 21 patients with left anterior descending coronary artery injuries survived, for a mortality of 76.2%. Two of these patients were noted to have high proximal left anterior descending coronary artery lesions with obvious ventricular dysfunction and presented with sufficient signs of life to warrant emergent coronary artery bypass. One of these patients survived. All seven injuries to the circumflex/obtuse marginal coronary artery were treated with ligation. The overall mortality in this group was 71.4%. There were eight right or posterior descending coronary artery injuries which were treated with ligation except for one treated with emergency coronary bypass. Five of these patients died resulting in an overall mortality of 62.5%.

Rea et al. (1969) in their analysis of 22 (4.4%) coronary artery injuries from 500 patients with penetrating heart wounds in which 12 were due to gunshot wounds and 10 were stab wounds. Of their 22 patients, seven were dead on arrival and five more ultimately died of their injury giving an overall mortality rate

of 55%. Of the seven who died on arrival, six were due to gunshot wounds. There were 12 patients with two more dying after reaching the hospital, for an overall mortality rate of 67%. This is in contrast to their 10 patients with stab wounds, where only one was dead on arrival and three died after admission, giving a mortality rate of 40%. This corresponds to all reported series of penetrating heart wounds, in which gunshot wounds were more often lethal.

## Wounds to Major Thoracic Vessels

Wounds to major vessels, particularly the aorta account for a large proportion of thoracic stab wounds. Unless prior chest drainage has been employed, the pathologist will find extensive bleeding into one or both thoracic cavities, usually comprising a mixture of large clots and fluid blood (Figures 8.16 and 8.17).

Perkins and Elchos (1958) emphasised in their paper that stab wounds to the aorta were more serious than wounds to the heart because they bled more profusely and rapidly. The reasons for this include the fact that there is a sustained high pressure in the aorta compared with low atrial and ventricular pressures. Secondly, the myocardium, which is thick, tends to quickly seal a wound compared to the much thinner walled aorta. In addition, the more distensible mediastinum surrounding the aorta offers less resistance to bleeding compared to the tougher pericardium.

Occasionally other objects than knives are used. Tamburrini et al. (2017) report the case of an 82-year-old woman who stabbed herself with a

◀ **Figures 8.16** Incised wound at the root of the ascending aorta.

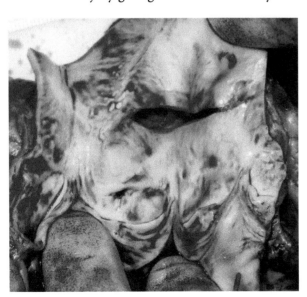

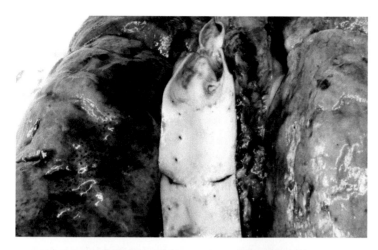

◄ **Figure 8.17** Partial transection of the descending thoracic aorta. Multiple wounds are also seen on the posterior lobes of both lungs.

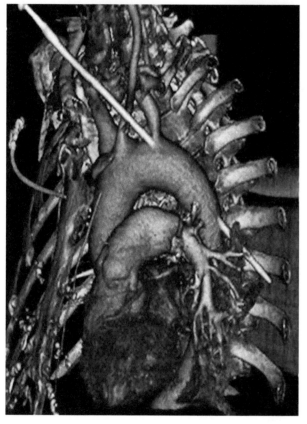

◄ **Figure 8.18** CT scan shows the needle penetrating the aortic arch at the origin of origin of the left subclavian artery. The exit point is in the descending aorta, corresponding T8 level. (The Annals of thoracic surgery, 103(2), e193 (Source figure 1); Used with permission and courtesy of Dr. Alessandro P. Tamburrini, Thoracic Surgeon at University Hospital, Southampton NHS Foundation Trust.)

163

knitting needle. The needle penetrated the aortic arch at the origin of the left subclavian artery exiting at the descending aorta, level with T8 and accompanied by a large left haemothorax and extensive mediastinal haemorrhages surrounding the aortic arch (Figure 8.18). Their patient was successfully treated.

A further case concerning a knitting needle described by Gettig et al. (2015) involves a four-year-old child who fell on to her mother's knitting bag. Radiography confirmed the impalement of an aluminium knitting needle which had entered the chest to a distance of just over 10 cm. There was concern for vascular injury but at operation, no injury was found to the major vessels. The tip of the needle was adjacent to the aortic arch, having displaced the trachea but there were no injuries to the pulmonary hilum, superior vena cava, or the oesophagus. The needle was removed and she made an uneventful recovery.

## Lung Injuries

Lung injuries are frequently seen in stabbing to the thoracic cavity (Figures 8.19, 8.20 and 8.21). The injuries to lungs include vascular trauma such as to

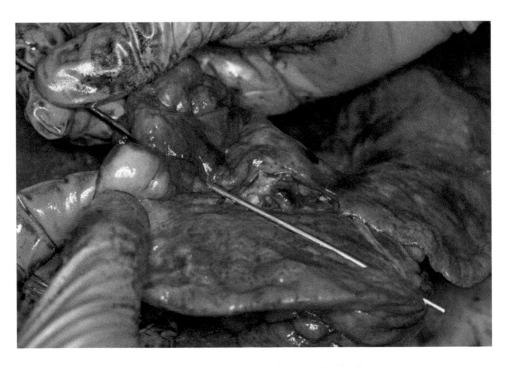

▲ **Figure 8.19** Stab wound track which has penetrated through the lung.

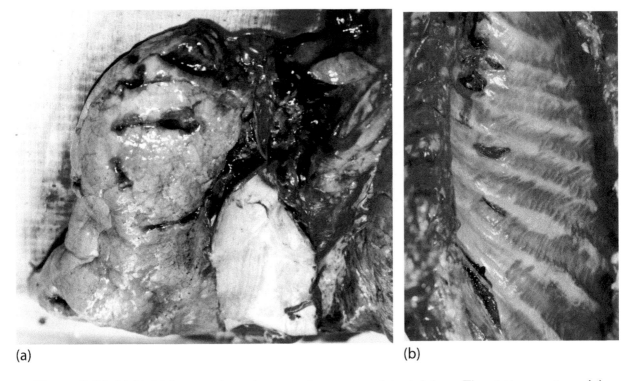

(a)                                                                    (b)

▲ **Figure 8.20** (a) Multiple wounds to the posterior aspect of the left lung. The victim was immobilised with blunt head injuries in a prone position and then sustained multiple stab wounds to his back and (b) Corresponding entry wounds at rib cage.

the pulmonary artery and branches, parenchyma, bronchi and other air passages. It is very common to see combined injuries to the heart in many cases. A resulting haemothorax and or pneumothorax is commonly present.

A pneumothorax is commonly produced when the track penetrates the chest, either by direct communication with the external surface by air being sucked in, or by communication to the pleural cavity from cut bronchi. Air within the enclosed intrathoracic space

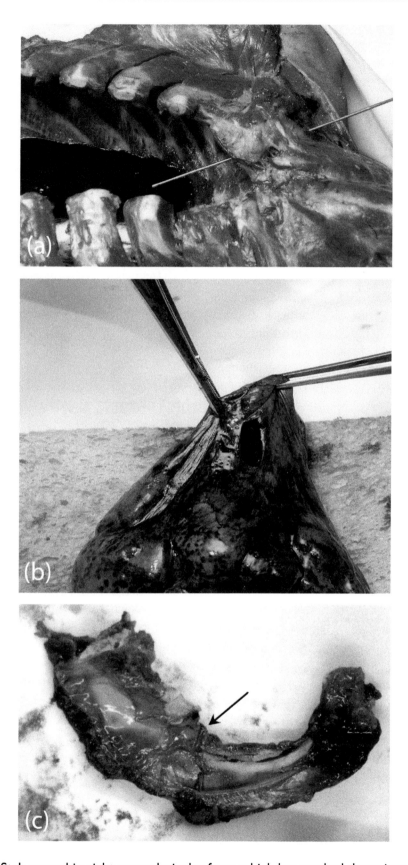

▲ **Figure 8.21** Stab wound in right supraclavicular fossa which has tracked down into the thoracic cavity. (a) Direction of track and right haemothorax. (b) Stab wound in right upper lobe near apex. (c) Inner aspect of first rib scored by knife (arrow).

applies pressure to the lung, which ultimately can lead to its collapse. Clinically there are several categories: simple pneumothorax, open pneumothorax and tension pneumothorax. A simple pneumothorax is defined as one that is non-expanding. An open pneumothorax is commonly seen in penetrating trauma as an unsealed opening in the chest wall. The most severe and potentially fatal type is the tension pneumothorax because high thoracic cavity pressure can cause rapid decompensation as a result of mediastinal shift, with lower blood return to the heart. For the detection of a pneumothorax at autopsy; see Chapter 5.

In addition to the more usual stab injuries from knives, instances involving other pointed instruments have been described including acupuncture needles. Jian et al. (2018) report the case of a 52-year-old man who underwent acupuncture for neck and back discomfort and was admitted to the hospital breathless some 30 hours later. The patient suddenly became unconscious and died despite attempts at resuscitation. Post-mortem computed tomography demonstrated bilateral lung collapse and mediastinal compression, confirmed by autopsy. More than 20 pinpricks were found on the skin of the back but not seen within the thoracic cavity. However, the authors were of the view that the use of fine needles may sometimes show no obvious internal injury; they suspected that the thoracic cavity had been penetrated in the paraspinal regions. The cause of death was concluded as acute respiratory and circulatory failure due to acupuncture-induced bilateral tension pneumothorax.

In the case described by Iwadate et al. (2003) in which they describe the collapse and death of a 72-year-old woman shortly after receiving acupuncture treatment; there was evidence of perforation of the thoracic cavity on a number of occasions. She was found to have bilateral tension pneumothorax due to perforation of the lungs by needle insertion into the thoracic cavity during treatment. Several ecchymoses were observed on the parietal pleura on both sides along the vertebral column, suggesting that the needles were inserted into the thoracic cavity and perforated the lungs.

## Emergency Thoracotomy and Other Medical Intervention

The pathologist is frequently faced with a deceased who has had an emergency clamshell thoracotomy as well as drainage to relieve a pneumothorax or haemothorax. It is essential where there has been life-saving treatment that the pathologist identifies injuries caused during the assault from drainage wounds and other incisions due to medical intervention. The survival rates following emergency thoracotomy are very low at 9%–12% for penetrating trauma and 1%–2% for blunt trauma (Farooqui et al. 2019). Occasionally the thoracotomy may incorporate the fatal stab wound, which frequently renders its assessment on the surface difficult (Figure 8.22). Furthermore, smaller drainage incisions, if the tubing has been removed and medical treatment information not available, may be mistaken for stab wounds.

## Position of Organs in the Thoracic Cavity

Ormstad et al. (1984) using computerised tomography, measured the distance between the anterior chest surface and intrapericardial surfaces of the heart and great blood vessels in 37 cases (seven with acute fatal haemopericardium) at autopsy and on 24 live persons. At autopsy, the apex of the heart was always closest to the skin surface except in cases with acute fatal haemopericardium, where the heart was displaced backwards by 10–40 mm. At computerised tomography, chest-heart distances were approximately 16 mm shorter than at autopsy. Changing the position of the patient from supine to prone decrease the distances by about 10 mm. The data presented demonstrate that the topography of the heart and great vessels is changing with the position of the body in vivo and that chest-heart distance tend to increase post-mortem; therefore, the depth of a stab wound in the anterior surface of the heart as measured at autopsy should be regarded as a maximum estimate of the length of the stabbing weapon actually having penetrated the tissues.

# Lower Thorax and Abdomen

The lower thorax is included with the abdomen, since some abdominal organs, including the liver and spleen, have a substantial amount of their structure located behind the lower ribs. Stab injuries to the thoraco-abdominal region can affect both the thoracic and upper abdominal organs (Figure 8.23)

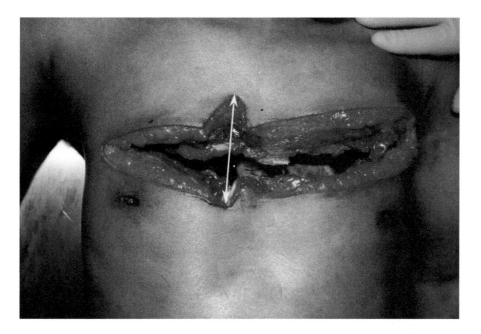

▲ **Figure 8.22a** Clamshell thoracotomy performed in young male with a cardiac stab wound. The wound on the surface crosses the thoracotomy (arrow).

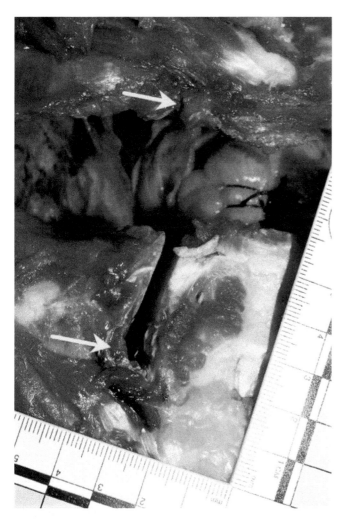

◀ **Figure 8.22b** Exposure of the rib cage reveals the wound which has cut through the cartilaginous part of the fourth rib just to the right side of the body of the sternum (arrows show the pointed upper end and a more rounded lower end).

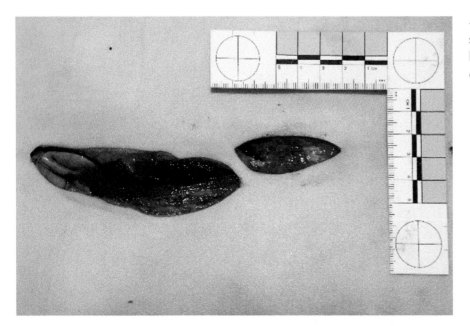

**◄ Figure 8.23a** Two stab wounds on the lower chest directed downwards.

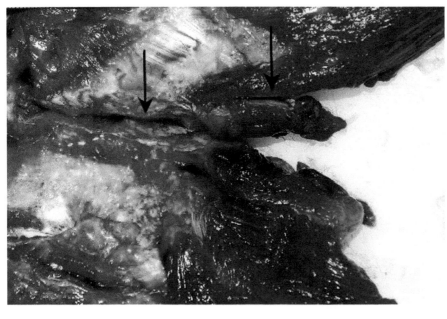

**◄ Figure 8.23b** There are two vertical cuts at the lower part of the body of the sternum and the xyphoid process (arrows).

and make assessment and management particularly challenging. The liver, and especially the spleen, may bleed extensively, causing a haemoperitoneum.

Bordoni et al. (2017) encountered 159 fatal abdominal stab cases from autopsies carried out in their institute from 2006 to 2011. The underlying cause of death was haemorrhage and its direct complications as well as trauma-related infections. The most damaged organs were the liver, followed by the stomach, the rest of the intestines and the kidneys. They found that 81% of the victims had lung injuries associated with the abdominal trauma. Abdominal vascular injuries due to penetrating trauma, especially those located in the upper portion of the abdomen, presented a high mortality rate (32%) because they produce massive haemorrhage and present a high incidence of associated lesions.

The jejunum was found to be the most commonly injured organ followed by the small bowel mesentery in a study of 201 stab injury cases by Stebbings et al (1987). Of their 47 abdominal wound cases, they occurred mainly in the upper abdominal quadrants (32 on the left, 68%) and were multiple in 8 cases (17%). Twenty-two patients (47%) had stab wounds in other sites as well, of which 12 (25%) were thoracic. All patients had erect abdominal X-rays, but only 3 of 28 (11%) had free air under the diaphragm radiologically. There was major arterial bleeding in four cases.

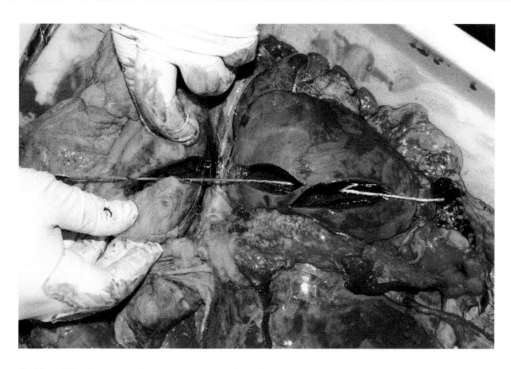

▲ **Figure 8.23c** The heart and liver are injured and both wounds have merged within the liver.

169

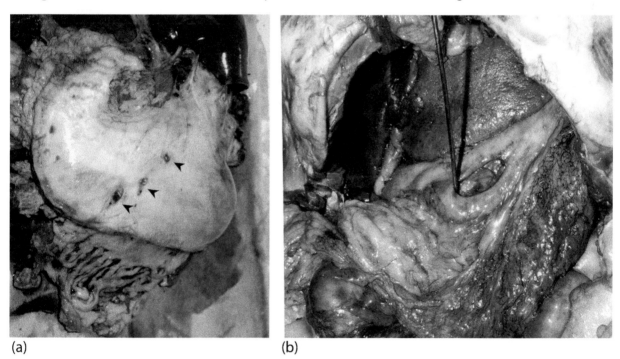

(a)          (b)

▲ **Figure 8.24** Stab wounds to the body of the stomach: (a) three wounds in line (arrows); (b) stab wound in a further case. The wound is enlarged and modified as a result of post-mortem change.

Concerning posterior abdominal stab wounds, Kong et al. (2015) in their 105 patients, from a South African hospital between January 2008 and December 2013, demonstrated a markedly different pattern of injury to that seen with the anterior abdomen. Colonic injury was most commonly encountered, followed by injuries to the spleen and kidney.

Pathologists at autopsy, occasionally encounter exteriorisation of part of the bowel through an abdominal wound. In a series of 379 patients who presented with abdominal stab wounds to the Trauma Centre at Groote Schuur Hospital in Cape Town, South Africa, between January 2005 and December 2007, 66 (17.4%) were with eviscerated bowel and/or omentum

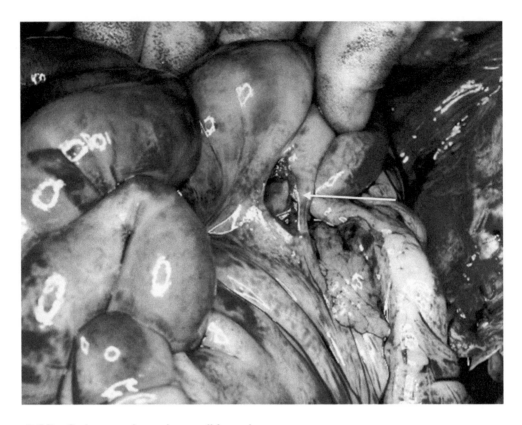

▲ **Figure 8.25a** Stab wounds to the small bowel mesentery.

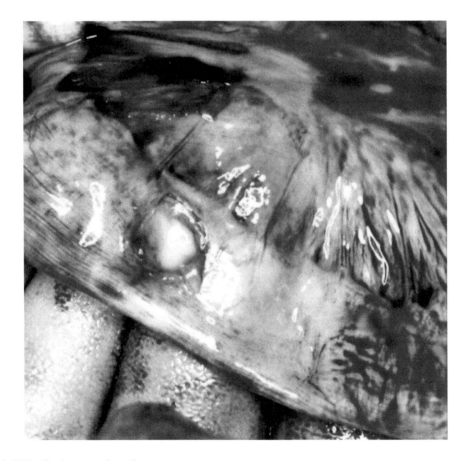

▲ **Figure 8.25b** Stab wound to ileum.

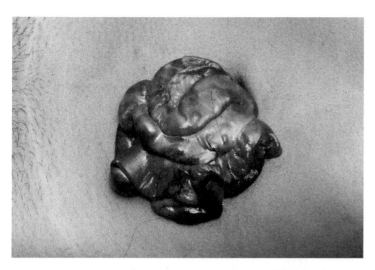

◀ **Figure 8.26** Exteriorisation of small bowel through an abdominal stab wound.

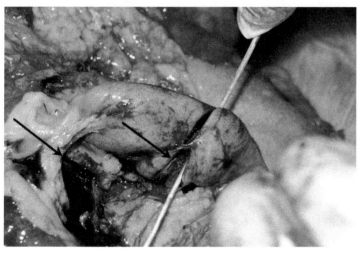

◀ **Figure 8.27** Stab wound through the central area of the kidney with exposure of renal vessels and haemorrhage in the peri-renal fat (arrows).

171

(da Silva et al 2009). They emphasise the high risk of mortality in such cases and the need for prompt surgical intervention. Exceptionally, they managed patients conservatively if only omentum had eviscerated and all other abdominal findings were benign.

Some examples of injuries to abdominal organs from stabbings that are commonly seen by pathologists are shown in Figures 8.24, 8.25, 8.26 and 8.27.

# Injuries to Extremities and Ano-genital Region

Thus far we have discussed injuries to the head, neck and trunk. This section deals with sharp force trauma to the remaining regions, namely the upper and lower extremities and the ano-genital area. Such injuries may be the sole cause of death or are more commonly seen in combination with injuries to other regions. Defence wounds which are seen principally on the upper limbs are described in chapter 9.

## Peripheral Vascular Injuries

Feliciano et al. (2011) in a position paper from members of the Western Trauma Association (WTA),

regarding the evaluation and management of peripheral vascular injury, found that in urban trauma centres in the United States, penetrating trauma accounted for 75–80% of cases. Approximately 30% of these were caused by stab wounds, although the majority 50% were caused by missiles from handguns with low muzzle velocity and low kinetic energy (1,000 ft. lbs). In countries where firearms are more difficult to obtain, stab injuries are much more common.

In the series of forensic autopsies examined by Bilgen et al. (2009), between 1996 and 2006, they

**Table 8.7** Limb injuries in homicide stab wound cases

| Limb | n (%) |
|---|---|
| Right lower | 10 (27) |
| Left lower | 23 (62.2) |
| Right upper | 2 (5.4) |
| Left upper | 2 (5.4) |
| Total | 37 (100) |

*Source:* Adapted from Bilgen et al. 2009

specifically surveyed cases where the primary cause of death was related to peripheral vascular injury and found 37 homicide cases, and a further three suicides described as cutting injuries. The distribution of the 37 stab wounds is shown in Table 8.7. Their findings showed that the left lower limb vessels were injured to cause exsanguination in just under two-thirds of the homicides. Their findings concur with a number of large series where injuries are found predominantly to the left side of the body (see Tables 8.1 and 8.2).

An example of a homicidal wounding of the femoral artery and vein is shown where the stabbing was to the left mid-thigh (Figure 8.28). With regard to suicidal wounding, the author of this book dealt with the case of a 37-year-old man who stabbed himself with a pen knife three times in the right upper thigh cutting through the femoral vein and artery causing death from exsanguination (Figure 8.29). He also

during this act managed to accidentally cut his own right hand as seen in Figure 8.31.

Vascular injuries to the upper limb in the clinical setting represent approximately 30% to 50% of all peripheral vascular injuries (Hunt and Kingsley 2000). The injuries are defined as those occurring distal to the lateral border of the first rib and including the axillary, brachial, radial, ulnar arteries and adjacent veins. The above authors found that the majority of injuries were to the brachial artery, and 90% of injuries were due to penetrating and 10% to blunt trauma (see also Chapters 9, 10 and 11).

## Buttock Injuries

Injuries to the buttock regions are surprisingly common; Campion and Cross (2017) found in their study at the Royal London Hospital Whitechapel that there had been an increasing trend over the past few years for stabbings in the gluteal and perineal regions. The prevalence had increased fourfold, from 27 cases in November 2012–2013, to 128 in November 2014–2015. Susmallian et al. (2005) in their series of stabbings to the gluteal region found that injury to this location accounted for 14% of all stab wounds seen and most frequently after chest and abdominal injuries. Although stabbing to this region usually results in minor trauma, the above authors from their series of 39 patients found nine with severe injuries and point out their potential life-threatening nature. They include bleeding from the superior and inferior

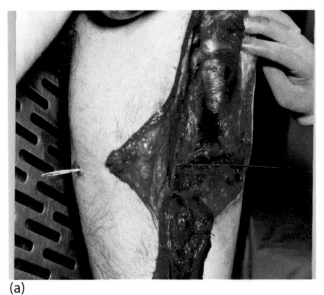

(a)

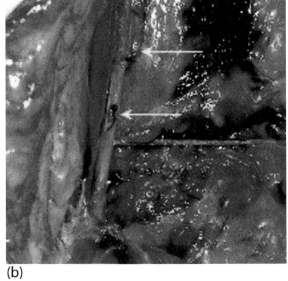

(b)

▲ **Figure 8.28** Homicidal stab wound in left mid-thigh partially cutting the femoral artery and vein. Detail of vascular injuries are seen on the right (femoral vein, upper arrow; femoral artery, lower arrow.

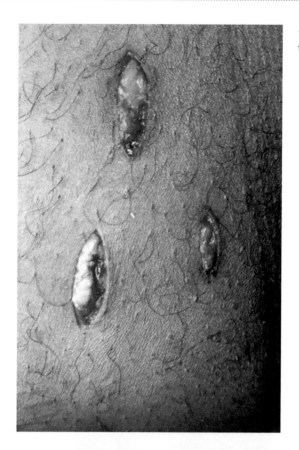

▲ **Figure 8.29a** Three self-inflicted stab wounds to right upper thigh directed medially.

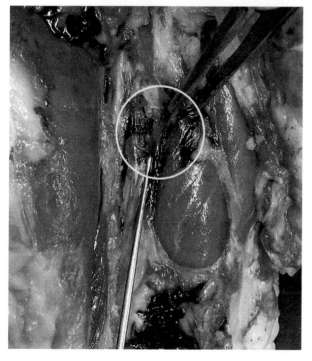

◀ **Figure 8.29b** Resulting cuts to both the right femoral artery and vein (circled).

gluteal and iliac vessels, damage of the sciatic or gluteal nerve, spinal cord penetration, urethral disruption and rectal and visceral perforation.

Feigenberg et al. 1992 report two cases involving boys aged 12 and 18 who were stabbed in the gluteal

region by three young men. They presented to hospital about 20 minutes later and were found to have sustained serious damage to internal organs. The 18-year-old boy presented as an acute abdomen following penetration of the rectum. In the other, there was tearing of retroperitoneal muscles and the internal iliac vessels causing hypovolaemic shock. Both were treated and made a full recovery.

Rutty and Busuttil (2000) report the case of a 51-year-old man who had been stabbed three times in the buttocks and died from necrotising fasciitis. He sought medical attention for the stab wounds which were sutured and dressed and then discharged. However, after three days the buttock wounds started to weep serosanguinous fluid and again he sought medical treatment; the wounds were redressed and he was started on antibiotics. He became increasingly unwell, was readmitted to hospital and diagnosed with necrotising fasciitis of the buttocks from which he died 3 days later. Autopsy examination confirmed necrotising fasciitis and microbiological culture grew Staphylococcus aureus which was not sensitive to penicillin, as well as beta-haemolytic streptococci (see also case described earlier in this chapter).

The buttock region is an unusual site for self-injury. Sauvageau et al. (2005) reported a suicidal stabbing to the right buttock with a piece of glass from a broken bottle which cut the right internal iliac artery leading to death from exsanguination. The deceased, a 38-year-old man, a month previously had tried to take his own life, whilst under the influence of alcohol, injuring himself with fragments of broken glass; he informed hospital staff that he wanted to perforate his right kidney.

## Genital Injuries

Sharp force injuries to the ano-genital region are unusual and in many instances are seen in sexually motivated assaults where they are frequently accompanied by other injuries elsewhere on the body. They are also seen from time to time in victims who have been tortured or as part of a ritualistic homicide. They may either be inflicted before or after death, including as part of dismemberment of the corpse

174

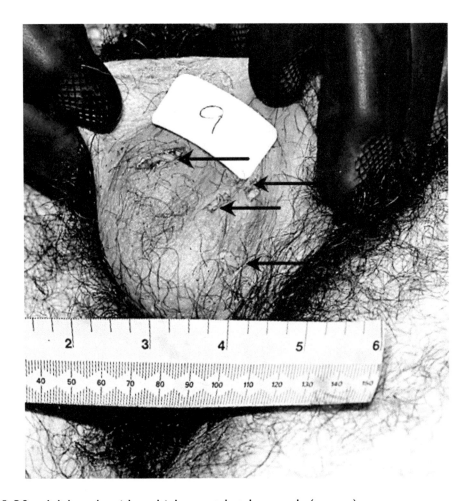

▲ **Figure 8.30a** Adult male with multiple scrotal stab wounds (arrows).

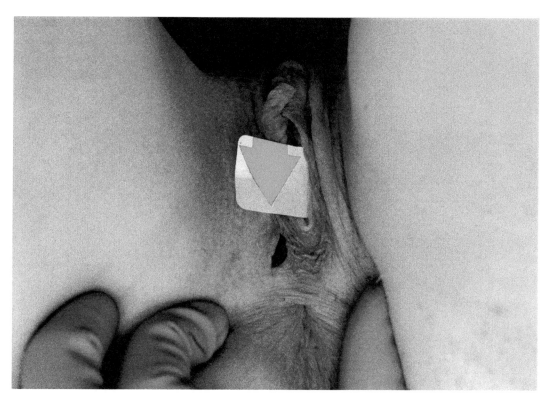

▲ **Figure 8.30b** Adult female with stab wound to the edge of the right posterior labia majorum. Both victims had died as a result of multiple stab wounds elsewhere.

or to retain as a *trophy*. In two of the author's cases of homicidal multiple stabbings, the genital area was also targeted (Figure 8.30). Self-mutilation and other circumstances such as accidents resulting in amputation of genitalia have been well described in the literature. Liu et al. (2019) reported on two cases of penile amputation; one was in a 41-year-old man who partially amputated his penis with a pair of sharp scissors during a family conflict, and the other involved a 53-year-old man whose penis was amputated by a threshing machine during farming. Both were treated successfully. The pathologist needs to be aware of the possibility of such injuries and needs to carefully evaluate any that are seen at autopsy, in the context of the circumstances surrounding the death.

Male and female circumcision, which are the most common types of genital mutilation, have been practised throughout history for cultural, religious and hygienic purposes. Female genital mutilation is found particularly in African, Middle Eastern or Asian populations. Less common male mutilations include subincisions (involving cutting the urethra) which are seen in Aboriginal tribes (Byard 2017). Discussion of the human rights and ethical issues involved in these practices is beyond the scope of this book.

## Accidental (Non-intentional) Self-inflicted Hand Wounds in Knife Users During Assaults and From Other Circumstances

In Karlsson's (1998) series of homicide cases in the Stockholm area between 1983 and 1992 there were 113 perpetrators physically examined shortly after the homicide, and it was found that 30 (27%) had evidence of sharp force injuries on their hands and four had injuries after para-suicides. It was established that in two further cases the perpetrator had injured himself to try and show that he had been attacked. Such accidental injuries are found on the flexor side of the knife-holding hand and typically may involve the index, middle ring and little fingers, most frequently at the proximal phalanx and interphalangeal joint. When the flexor tendons of the fingers are also severed and the tendon stumps are strongly retracted, this indicates that the fist was firmly closed at the time of the injury (Schmidt et al. 2004). Schmidt in a later 2010 publication, discussed the differences in the characteristics of defence injuries and those caused in an accidental manner in a perpetrator, in which the knife blade causes injury by slipping back

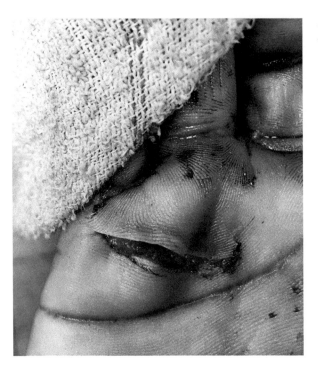

◀ **Figure 8.31** Palm of right hand showing a flapped incised wound which is on the radial side. Its position indicates that the blade of the knife had been protruding from the radial side of the hand.

onto the hand in which the knife is held. Clearly such accidental self-injury will depend on how the perpetrator had been holding the knife and from which side of the hand the blade was protruding, whether from the radial or ulnar side.

In the completed suicide case seen by the author of the text, the deceased accidentally incised his own hand. The wound was found in the palm of his right hand proximal to the fourth and fifth digits and distal to the palmar crease (Figure 8.31).

# References

Asirdizer, M., Yavuz, M. S., Buken, E., Daglar, S., & Uzun, I. (2004). Medicolegal evaluation of vascular injuries of limbs in Turkey. *J Clin. Forensic Med.*, 11, 59–64.

Bartoloni G, Trio F, Bartoloni A, Giorlandino A, Pucci A. (2013). A fatal stab wound causing selective injury to the left anterior descending coronary artery, myocardial infarction and delayed cardiac tamponade. *Forensic Sci Int* 229, e16–18.

Bauer M, Patzelt D. (2002). Intracranial stab injuries: case report and case study. *Forensic Sci Int* 129, 122–127.

Beer-Furlan AL, Paiva WS, Tavares WM, de Andrade AF, Teixeira MJ. (2014). Brown-Sequard syndrome associated with unusual spinal cord injury by a screwdriver stab wound. *Int J Clin Exp Med* 7, 316–319.

Bhootra BL. (2007). Retained intra cranial blade—medicolegal perspectives. *J Forensic Leg Med* 14, 31–34.

Bilgen S, Türkmen N, Eren B, Fedakar R. (2009). Peripheral vascular injury-related deaths. *Ulus Travma Acil Cerrahi Derg* 15, 357–361.

Bordoni PHC, Santos DMMD, Teixeira JS, Bordoni LS. (2017). Deaths from abdominal trauma: analysis of 1888 forensic autopsies. *Rev Col Bras Cir* 44, 582–595.

Burney RE, Maio RF, Maynard F, Karunas R. (1993). Incidence, characteristics, and outcome of spinal cord injury at trauma centers in North America. *Arch Surg* 128, 596–599.

Byard RW. (2017). Implications of genital mutilation at autopsy. *J Forensic Sci* 62, 926–929.

Campbell NC, Thomson SR, Muckart DJ, Meumann CM, Van Middelkoop I, Botha JB. (1997). Review of 1198 cases of penetrating cardiac trauma. *Br J Surg* 84, 1737–1740.

Campion T, Cross S. (2017). The spectrum of injuries in buttock stab wounds. *Clin Radiol* 72, 543–551.

Chui M, de Tilly LN, Moulton R, Chui D. (2002). Suicidal stab wound with a butter knife. *CMAJ* 167, 899.

Cosan TE, Arslantas A, Guner AI, Vural M, Kaya T, Tel E. (2001). Injury caused by deeply penetrating knife blade lodged in infratemporal fossa. *Eur J Emerg Med* 8, 51–54.

Davis NL, Kahana T, Hiss J. (2004). Souvenir knife. A retained transcranial knife blade. *Am J Forensic Med Pathol* 25, 259–261.

Deb S, Acosta J, Bridgeman A, Wang D, Kennedy S, Rhee P. (2000). Stab wounds to the head with intracranial penetration. *J Trauma* 48, 1159–1162.

Demetriades D. (1986). Cardiac wounds. Experience with 70 patients. *Ann Surg* 203, 315–317.

Demetriades D, Theodorou D, Cornwell EE, Berne TV, Asensio J, Belzberg H, Velmahos G, Weaver F, Yellin A. (1997). Evaluation of penetrating injuries of the neck: prospective study of 223 patients. *World J Surg* 21, 41–48.

Dempsey LC, Winestock DP, Hoff JT. (1977). Stab wounds of the brain. *West J Med* 126, 1–4.

DiMaio VJ, DiMaio D. (2001). *Forensic pathology*, 2nd ed., p 207. CRC Press, Boca Raton.

Farley HH, Nixon R, Peterson TA, Hitchcock CR (1964). Penetrating wounds of the neck. *Am J Surg*, 108, 592–596.

Farooqui AM, Cunningham C, Morse N, Nzewi O. (2019). Life-saving emergency clamshell thoracotomy with damage-control laparotomy. *BMJ Case Rep* Mar 4, 12.

Feigenberg Z, Ben-Baruch D, Barak R, Zer M. (1992). Penetrating stab wound of the gluteus—a potentially life-threatening injury: case reports. *J Trauma* 33, 776–778.

Feliciano DV, Moore FA, Moore EE, West MA, Davis JW, Cocanour CS, Kozar RA, McIntyre RC Jr. (2011). Evaluation and management of peripheral vascular injury. Part 1. Western Trauma Association/critical decisions in trauma. *J Trauma* 70, 1551–1556.

Gee DJ. (1972). Two suicidal transfixions of the neck. *Med Sci Law* 12, 171–172.

Gettig K, Lawson KA, Garcia NM, Fox KA. (2015). Penetrating knitting needle through the mediastinum in a child. *J Trauma Nurs* 22, 132–135.

Giles C. (1956). Suicidal laryngectomy. *J Forensic Med* 3, 91–93.

Gluncic I, Roje Z, Tudor M, Gluncic V. (2001). Unusual stab wound of the temporal region. *Coratian Med J* 42, 579–582.

Hasekura H, Fukushima H, Yonemura I, Ota M. (1985). A rare suicidal case of a ten-year-old child stabbing himself in the throat. *J Forensic Sci.*, 30, 1269–1271.

Hewett KM, Mellick L. (2012). A case of penetrating neck trauma in a child. *Pediatr Emerg Care* 28, 49–51.

Hirt M, Karger B. (1999). Fatal brain injury caused by the free-flying blade of a knife—case report and evaluation of the unusual weapon. *Int J Legal Med* 112, 313–314.

Hunt CA, Kingsley JR. (2000). Vascular injuries of the upper extremity. *South Med J* 93, 466–468.

Iwadate K, Ito H, Katsumura S, Matsuyama N, Sato K, Yonemura I, Ito Y. (2003). An autopsy case of bilateral tension pneumothorax after acupuncture. *Leg Med (Tokyo)* 5, 170–174.

Iwakura M, Kawaguchi T, Hosoda K, Shibata Y, Komatsu H, Yanagisawa A, Kohmura E. (2005). Knife blade penetrating stab wound to the brain. *Neurol Med Chir* 45, 172–175.

Jian J, Shao Y, Wan L, Zhang M, Liu N, Zhang J, Chen Y. (2018). Autopsy diagnosis of acupuncture-induced bilateral tension pneumothorax using whole-body postmortem computed tomography: a case report. Medicine (Baltimore) 97, e13059.

Karin E, Greenberg R, Avital S, Aladgem D, Kluger Y. (2001). The management of stab wounds to the heart with lacerationof the left anterior descending coronary artery. *Eur J Emerg Med* 8, 321–323.

Karlsson T. (1998). Sharp force homicides in the Stockholm area, 1983–1992. *Forensic Sci Int* 94, 129–139.

Karmy-Jones R, VanWijngaarden V, Talwar M, Lovoulos C. (1997). Penetrating cardiac injuries. *Injury* 28, 57–61.

Karnecki K, Jankowski Z, Kaliszan M. (2014). Direct penetrating and indirect neck trauma as a cause of internal carotid artery thrombosis and secondary ischemic stroke. *J Thrombosis Thrombolysis*, 38, 409–415.

King. (1885). Wound of vertebral artery; recovery. *Lancet* 126(3248), 993.

Kong VY, Oosthuizen GV, Clarke DL. (2015). The spectrum of injuries resulting from posterior abdominal stab wounds: a South African experience. *Ann R Coll Surg Engl* 97, 269–273.

Krywanczyk A, Shapiro S. (2015). A retrospective study of blade wound characteristics in suicide and homicide. *Am J Forensic Med Pathol* 36, 305–310.

Lord JM, Midwinter MJ, Chen YF, Belli A, Brohi K, Kovacs EJ, Koenderman L, Kubes P, Lilford RJ. (2014). The systemic immune response to trauma: an overview of pathophysiology and treatment. *Lancet (London, England)*, 384, 1455–1465.

Liu X, Liu Z, Pokhrel G, Li R, Song W, Yuan X, Guo X, Wang S, Wang T, Liu J. (2019). Two cases of successful microsurgical penile replantation with ischemia time exceeding 10 hours and literature review. *Transl Androl Urol* 8(Suppl 1), S78–S84.

Low GM, Inaba K, Chouliaras K, Branco B, Lam L, Benjamin E, Menaker J, Demetriades D. (2014). The use of the anatomic 'zones' of the neck in the assessment of penetrating neck injury. *Am Surg* 80, 970–974.

Mitton L, du Toit-Prinsloo L. (2016). Sharp force fatalities at the Pretoria Medico-Legal laboratory, 2012–2013. *S Afr J Surg* 54, 21–26.

Mohan AL, Slim M, Benzil DL. (2005). Knife wound of the posterior fossa in a child. *Child Nerv Syst* 21, 255–258.

Moreno C, Moore E, Majure JA, Hopeman AR. (1986). Pericardial tamponade. A critical determinant for survival following penetrating cardiac wounds. *J Trauma* 26, 821–825.

Nagpal K, Ahmed K, Cuschieri R. (2008). Diagnosis and management of acute traumatic arteriovenous fistula. *Intern J Angiol: Official Publ Intern College Angiol, Inc*, 17, 214–216.

Naouli H, Jiber H, Bouarhroum A. (2015). False aneurysm of perforating branch of the deep femoral artery-report of two cases. *Int J Surg Case Rep* 14, 36–39.

Neblett A, Williams NP. (2014). Sharp force injuries at the University Hospital of the West Indies, Kingston, Jamaica: a seventeen-year autopsy review. *West Indian Med J* 63, 431–435.

Ormstad K, Rajs J, Calissendorff B, Ahlberg NE. (1984). Difference between in vivo and postmortem distances between anterior chest and heart surface. A combined autopsy and in vivo computerized tomography study. *Am J Forensic Med Pathol* 5, 31–35.

Park JJ, Shim HS, Jeong JH, Whang SH, Kim JP, Jeon SY, Kwon OJ. (2007). A case of cerebellar infarction caused by vertebral artery injury from a stab wound to the neck. *Auris Nasus Larynx* 34, 431–434.

Patel F. (1998). Vasovagal death from screwdriver stabbing of the neck case report. *J Clin Forensic Med* 5, 205–206.

Peacock WJ, Shrosbree RD, Key AG. (1977). A review of 450 stab wounds of the spinal cord. *S Afr Med J* 51, 961–964.

Perkins R, Elchos T. (1958). Stab wound of the aortic arch. *Ann Surg* 147, 83–86.

Polson CJ, Gee DJ, Knight B. (1985). *The essentials of forensic medicine*. 4th Edition. Pergamon Press, Oxford, pp 179–180.

Pratt LW. (1985). Chain saw injuries of the head and neck. *Ear Nose Throat J* 64, 215–222.

Rao D. (2015). An autopsy study of 74 cases of cut throat injuries. *Egyptian J Forensic Sci* 5, 144–149.

Rea WJ, Sugg WL, Wilson LC, Webb WR, Ecker RR. (1969). Coronary artery laceration: an analysis of 22 patients. *Ann Thorac Surg* 7, 518–528.

Robbs JV, Carrim AA, Kadwa AM, Mars M. (1994). Traumatic arteriovenous fistula: experience with 202 patients. *Br J Surg.*, *81*, 1296–1299.

Rothschild MA, Karger B, Schneider V. (2001). Puncture wounds caused by glass mistaken for with stab wounds with a knife. *Forensic Sci Int* 121, 161–165.

Rouse DA. (1994). Patterns of stab wounds: a six year study. *Med Sci Law* 34, 67–71.

Rubin G, Tallman D, Sagan L, Melgar M. (2001). An unusual stab wound of the cervical spinal cord: a case report. *Spine* 26, 444–447.

Rutty GN, Busuttil A. (2000). Necrotizing fasciitis: reports of three fatal cases simulating and resulting from assaults. *Am J Forensic Med Pathol* 21, 151–154.

Saeidiborojeni HR, Moradinazar M, Saeidiborojeni S, Ahmadi A. (2013). A survey on spinal cord injuries resulting from stabbings: a case series study of 12 years' experience. *J Inj Violence Res* 5, 70–74.

Sauvageau A, Yesovitch R, Racette S. (2005). An unusual case of suicide by broken glass pierced through the buttocks: a case report. *Med Sci Law* 45, 81–84.

Schuessler WW. (1944). Self -infliction excision of the larynx and thyroid and division of the trachea and oesophagus with recovery. *J Am Med Assoc* 125, 551–552.

Schulz F, Colmant HJ, Trtübner K. (1995). Penetrating spinal injury inflicted by screwdriver: unusual morphological findings. *J Clin Forensic Med* 2, 153–155.

Shirkey AL, Beall AC, DeBakey ME. (1963). Surgical management of penetrating wounds of the neck. *Arch Surg* 86, 955–963.

Shiroff AM, Gale SC, Martin ND, Marchalik D, Petrov D, Ahmed HM, Rotondo MF, Gracias VH. (2013). Penetrating neck trauma: a review of management strategies and discussion of the 'no zone' approach. *Am Surg* 79, 23–29.

da Silva M, Navsaria PH, Edu S, Nicol AJ. (2009). Evisceration following abdominal stab wounds: analysis of 66 cases. *World J Surg* 33, 215–219.

Schmidt U, Faller-Marquardt M, Tatschner T, Walter K, Pollak S (2004)., Cuts to the offender's own hand—unintentional self-infliction in the course of knife attacks. *Int J Legal Med* 118, 348–354.

Schmidt U (2010). Sharp force injuries in "clinical" forensic medicine. *Forensic Sci Int*. 195, 1–5.

Stebbings WSL, Chalstrey LJ, Gilmore OJA, Shand WS, Staunton MD, Thomson JPS. (1987). Stab injury-the experience of an East London Hospital 1978–1983. *Postgrad Med J* 63, 81–84.

Susmallian S, Ezri T, Elis M, Dayan K, Charuzi I, Muggia-Sullam M. (2005). Gluteal stab wound is a frequent and potentially dangerous injury. *Injury* 36, 148–150.

Tamburrini A, Rehman SM, Votano D, Malvindi PG, Nordon I, Allison R, Miskolczi S. (2017). Penetrating trauma of the thoracic aorta caused by a knitting needle. *Ann Thorac Surg* 103(2), e193.

Du Trevou MD, van Dellen JR. (1992). Penetrating stab wounds to the brain: the timing of angiography in patients presenting with the weapon already removed. *Neurosurgery* 31, 905–912.

Vanezis P, West IE. (1983). Tentative injuries in self stabbing. *Forensic Sci Intern*, 21, 65–70.

Vanezis P. (1989). *Pathology of neck injury* Ch. 4, p37. Butterworths, London.

Vassalini M, Verzeletti A, De Ferrari F. (2014). Sharp force injury fatalities: a retrospective study (1982–2012) in Brescia (Italy). *J Forensic Sci* 59, 1568–1574.

De Villiers JC, Grant AR. (1985). Stab wounds of the craniocervical junction. *Neurosurgery* 17, 930–936.

De Villiers JC, Sevel D. (1975). Intracranial complications of transorbital stab wounds. *Br J Ophthal* 59, 52–56.

Wall MJ Jr, Mattox KL, Chen CD, Baldwin JC. (1997). Acute management of complex cardiac injuries. *J Trauma* 42, 905–912.

Zaldivar-Jolissaint, J. F., Bobinski, L., Van Dommelen, Y., Levivier, M., Simon, C., & Duff, J. M. (2015). Delayed presentation of deep penetrating trauma to the subaxial cervical spine. *Eur Spine J: Official Publi Eur Spine Soc, Eur Spinal Deformity Soc, Eur Sec Cervical Spine Res Soc.*, 24 Suppl 4, S540–S543.

# ▮ Chapter 9
# Defence Injuries

## Introduction

Defence wounds are injuries which are received by a victim trying to defend themselves or occasionally defend another person, against an assailant. There are a number of different types of such injuries, depending on the implement being used to attack the victim, ranging from different types of sharp or blunt trauma or a combination of the two. In this chapter, injuries caused by sharp force trauma are considered, in terms of their morphology, pattern, distribution and other relevant factors.

## General Considerations in the Investigation of Defence Injuries

### How Are They Caused?

There are a number of ways in which a person may sustain defence injuries in an attack from an object such as a knife. It is also important to appreciate that such injuries are found in less than half of all homicidal stabbing cases and therefore it should be understood that if an assailant is threatening someone or actively stabbing them, and the victim is trying to defend themselves, it does not necessarily follow that the attacking knife will inevitably cause a defence injury to the victim. The chances of doing so, however, do increase with the length of time of an attack as well as the number of stab wounds inflicted. Among the more understandable reasons why defence wounds may be absent are that the victim is immobilised and/or unconscious for whatever reason or unaware of trauma being inflicted (taken by surprise).

In terms of their appearance, defence injuries are in most instances incised wounds of variable depth although some stab wounds may also be seen. A combination of the two types is not unusual. Furthermore, in many instances, careful examination of the wounds may assist in assessing the type of blade, whether serrated or smooth edged.

In relation to reconstruction of events, the pathologist, in addition to considerations such as the scene and overall pattern of injury, will find that defence injuries, when they are present, will frequently add useful information by clarifying some of the issues relating to the dynamics of the stabbing, taking into account their location, distribution, number and characteristics.

There are a number of ways in which defence injuries may be sustained. A common defensive action to ward off an attack involves blocking the movement of a knife with the arms. Wounds from blocking, in particular, are seen to the back of the hands and forearms. Less often the upper arms and shoulders are injured.

Attempting to take hold of the weapon from the assailant's hand or by blocking the weapon with the open hand are also quite common defensive actions. In such a situation, injuries are seen to the palms and flexor surfaces of the fingers resulting from the grasping action of the hand with the fingers and thumb in apposition. The pattern of injuries seen will depend on the position of the knife within the hand, the orientation of the sharp side of the blade, as well as the movement of the hand whilst the weapon is being held.

Injuries may also be seen as a result of attempting to cover up the targeted area by placing the hands or arms to that region, e.g. placing the hands directly over the face or head or occasionally doubling or folding the legs to cover the groin or abdomen.

Occasionally defence wounds may be seen to the side of the body or the back which are unusual sites for such injuries. They may occur if the victim takes avoiding action by turning his/her body to present an assumed non-vital area to the assailant. It should also be appreciated that defence injuries may be sustained when another person is trying to protect an individual during the course of an assault. A good example would be a bodyguard protecting a dignitary from assassination by acting as a human shield. Examples of a variety of defence injuries are shown in Figures 9.1–9.9.

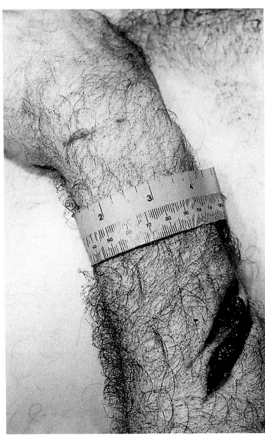

◀ **Figure 9.1a** Defensive incised wounds of the extensor (posterior) surface of the right forearm.

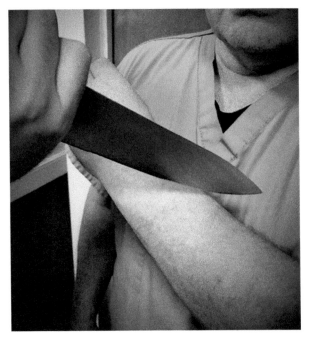

◀ **Figure 9.1b** The type of position in which the arm is raised to block a knife to result in such injury.

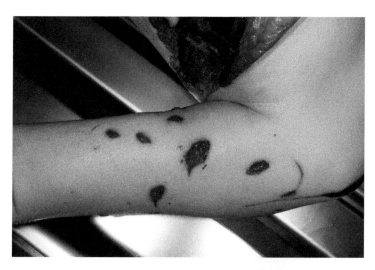

◀ **Figure 9.2** Multiple stab wounds to the left upper arm and shoulder caused by the victim trying to ward off the knife by lifting his arm.

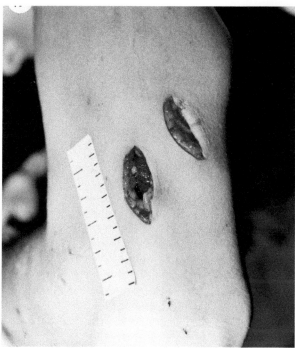

◀ **Figure 9.3a** Two stab wounds on the left upper arm caused by the victim lifting his arm to ward off the attacker's knife.

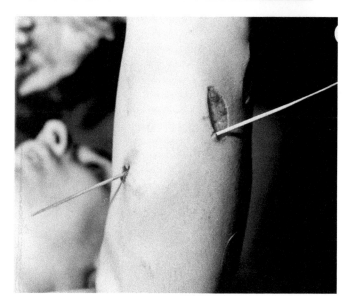

◀ **Figure 9.3b** The upper wound has penetrated the arm and produced an exit wound. A probe is used to show the direction of the track.

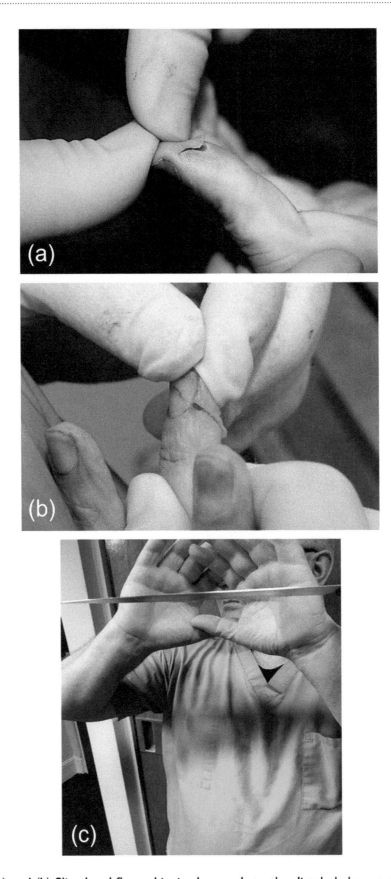

▲ **Figure 9.4** (a) and (b) Sliced and flapped incised wounds to the distal phalanges of the thumb and middle finger caused by raising the hands to ward off a knife. (c) Typical stance in which hands might be held to block a knife, with the palms facing the weapon in a defensive motion.

## Active or Passive Defence Injuries?

A distinction is frequently made between warding off/blocking an attack and grabbing the assailant's weapon. The former is described as a defence injury which is "passive" and the latter as "active". In the study by Katkici et al. (1994), of 195 stabbing homicides 39.7% defence wounds were classed as "active" and 40.5% as "passive." In reality this distinction does not accurately convey the dynamics between the assailant and victim, including the length of struggle between them and the force used by the victim in trying to protect themselves. It therefore does not give us a true picture of what occurred and indeed may be somewhat misleading in the interpretation one places on the extent of resistance offered by the victim when reconstructing the assault.

## Distribution of Defence Wounds

Most defence wounds as stated above are located on body extremities, particularly the upper limbs but may occasionally be found on the thighs, lower legs or feet. Where there is a glancing avoiding action, the wounds may well be elsewhere on the body including the back. Racette et al. (2008) noted that most commonly, defence wounds were found on the hands, followed by the upper arms then forearms.

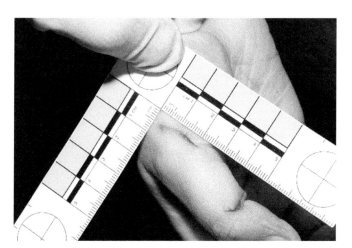

◀ **Figure 9.5a** Two linear incised wounds, one at the base of the right thumb and the other at the interphalangeal joint.

183

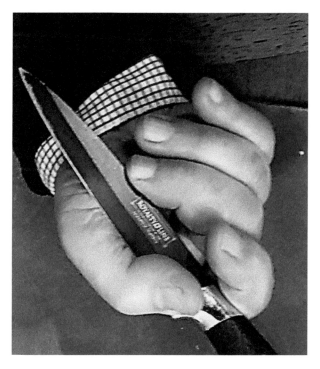

◀ **Figure 9.5b** Reconstruction to show how such wounds can be caused by closing the thumb in attempting to grip the knife blade.

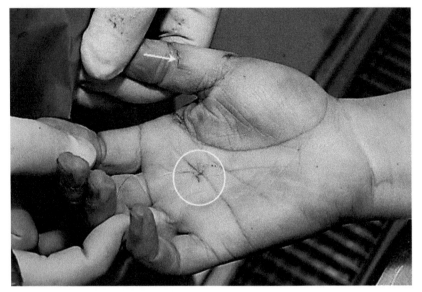

**◄ Figure 9.6a** Superficial stab wound to palm of right hand (circled) with wounds to the right proximal phalanx of the thumb near the interphalangeal joint (arrow), radial surface of the palm and a further wound distal to the metacarpophalangeal joint; all caused by stabbing the palm as the knife is being gripped by the victim.

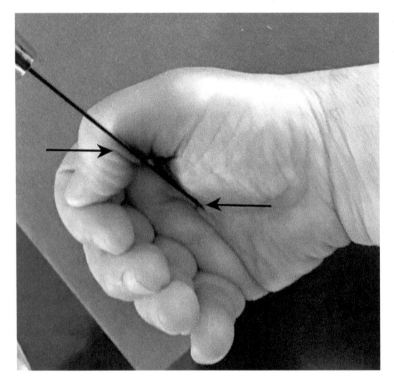

**◄ Figure 9.6b** The reconstruction shows the direction of the blade with the corresponding points of two of the injuries (arrows).

Kemal et al. (2013), in their series of 109 homicide victims (31% of all stabbings), in which they found defensive-type wounds, observed that 264 were to the hands (77%), most commonly on the palm (62%) and 79 were to the forearms (23%). Of the forearm injuries, they were more commonly seen on the extensor surface (posteriorly) (61%). They are also seen on both upper limbs in around half the cases.

Regarding the side of the body, most series have demonstrated that more defensive injuries are seen on the left upper extremity in keeping with being attacked more towards their left side since most of the population are right handed and most attacks are from frontal confrontations. The victim in general attempts to defend themselves with their arm nearest the side from which they are being attacked (Katkici et al. 1994; Chattopadhyay and Sukul 2013). This also appeared to be the case in the skeletal remains of a 19-year-old male who was alive in Gloucester in the sixteenth century (Valoriani et al. 2017). Three sharp force injuries were found to the skeleton that were caused by cuts; to the cranium, right scapula and left radius. The cut on the radius (Figure 9.10) was a typical defence injury caused by

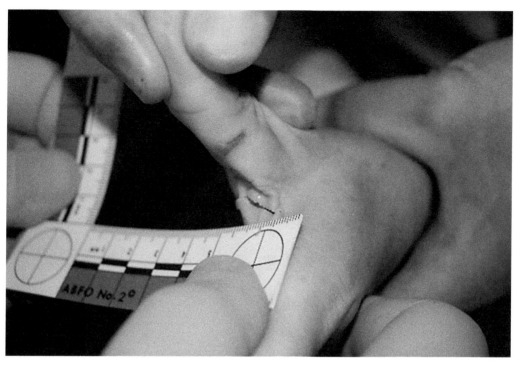

▲ **Figure 9.7** Incised wounds in the web between the right thumb and forefinger, close to the base of the opposing forefinger caused as the assailant's knife was being gripped by the victim.

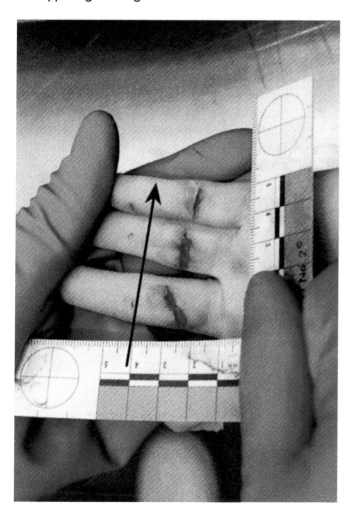

◀ **Figure 9.8** Incised wounds across the forefinger, middle and ring finger of the left hand caused by gripping the knife when being attacked by an assailant. The blade of the weapon has come from the direction of the forefinger and thumb (arrow) with the depth and length of each wound decreasing from the forefinger to the ring finger.

185

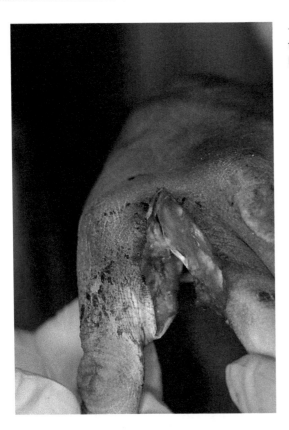

◄ **Figure 9.9** Deep cut through web between the left thumb and forefinger caused by a large kitchen knife.

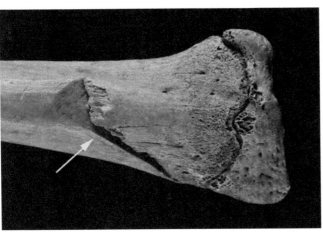

◄ **Figure 9.10** Close-up of the trauma to the posterior distal radius. Note the partially fused epiphysis (Valoriani, Eliopolos and Borrini, (2017). Sharp Force Trauma Death in a Young Individual From Medieval Gloucester. *Am J Forensic Med Pathol* 38, 111–114 (Source figure 3); used with permission and courtesy the *American Journal of Forensic Medicine and Pathology*. Wolters Kluwer).

the male raising his arm to ward off what appeared to have been a long heavy sharp weapon. It was concluded that the young man was a victim of interpersonal violence.

A further reason why defence wounds are seen more on the left side is that many attacks are aimed at the heart towards the precordial region.

# Other Demographic Factors

## Incidence of Defence Injuries in Homicide Cases

The number of defence wounds tends to increase, as the number of stab wounds to the body increases and the overall incidence in all stab wound cases in three series (Table 9.1) ranged from 38.5% to just over 45%. However, the absence of defence injuries is not by any means unusual. Such injuries may be absent if the victim is not

**Table 9.1** Percentage incidence of defence wounds in relation to numbers of stab wounds inflicted

| Number of stab wounds inflicted on each victim | 1 | 2 | 3-9 | 10 + | 20+ | Percentage from all cases in series |
|---|---|---|---|---|---|---|
| Katkici et al (1994) | 3.3 | 9.1 | 65.1 | 74.4 | | 38.5 |
| Karlsson (1998) | | | - | | | 41 |
| Rouse (1994) | | 42.1 | | 56.1 | 62.5 | 45.2 |

*Source:* Data taken from three studies

**Table 9.2** Gender differences in incidence of defensive injuries

| Authors | Percentage incidence of defence injuries | | Total number of cases in each series |
|---|---|---|---|
| | Female | Male | |
| Hunt and Cowling (1991) | 55 | 27.3 | 100 |
| Katkici et al. (1994) | 54.5 | 35.2 | 195 |
| Rogde et al. (2000) | 79 | 36 | 141 |
| Racette et al. (2008) | 71 | 54 | 149 |

able to defend themselves, particularly in the case of a very young or elderly person; they may have been rapidly immobilised for any reason or caught unaware and collapsed very rapidly. Indeed, as can be seen from different authors' series, defence wounds in stabbing homicides overall are found in less than 50% of cases.

Schmidt and Pollak (2006), in their series of 158 victims surviving bodily injury, found that 45.9% had defence injuries. In surviving victims with only one singular stab wound to the trunk, defence injuries on the hands and/or forearms were significantly higher (28.3%) than in autopsy studies. Schmidt (2010) discussed the differences between the characteristics of defence injuries and those caused in an accidental manner in a perpetrator (see Chapter 8).

## Effect of Alcohol and/or Drugs

Defence wounds according to Katkici et al. (1994) are less likely to be seen if the victim was drunk, or had used drugs or was unconscious because of other secondary physical trauma. They found that the rate of occurrence of defence wounds was lower in cases where alcohol had been consumed, and it is believed that being drunk before the stabbing played an important role as a resistance-breaking factor.

Racette et al (2008) found that in homicide victims, defence wounds were absent in cases where the blood alcohol was above 250 mg/100ml. Since important loss of coordination and reflexes is generally observed over 200 mg/100 ml, the absence of defence wounds can be explained by the victim's decreased defensive capabilities.

## Gender

Female homicide victims of stabbings have been shown to have a higher incidence of defensive injuries than their male counterparts (Table 9.2). Although to some the reasons for this difference appears unclear, Hunt and Cowling (1991) have ventured that this difference might be explained by the fact that a greater number of females are involved in long domestic arguments with their assailants and therefore have more time to defend themselves.

## Age

Defence wounds may be few or absent in the very young and very old where immobilisation may be rapid because of inability to resist because of infirmity and in the very young where they lack the strength to resist an assault. They greatest incidence

187

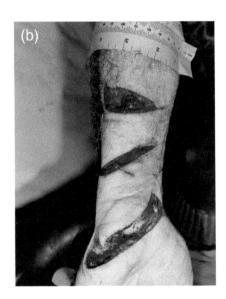

▲ **Figure 9.11** Defensive incised wounds to (a) the anterior aspect of left wrist and forearm (flexor surface) and (b) the right wrist and forearm. Such injuries might be mistaken for being self-inflicted.

of defence injuries is seen in young adults of both sexes. Chattopadhyay and Sukul (2013) in their series found the greatest incidence was in males aged 30–44 and in females aged 15–29.

## Differentiation of Defence Wounds from Self-inflicted Injuries

In the vast majority of cases there is no difficulty in identifying and correctly classifying wounds as defensive because of the other associated wounds found on the body and other factual circumstances in the vast majority of cases. However, one should always be aware of the possibility when injuries are confined to the extremities (mostly the upper limbs) that defence or homicidal wounds may be difficult to differentiate from each other (Figure 9.11).

O'Donovan et al. (2018) report on a case involving a 39-year-old woman who was found deed with incised wounds which resembled defence injuries to the back of both hands. The flexor surfaces of both wrists, however, revealed horizontal incised wounds typical of self-infliction. They appear to have been caused by the use of razor blades. The authors perfused the subclavian arteries and leakage of water from peripheral veins was seen within the wounds on the back of both hands as well as the flexor surface of the right wrist. There were no other associated injuries or other significant findings to the body to indicate that she had been assaulted.

## Defence Injuries in Non-Fatal Wounding

In certain situations, the victim may sustain only defence injuries when the weapon has been used in a threatening manner or the victim has been able to ward off a stabbing attempt by using their arms and/or hands. According to Schmidt (2010) this situation may arise when the weapon is used only to threaten the victim or limited in some other way to inflict other types of wounds to the victim.

As part of the assessment in an investigation of a homicide, it is important that the pathologist be

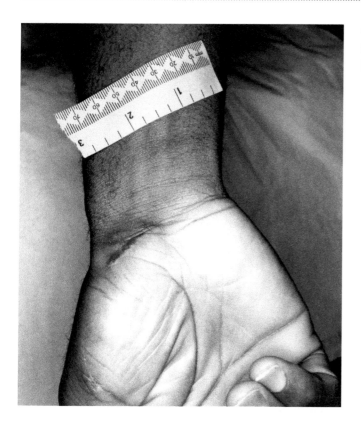

◀ **Figure 9.12** Right hand showing a defensive injury scar at the junction of the radial border and thenar eminence.

aware of the possibility that the victim may have been involved in previous non-fatal assaults involving

sharp weapons and sustained previous healed wounds including defensive injuries (Figure 9.12).

# Perpetrator Injuries

Care should be taken to differentiate between injuries caused by the knife slipping through the hand of the assailant thus injuring his own hand, from

a genuine defence injury suffered by the victim. Accidental injuries to the hand from perpetrators of assaults are discussed in chapter 8.

# Other Injuries that Might be Misinterpreted as Defensive

## Fraudulent and Other Criminal Motive

Occasionally one sees cases in living subjects who have deliberately harmed themselves in order to incriminate another person or for other fraudulent reasons. These injuries are described in Chapter 10.

## Attempted Dismemberment

A case seen by the author was of an elderly woman with multiple stab wounds, who had a number of defence injuries to the upper limbs. In addition, on her right forearm and hand there were a number of parallel cuts where the perpetrator it appears, tried to dismember her beginning with cuts to the right forearm but abandoned the attempt and fled the scene. Such wounds could have been misinterpreted as defence injuries (Figure 9.13).

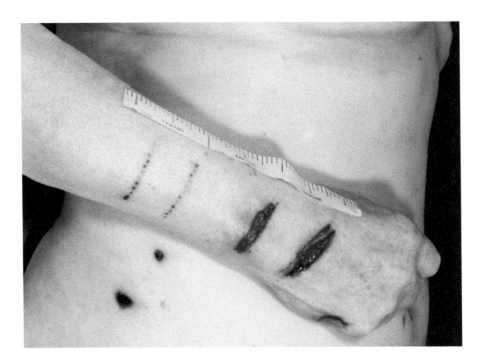

▲ **Figure 9.13a** The right hand and posterior aspect of forearm show regular and parallel incised wounds that resemble defence injuries. These appear to have been caused after death in an attempt to remove the hand. The left hand and wrist of the victim show a number of defence wounds.

190

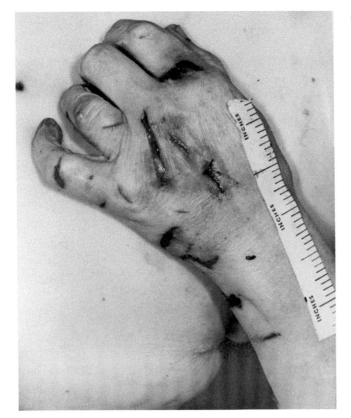

◄ **Figure 9.13b** Dorsal surface.

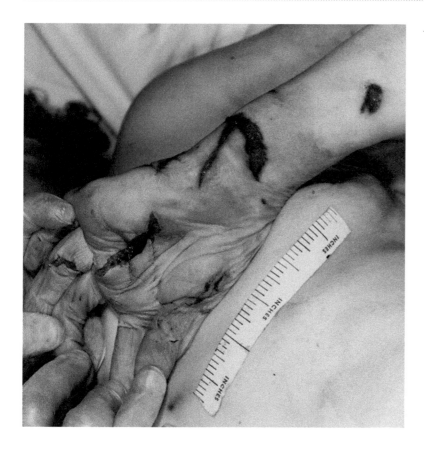

**◀ Figure 9.13c** Palmar aspect.

191

## References

Chattopadhyay S, Sukul B. (2013). Pattern of defence injuries among homicidal victims. *Egypt J Forensic Sci* 3, 81–84.

Hunt AC, Cowling RJ. (1991). Murder by stabbing. *Forensic Sci Int* 52, 107–112.

Karlsson T. (1998). Homicidal and suicidal sharp force fatalities in Stockholm, Sweden. *Forensic Sci Int* 93, 21–32.

Katkici Ü, Özkök MS, Örsal M. (1994). An autopsy evaluation of defence wounds in 195 homicidal deaths due to stabbing. *J Forensic Sci Soc* 34, 237–240.

Kemal CJ, Patterson T, Molina DK. (2013). Deaths due to sharp force injuries in Bexar County, Texas, with respect to manner of death. *Am J Forensic Med Pathol*, 34, 253–259.

O'Donovan S, Langlois NEI, Byard RW. (2018). "Defense" type wounds in suicide. *Forensic Sci Med Pathol* 14, 402–405.

Racette S, Kremer C, Desjarlais A, Sauvageau A. (2008). Suicidal and homicidal sharp force injury: a 5-year retrospective comparative study of hesitation marks and defense wounds. *Forensic Sci Med Pathol* 4, 221–227.

Rogde S, Hougen HP, Poulsen K. (2000). Homicide by sharp force in two Scandinavian capitals. *Forensic Sci Int* 109, 135–145.

Rouse DA (1994). Patterns of stab wounds: a six year study. *Med Sci Law* 34, 67–71.

Schmidt U. (2010). Sharp force injuries in "clinical" forensic medicine. *Forensic Sci Int* 195, 1–5.

Schmidt U, Pollak S. (2006). Sharp force injuries in clinical forensic medicine—findings in victims and perpetrators. *Forensic Sci Int* 159, 113–118.

Valoriani S, Eliopoulos C, Borrini M. (2017). Sharp force trauma death in a young individual from medieval Gloucester. *Am J Forensic Med Pathol* 38, 111–114.

# ▌Chapter 10
# Intentional Self-inflicted Injuries

## Introduction

In this chapter are described the appearance and distribution of self-inflicted injuries, and the differences from injuries caused by other means, either in an assault or accidentally. Injuries which are intentionally self-inflicted should be distinguished from those that are sometimes self-inflicted but caused accidentally, for example falling through a glass door; accidental injuries are described in detail in Chapter 10.

The motive for intentionally self-inflicted wounds is, in most cases, for the purpose of committing suicide or at least harming oneself to a lesser degree, during a state of "mental anguish." In a few cases however, the production of such wounds may be for a number of fraudulent reasons by simulating injury to incriminate another person, for financial gain or for attention seeking.

## Incidence of Self-inflicted Sharp Force Trauma

The World Health Organisation data from August 2018 reveals that close to 800,000 people die due to suicide every year, which is one person every 40 seconds. Suicide is the second leading cause of death among 15–29-year-olds globally. Rates vary from country to country and are influenced to a great extent by local culture, religious beliefs, social and economic situation (much higher in lower middle-income countries). Worldwide, suicide accounted for 1.4% of all deaths in 2016, making it the 18th leading

cause of death in that year. When considering sharp force trauma, in the past it was a classic form of suicide, whereas in modern times it is quite rare, constituting only 2–3% of all self-inflicted deaths (WHO 2019). Assessing the profile of the victim is important, including their age, sex, whether mental illness is present, suicidal ideation, lifestyle circumstances including use of alcohol and drugs and motivation for self-harm.

## The Scene

Most locations where the deceased is discovered are at home, and most commonly in the bedroom. Other places may include the home of a relative, workplace or usually in a setting where interruption is unlikely. As stated, the vast majority of cases are at a domestic setting and household implements such as kitchen

knives or tools which are present are frequently used (Watanabe et al. 1973; Karlsson et al. 1988; Start et al. 1992; Karlsson 1998). Scene examination, which is key to assisting in the differentiation between homicidal, suicidal and accidental sharp force trauma, is discussed in detail in Chapter 4.

## Pattern, Morphology, Distribution and Demographic Factors

### Types of Sharp Force Trauma

The main types of sharp force trauma which are recognised in self-inflicted deaths can be, unsurprisingly,

divided into stabbing or incised wounds most commonly from knives, occasionally involving glass and rarely other sharp-sided implements.

These categories are by no means mutually exclusive and stabbing and incised wounds may both be seen in combination.

## Deaths from Self-stabbing

As has been stated, the incidence of self-stabbing is low compared to all other forms of sharp force trauma, ranging from approximately 5% of all sharp force trauma types (Rouse 1994) to around 10% from 273 cases (Start et al 1992). Its low incidence in comparison to homicidal wounding should be borne in mind when the pathologist is dealing with such a case even though the circumstances and scene visit may indicate very clearly the manner of death. Many authorities would not only advise great caution in the examination of such deaths, but even adhere to the policy that such deaths should be treated as homicide at least until there is sufficient evidence found to indicate otherwise. Such evidence will rely on a number of aspects including scene examination, the appearance and distribution of the wounds, the presence of hesitation (tentative wounds), the presence of a recorded message or notes indicating the deceased's intention and other important associated demographic factors in common with other similar deaths.

## Number of Stab Wounds

In most series, a single or two stab wounds were the most common findings (Table 10.1). The combined findings from the four series in the table demonstrate that single stab wounds followed by two to five wounds are the most expected in suicidal

stabbing. Start et al 1992; Rouse 1994; Kraniotis et al 2017 also noted cases with over twenty stab wounds.

The author of this book has examined a case involving a female in her 50s with 34 stab wounds to her chest, abdomen and both thighs, in addition to incised wounds to the hands and right forearm. The fatal wound was to her left side of chest into the lung and heart. A further wound in the right side of the lower chest had injured the liver. All other wounds did not enter body cavities. She was fully clothed and had stabbed herself through clothing. The case was treated with suspicion until the evidence demonstrated that it was a clear case of self-infliction (Figure 10.1).

A further case seen by the author was of a 20-year-old depressed foreign student studying at an English University. He was found in his room on the campus with three stab wounds to his lower chest and abdomen with a knife by his side (Figure 10.2).

Occasionally one sees a combination of stab wounds together with incised wounds to the neck region. In a case seen by the author there were two merged midline upper abdominal stab wounds with the knife that had been used present in the wounds. The direction of the thrust was upwards, causing a gaping injury to the left ventricle. In addition, he had also incised his neck severing his major neck vessels and his trachea. As in the previous case, the clothes had been lifted above the wounds. The blood pattern on his body and nearby at the scene indicated that he had been in a sitting or crouching position when he caused the injuries (Figure 10.3).

**Table 10.1** Number of stab wounds seen in suicidal stabbing cases from four studies

| Number of wounds seen in each case (% in parenthesis in each category from each series) | 1 | 2–5 | 6–10 | 11–19 | >20 | Total number of cases in each series |
|---|---|---|---|---|---|---|
| Start et al. (1992) | 18 (64) | 6 (21) | 1 (4) | 1 (4) | 2 (7) | 28 |
| Rouse (1994) | 3 (38) | 2 (25) | 1 (12.5) | 1 (12.5) | 1 (12.5) | 8 |
| Karger (2000) | 13 (54) | 8 (33) | 1 (4) | 2 (8) | - | 24 |
| Kranioti et al. (2017) | 6 (60) | 1 (10) | 1 (10) | - | 2 (20) | 10 |
| Combined series total | **40 (57)** | **17 (24)** | **4 (6)** | **4 (6)** | **5 (7)** | **70** |

*Note:* Percentages in each category in parenthesis

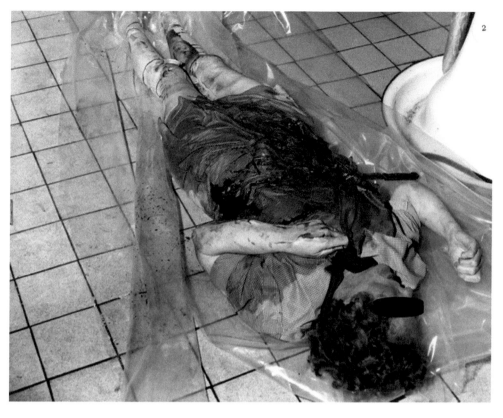

▲ **Figure 10.1a** Fully dressed adult female with knife in situ on right side of chest. Most stab wounds were through her clothing.

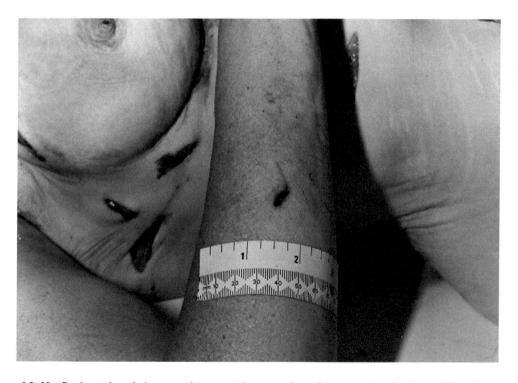

▲ **Figure 10.1b** Right side of chest and arm with wound on forearm simulating a defensive injury.

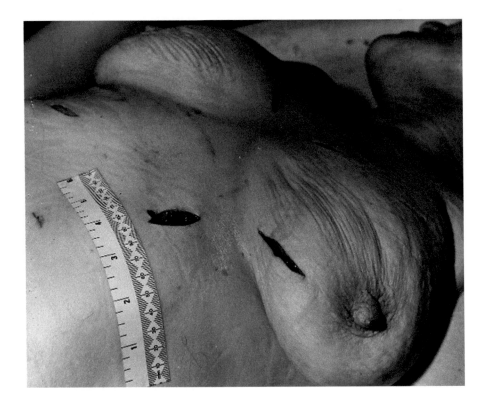

▲ **Figure 10.1c** Front of chest and upper abdomen.

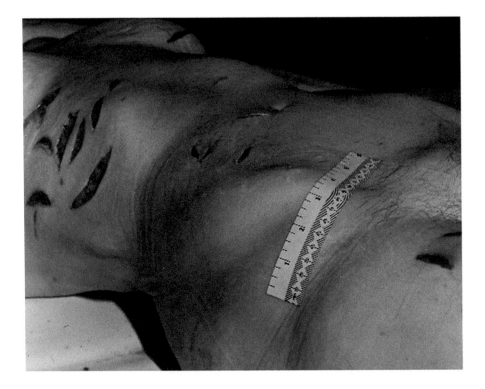

▲ **Figure 10.1d** Right side of the trunk and upper right thigh.

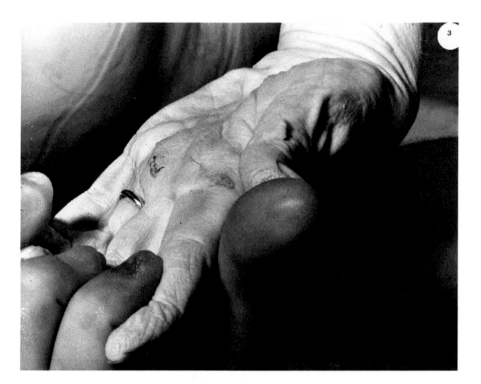

▲ **Figure 10.1e** Palmar side of both hands show incised wounds from accidental self-injury from the knife blade.

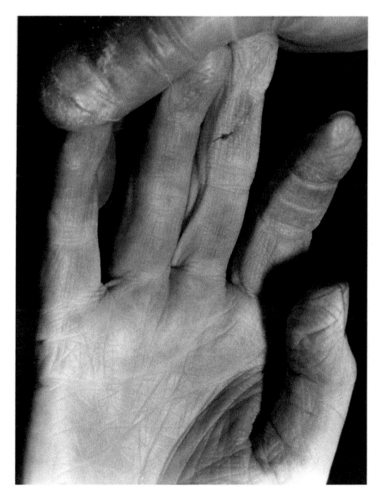

◀ **Figure 10.1f** Palmar side of both hands show incised wounds from accidental self-injury from the knife blade.

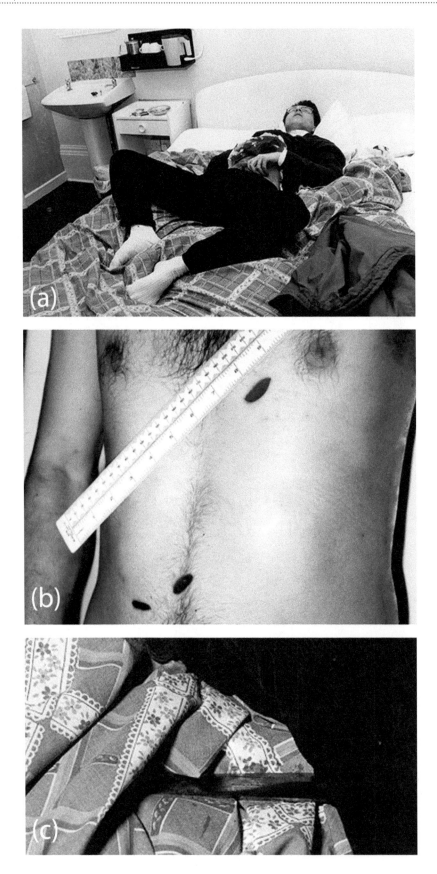

▲ **Figure 10.2** Self-inflicted stab wounds to the lower chest and abdomen in a young man. (a) Clothes have been lifted above area stabbed. (b) Unclothed body showing distribution of three stab wounds. (c) Knife blade partly concealed under right trouser leg.

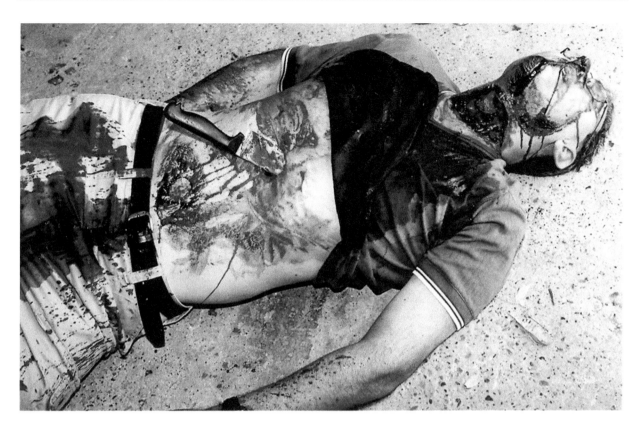

▲ **Figure 10.3a** Adult male found at home with a large kitchen knife in situ in the upper abdomen. The blood pattern indicates that he had been sitting or crouching when the wounds were inflicted. He had also incised his neck.

# Location of Stab Wounds on the Body

*Chest, Head and Neck*

The most frequent number of suicidal stab wounds as discussed, are single and in most published series are situated on the front of the chest (Table 10.2), (Vanezis and West 1983; Start et al 1992; Rouse 1994; Fukube et al 2008) with most being to the left side. Kranioti et al. (2017) in their small series of 12 cases, found the neck to be the more common location of injury, followed by the chest.

The front of the chest was the location for the stab wounds in two elderly identical twin brothers seen by the author of this book. The following case also illustrates the close similarity of the injuries produced by both siblings. The brothers aged 79 who were suffering from prostatic carcinoma were found in their shared home lying on twin beds next to each other with two kitchen knives (one on each bed). Both were unclothed above the waist. It became apparent that they had earlier in the day purchased

the two kitchen knives. Both decedents were found to have wounds similarly located, just to the left side of the lower chest near the xyphisternum. It appears that they had stabbed themselves more than once, through or very close to the main wound, resulting in one large and a number of smaller wounds to the heart (Figures 10.4 and 10.5).

Facial and neck injuries were seen in a case by the author of this book involving a 44-year-old male who had financial problems. He stabbed himself through the left side of the mouth and incised the right internal carotid. A number of hesitation marks were found on his neck (Figure 10.6).

*Abdomen*

Self-inflicted stab wounds in the abdominal region are also quite commonly seen, with the highest number seen in Start et al.'s series (1992). Most are seen in the umbilical and epigastric region, aimed usually in an upward direction as seen in the case reported by Atreya et al. (2017). Kharbach et al. (2014) described the case of a 56-year-old Moroccan

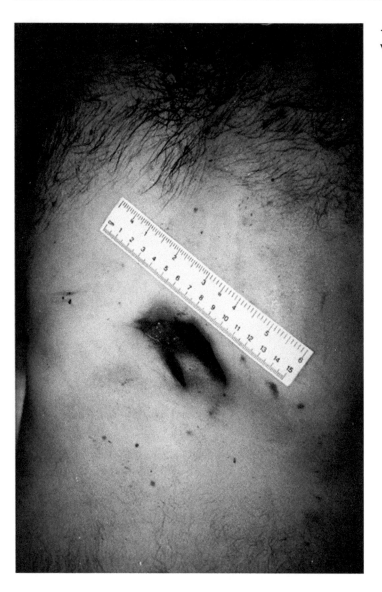

◀ **Figure 10.3b** Abdominal stab wounds.

man known to have untreated paranoid schizophrenia and a history of several previous suicide attempts who stabbed himself with a 15cm sewing needle in the hypogastric region of the abdomen and penetrated his urinary bladder. The patient made a full recovery following surgery.

*Other Regions*

In the extremities, stab wounds are very uncommon. Another occasional finding, although not dictated by common sense, is for the stabber to use a knife on his/her back. Such cases require very careful consideration before a homicide can be ruled out (Figure 10.7).

In a further stabbing case the knife was held in the right hand and the tip of the blade had broken off and became embedded in the cervical vertebral column (Figure 10.8).

## Clothing

Pulling clothes aside or lifting it to expose an area for stabbing is very helpful in indicating self-injury but the inexperienced should be aware of the possibility of the clothes being pulled up or rearranged in some way during a fight between two individuals rather than deliberately altered by the victim. On the other hand, it should not be assumed that the manner of death was homicidal if stabbing through clothing is found to be the case. There are many publications which show that perforation of clothing in self-stabbing is not at all unusual (Start et al. (1992) found 28% from 24 cases; Fukube et al. (2008) 38.5% from 26; Karger et al. (2000) 52% from 31).

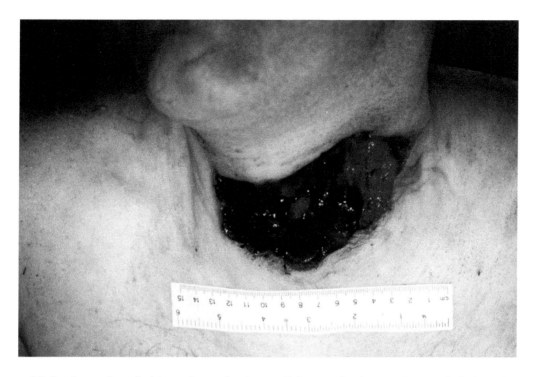

▲ **Figure 10.3c** Incised neck. Note the multiple parallel superficial incised wounds below the gaping wound.

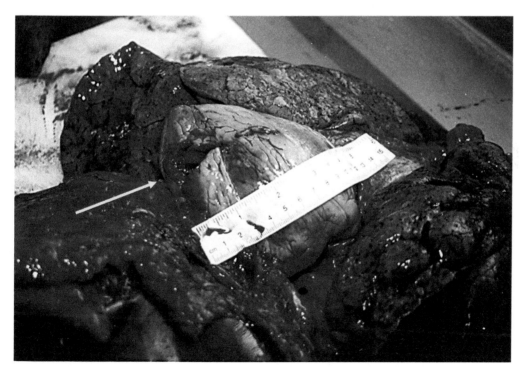

▲ **Figure 10.3d** Heart wound produced by the upward thrust of the knife.

## Hesitation Wounds

Hesitation wounds are synonymous with tentative wounds. Such wounds when they are present are virtually diagnostic of self-stabbing, except in situations where the assailant may have deliberately produced injuries of similar characteristics, either as a form of torture or as part of a bizarre ritualistic practice. Hesitation wounds are typically grouped together and produced in

**Table 10.2** Stab wound locations on the body (more than one fatal stab wound) in two cases.

| Studies | Head | Neck | Neck and Chest | Chest | Chest and Abdomen | Abdomen | Upper limb | Lower limb | Multiple sites | Total number of cases |
|---|---|---|---|---|---|---|---|---|---|---|
| Vanezis and West (1983) | 2 | 2 | 2 | 11 | 2 | 8 | 1 | - | 2 | 29 |
| Start et al. (1992) | - | 2 | - | 17 | - | 10 | - | 2 | 2 | 33 |
| Karger (2000) | - | 10 | - | 31 | - | 8 | - | - | - | 49 |
| Fukube et al. (2008) | 1 | 10 | - | 17 | - | 7 | - | - | - | 35 |
| Kemal et al. (2013) | - | 3 | - | 11 | - | 3 | - | - | - | 17 |
| Kranioti et al. (2017) | - | 5 | - | 3 | - | 2 | 1 | - | - | 10 |
| **Combined studies (%)** | **3 (2)** | **32 (18)** | **2 (1)** | **90 (52)** | **2 (1)** | **38 (22)** | **2 (1)** | **2 (1)** | **4 (2)** | **174** |

a repetitive manner over one or more locations on the body. They are frequently near the final and fatal wound although they can be on a completely different and distant part of the body. In self-stabbing cases, most hesitation wounds comprise small punctures in the skin, surrounded by bruising. They are generally superficial, but may vary in depth, penetrating into subcutaneous fat or may be confined to the epidermis alone. They may also be linear incised wounds, again of variable depth and may be found in combination with the puncture wounds. Self-harm but non-fatal wounds particularly on the wrists and forearms may also be described as tentative, even though a final fatal wound was not produced.

Hesitation wounds are by no means found in every case of self-stabbing. Vanezis and West (1983), in their series of 29 cases found them in 15. They were more commonly associated with more than one stab wound to the chest, being present in 7 of 11 such cases, whereas they were seen in only one case in four single chest stab wounds. In addition, they were found only on clothing but not associated with an injury to the skin in two further cases. Karger et al. (2000) in their series found hesitation injuries in the form of superficial cutting or stab injuries in 50 from 65 fatalities (77%). In 42 of these, the tentative marks and the fatal injury were located in close proximity. They also found that the number of hesitation marks per case correlated positively with the number of severe injuries.

Karakasi et al. (2006) reviewed the relevant literature on the incidence, distribution, character, and function of hesitation wounds as well as their sociodemographic variables. They particularly stress the importance of considering the interpretation and motivation for the production of such wounds from the psychopathological point of view. The overall incidence of hesitation injuries from their literature review adapted here omitting two series with less than ten cases, is 60%, with the individual series ranging from 35 to 77% (Table 10.3).

The author examined the case of a 70-year-old female found on the floor in her hallway by her brother. The Ambulance Service was called and on arrival they pronounced life extinct. The police found numerous self-harm marks on her body, some of which appeared deeper than others. There was a large amount of blood in the bathroom and on her duvet. Although she did not suffer from mental health problems, her general practitioner thought that she was very "fed up" with being unwell. She had lumbar back pain and was taking various analgesics. The autopsy revealed multiple stab, incised and tentative wounds. She had bled profusely from her wounds and died of exsanguination. Tentative wounds comprising multiple puncture wounds with surrounding bruising were present in a number of areas over her body. The fatal injuries were a combination of multiple deep stab wounds to her legs and deep incised wounds to her left wrist (Figure 10.9).

## Age and Gender

There is a much higher male to female ratio varying in three series from 3:1 – 3.6:1 (Karger et al 2000;

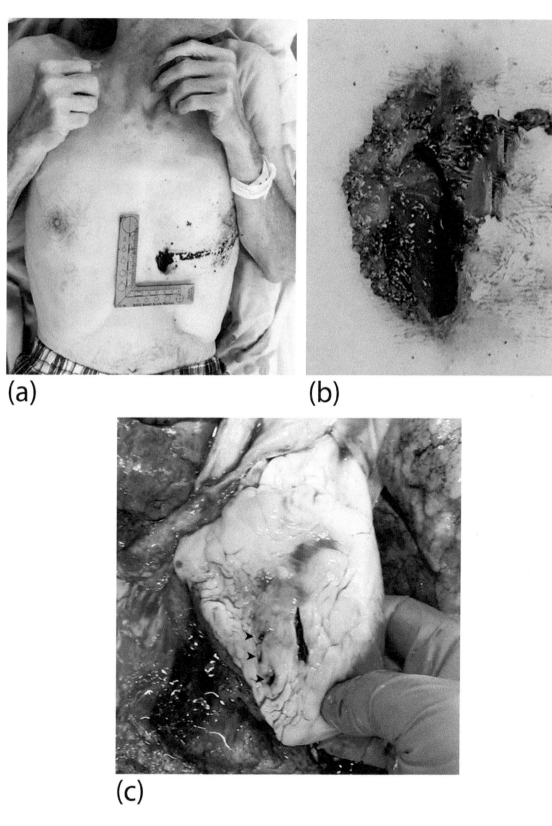

(a)

(b)

(c)

▲ **Figure 10.4** Twin A. a. Wound just to the left of xyphisternum and next to costal margin. b. Close up showing vertically orientated wound with the pointed part of the wound at the upper end in keeping with the knife being held with the sharp-edge uppermost and thrust into the body with a slightly upward motion into the thorax. c. Major stab wound in left ventricle with three minor wounds (arrowed), nearby. (Source: Author)

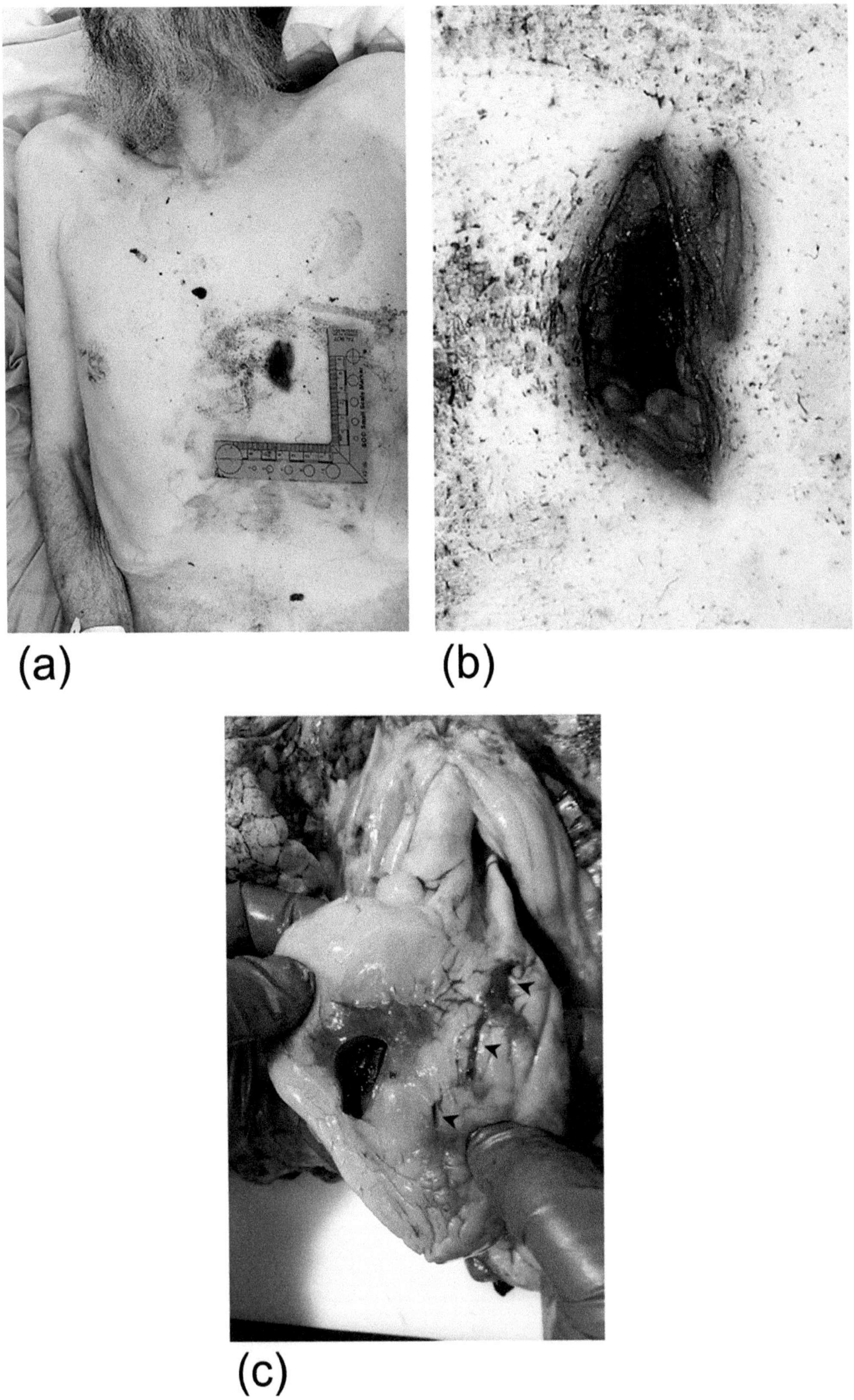

(a)

(b)

(c)

▲ **Figure 10.5** Twin B. a. Wounds at the left parasternal edge. b. Close-up showing one large and smaller parallel wound; both are vertically orientated and the edges are dried. c. Major heart wound in the right atrio-ventricular region and three further wounds nearby (arrows). (Source: Author)

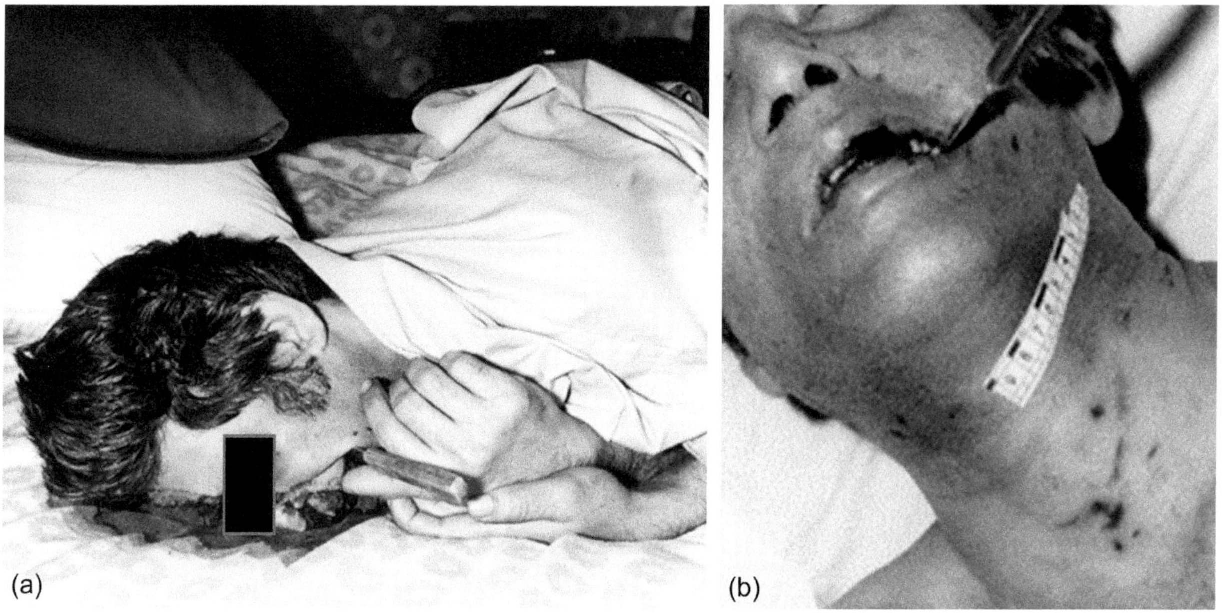

▲ **Figure 10.6** (a) View of deceased at the scene with the knife impaled within his mouth.
(b) Hesitation marks can be seen on the neck.

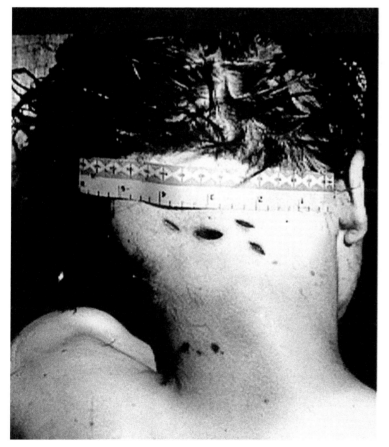

◀ **Figure 10.7a** Young man with
four self-inflicted stab wounds to the
occipital region and some smaller
hesitation wounds below them.
All wounds were in reach of the
deceased's right hand.

205

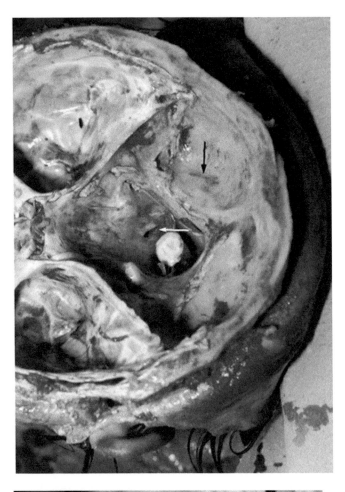

◀ **Figure 10.7b** View of the base of the skull showing knife marks just above the foramen magnum and the right occipital fossa (arrows).

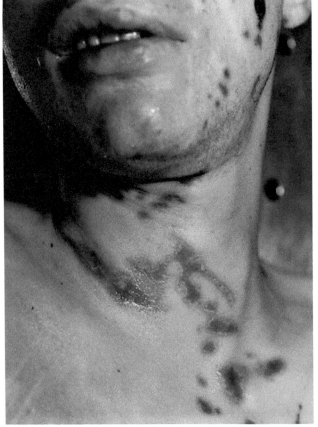

◀ **Figure 10.7c** Further hesitation wounds were found on the front of his neck.

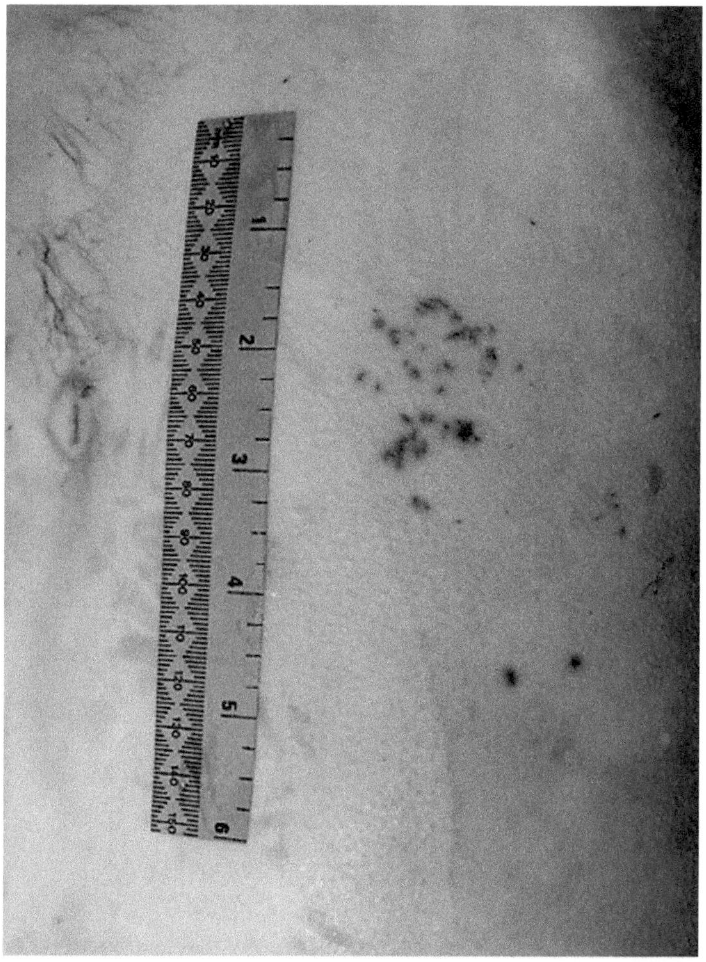

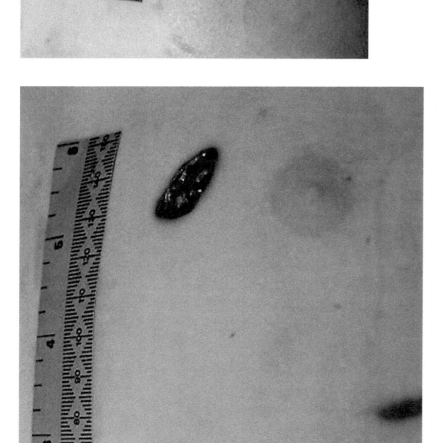

◀ **Figure 10.7d** The left lower abdomen.

◀ **Figure 10.7e** The fatal wound to the heart.

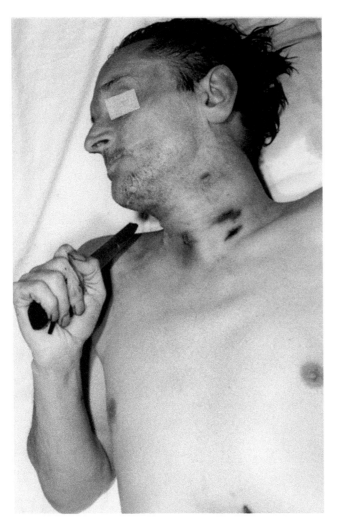

◀ **Figure 10.8a** Self-inflicted stab wounds to the neck. There were also five wounds on the abdomen. The knife was held firmly in the right hand and its tip broken.

Fukube 2008 and 3.6:1 and Karlsson 1998). Karlsson et al. (1988) in their series of 89 cases, found the most common age group for suicide victims to be 40–49 years. The age distribution in a further study carried out by Karlsson (1998) among suicide victims differed only slightly from the earlier series.

## Mental Health Issues/ Drugs and Alcohol

A psychiatric diagnosis had been ascribed in 22 of Karlsson et al's (1988) cases, and addiction to drugs or alcohol in 23. Toxicological analysis was positive for drugs in 22 and for alcohol in 27 cases. Blood alcohol levels were roughly similar to those found in victims of homicidal sharp force, whereas drug levels tended to be lower or higher in suicides.

## Cultural and Historical Influence – Suicide by Hara-Kiri (Seppuku)

Hara-kiri is a traditional Japanese method of attempting suicide, originally by the samurai and followed by other Japanese, aimed at maintaining honour or taking responsibility (see also Chapter 1). The practice of hara-kiri primarily stems from the manners and customs that a samurai held in the Heian Period (794–1185). Hara-kiri was firmly established for self-determination of samurais after the Kamakura Period (1185–1333) and has subsequently been considered to be a form of honourable death in Japan. It was formally abolished in 1837, but the tradition is still part of Japanese culture, even though its form has changed since the times of the samurai.

The method in hara-kiri involves stabbing the left side of the abdomen with a knife and drawing

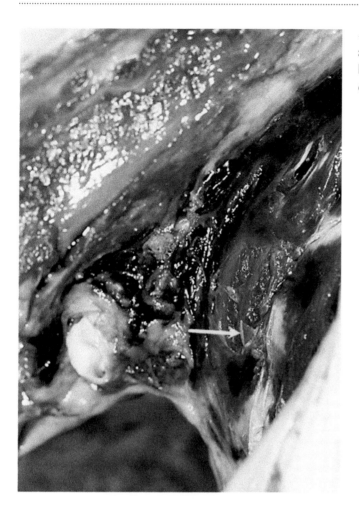

◀ **Figure 10.8b** Anterior aspect of the neck after removal of the larynx. The tip of the blade was embedded in the cervical vertebral column (arrow).

209

**Table 10.3** Incidence of hesitation wounds from a number of authors' series

| Study | Number of suicide cases | Presence of hesitation marks | Percentage of suicide cases |
|---|---|---|---|
| Vanezis and West (1983) | 29 | 15 | 52 |
| Start et al. (1992) | 28 | 18 | 64 |
| Karlsson (1998) | 105 | 65 | 62 |
| Karger et al. (2000) | 65 | 50 | 77 |
| Gill and Catanese (2002) | 17 | 11 | 65 |
| Byard et al. (2002) | 51 | 23 | 54 |
| Fukube et al. (2008) | 65 | 37 | 57 |
| Racette et al. (2008) | 58 | 43 | 74 |
| Kemal et al. (2013) | 54 | 19 | 35 |
| **All series** | **472** | **281** | **60** |

*Source:* Adapted from Karakasi et al. (2006)

the blade across to the right side. This procedure originates from an ancient belief that the human soul and love dwell in the abdomen and that the act of bravely cutting one's abdomen was considered an appropriate method of ending one's life in the tradition of Bushido, the "way of the warrior-knight" (Kato et al. 2014).

The latter authors investigated the clinical features of 647 patients who had attempted suicide by hara-kiri. Clinical features were compared between

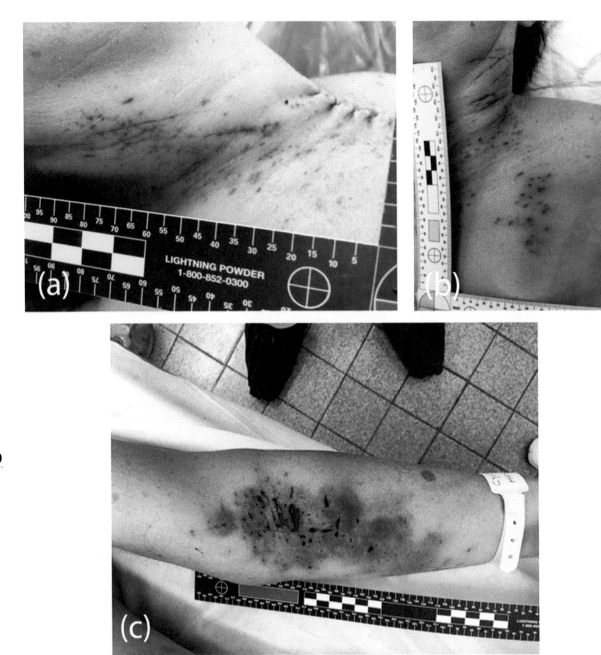

▲ **Figure 10.9** Multiple self-inflicted stab and incised wounds are seen in various parts of the front of the trunk and upper and lower limbs. a. Upper chest and neck showing small puncture marks typical of hesitation marks. b. Superficial and small puncture (hesitation) marks to right side of neck. c. Extensive bruising, incised and puncture wounds seen on left arm. d. Similar marks to (b) found on upper abdomen. e. detail of incised wounds to left wrist. f. Incised wounds on left thigh. g. Multiple stab and more superficial puncture wounds on both lower legs. (Source: Author)

those who had employed hara-kiri and those who had used other methods. Twenty-five of the 647 subjects had attempted suicide by hara-kiri (3.9%). The ratio of men to women and the proportion of patients with mood disorders were significantly higher in the hara-kiri group than in the other methods group. The average length of stay in either the hospital or in the intensive care unit was also longer in the hara-kiri group than in the other methods group.

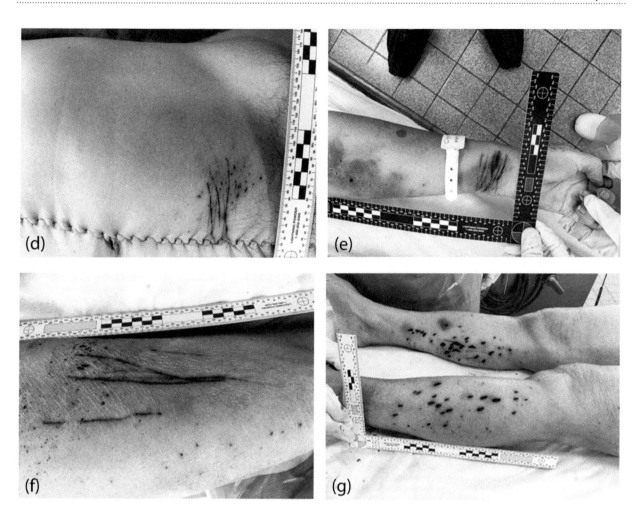

(d)

(e)

(f)

(g)

▲ **Figure 10.9** (Continued)

# Self-inflicted Injuries from Other Sharp Objects than Knives

Other sharp objects such as needles may be inserted, particularly into the chest and cause cardiac or lung injury with sometimes fatal consequences. Di Paolo et al. (2015) report the case of a patient from a local prison who was admitted to the emergency department with an initial suspicion of acute coronary syndrome, deteriorated and died. Insertion of foreign objects was not initially suspected. A forensic autopsy was carried out and multiple needles were found in the chest and two in the abdomen. The longest was 9 cm which had transfixed the heart. There was a significant mediastinal haematoma and cardiac tamponade. Further information from the prison reported previously diagnosed psychosis, with self-introduction of foreign objects into the chest and abdomen.

## Scissors

A case of historical interest involves the death of the Sultan of the Ottoman Empire Abdul Aziz on 30 May 1876 (Figure 10.10). He was found dead in a bath with both blood vessels cut below the antecubital fossae. It was thought that he had committed suicide and that the wounds were caused by a pair of embroidery scissors belonging to one of the ladies of the harem. His mother was said to have brought him the scissors and mirror so that he could trim his beard.

There was incredulity in Western countries as to the manner of his death. Dickson (1876). The following

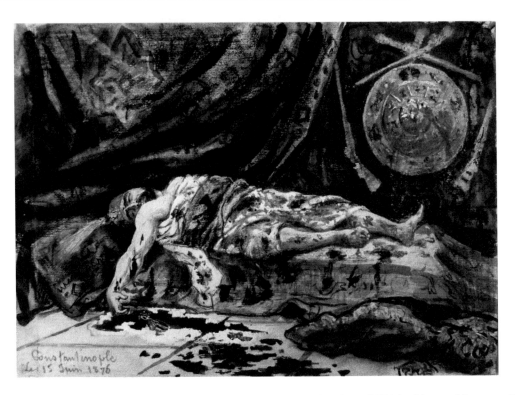

▲ **Figure 10.10** Sultan of the Ottoman Empire Abdul Aziz's death in 1876 by Victor Masson. (Public domain)

212

extract from the *British Medical Journal* entitled, The death of the Sultan Abdul Aziz 1876) echoes the reaction to the official Turkish medical report and the view that in such a case of high importance a thorough post-mortem examination should have been made:

*we have a loose description of the appearances presented by the outside of the body only….. wound, two inches long below the bend of the left arm…….had cut through the superficial veins, and partially divided the ulnar artery…At the bend of the right arm……slight oblique wound, less than an inch ……divided the small vein only, leaving the main artery untouched…..A pair of scissors, four inches long produced, and ….very sharp, stained with blood……no account of the amount of blood found near the body – one of the most important elements in forming an opinion of death from haemorrhage. No description of the interior of the body – whether, drained of blood, whether death caused by asphyxia from the thrusting of a plug into the throat, or by any other mechanical cause to obstruct breathing.*

The writer further stated that on the basis of such an unsatisfactory examination, 19 physicians came to the unanimous view that death was caused by haemorrhage from the ulnar artery; that the scissors *might* have produced the wounds found on the arms, and that the direction and nature of the wounds, as well as the instrument, led them to the belief that it was a case of suicide.

The author of the article only agrees that the wounds **might** have been produced by the scissors and continues…

*A wound of the ulnar artery may prove fatal, but it would not produce rapid death; and if haemorrhage had really been the cause of death (as the bleeding would go on so long as the person lived), a large quantity of blood should have been found near the dead body. The wounds in the arm do not furnish, either by direction or position, any proof whatever of suicide. Any other person might have produced them with the scissors found near the body. The evidence of two competent men, with an examination of the interior of the body, would have done more to satisfy the public mind respecting suicide or homicide*

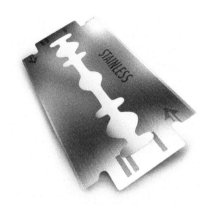

◀ **Figure 10.11** Safety razor blade. (Public domain)

*than the unanimity of nineteen physicians, who could certify that this was an act of suicide from such imperfect data. As it is, their report will only excite serious doubts of the real cause of death.*

It was suspected that either his suicide had been *arranged* by his political adversaries, supplying him with the scissors or that he was killed in some other way and the wounds were produced after death; one theory being that he had been smothered.

A rare case of suicide involving the use of scissors is reported by Jo and Lee (2015). The deceased, a 76-year-old man who had terminal gastric cancer, had made four cuts in his tongue with a pair of scissors, apart from cutting his finger-tip and stabbing his abdomen with the same implement.

## Razor

Rautji et al. (2004) reported the unusual case of a 29-year-old man who cut his throat using a safety razor blade similar in type to that shown in Figure 10.11. Such a razor blade is difficult to hold with bare hands and as a result he, not surprisingly, sustained three incised wounds, on the palmar aspect of the right index finger. A further case reported by Durmić et al. (2018) was that of a 69-year-old woman who committed suicide by cutting her lower legs with a safety razor blade. At autopsy there were horizontal deep wounds around the circumference of the legs at mid-calf level, causing severance of vessels and musculature. She died from exsanguination.

A case seen by the author of this text involved a 56-year-old man who suffered from schizophrenia and had a history of self-harming. Although he died from natural causes he was found to have multiple healing superficial incised wounds to both sides of his face caused by a safety razor (Figure 10.12).

## Mechanised Saw

The use of mechanised saws is occasionally seen and most are self-inflicted. Accidental and homicidal manners of death are more unusual. Janík et al. (2016) report the suicide of a 79-year-old man using a self-made circular table saw. Autopsy confirmed that that he sustained multiple saw-type wounds to the head and neck resulting in complete amputation of the upper skull and partial beheading.

In regard to chainsaws, most injuries occur as a result of accidents, whilst rarely used to commit suicide. Schyma et al. (2013) report the case of an adult male who killed his young son with a chainsaw then fatally injured himself by applying the saw to his neck. The motive involved custody issues during a divorce.

Another situation when a mechanised saw may be used is for dismemberment following homicide, to facilitate removal and disposal of the victim's body (see Chapter 12).

## Crossbow

The author of the text has seen a case where a crossbow was used. The deceased was a young man with depression. No note had been left. It appears he used his foot to release the bolt whilst sitting in the chair (Figure 10.13).

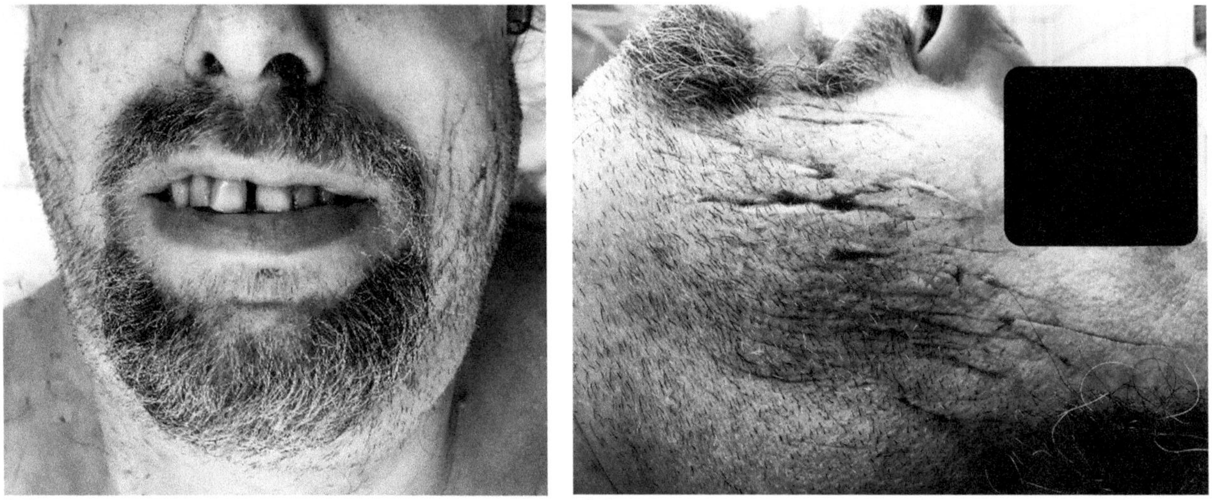

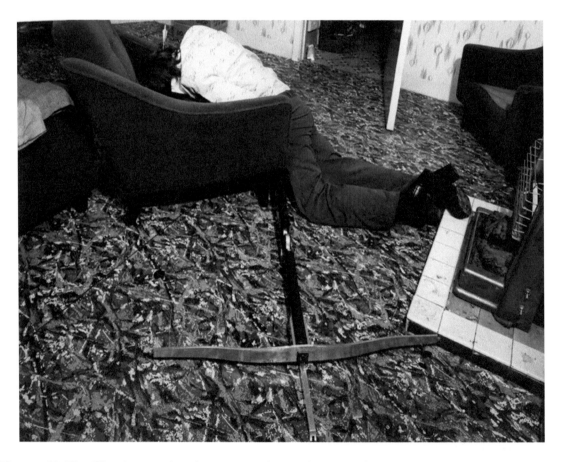

(a)                                                              (b)

▲ **Figure 10.12** Healing multiple incised wounds. a. Front of face showing wounds on both sides. b. View of left side of face. (Source: Author)

▲ **Figure 10.13a** The deceased at the scene with crossbow nearby.

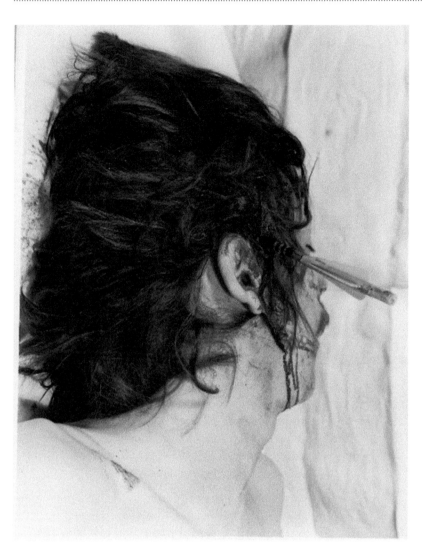

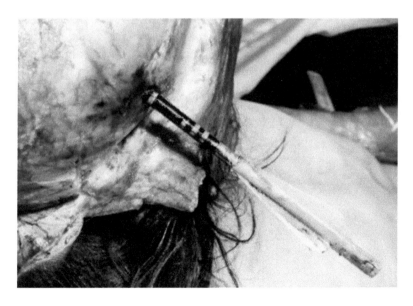

◀ **Figure 10.13c** Reflected scalp.

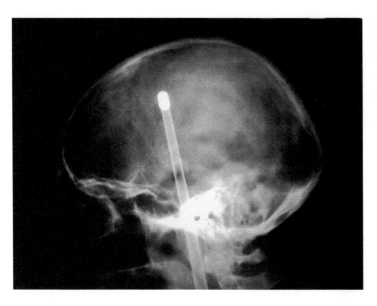

◄ **Figure 10.13d** Radiograph of the skull. The photographs demonstrate that the crossbow bolt could have been fired from a lower height to his head and consistent with crossbow trigger being released by his foot.

# Incised Wounds to the Neck (Cut Throat Wounds)

Such injuries are either homicidal, suicidal or occasionally, accidental. Accidental wounds are seen particularly in vehicular accidents where such injuries are caused by fragments of glass. In the United Kingdom most deaths resulting from incised wounds to the neck are due to self-infliction but in other parts of the world at least as many or the majority of such deaths are homicidal (Bhattacharjee et al. 1997).

The distinction between homicidal and suicidal wounds may be difficult if not impossible to make on post-mortem examination alone. It is essential before an opinion is given that account is taken of the circumstances surrounding the deceased's movements shortly before death, his personal history and a thorough examination of the scene of discovery of the body (Figure 10.14).

There are, however, a number of features in the character and distribution of such wounds that will frequently be of some assistance to the pathologist in making the distinction between self-infliction and attack by an assailant. Self-inflicted injuries when made by right-handed persons, normally begin high on the left side of the neck and pass downward across the front to end on the right side. They are deeper at their origin and then tail off on the right. Such wounds may also be horizontal, lying across the front of the neck. They are usually linear and clean cut, since the skin is likely to be put under tension. Separate shallow wounds – "tentative" or "hesitation" wounds – are strongly indicative of self-infliction. There are quite

often accompanying incised wounds to the wrist or occasionally elsewhere. Some self-inflicted incised wounds may be extremely deep, leaving multiple pronounced score marks on the cervical vertebrae. It is also not unheard of for a victim to excise his own larynx (Giles 1956; Schuessler 1944).

Homicidal wounds as a rule do not have the regular planned appearance of those that are self-inflicted and they are unaccompanied by tentative injuries (Figure 10.15). Nevertheless, they are frequently accompanied by incised wounds that may be difficult to interpret without accompanying obvious self-inflicted injuries. As a rule they are more haphazardly placed on the neck and, in some cases, have more irregular edges. In addition, such wounds tend to be deeper, although this is by no means invariably so. Accompanying stab wounds may also be present on the neck and other parts of the body, as well as defence cuts to the backs of the arms and hands. There may also be non-cutting injuries to the body which may have contributed to the cause of death.

Ozdemir et al. (2013) in their series of 15 honour killings in Eastern Turkey, found an approximately fivefold greater number of wounds compared to other homicides and suicides. Not unreasonably, their view is that the significantly greater number of wounds in honour killings is associated with more impulsive action due to intense stress the killer is under and losing control owing to extreme anger.

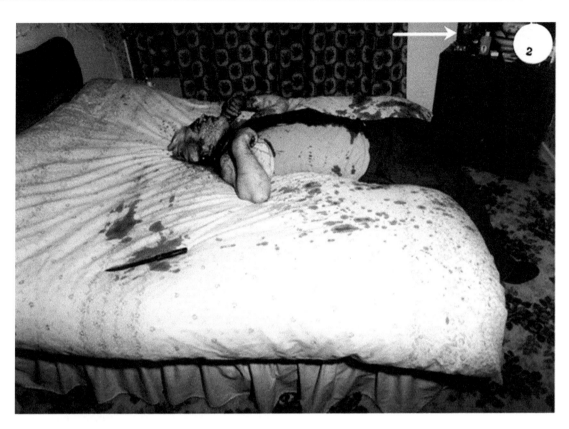

▲ **Figure 10.14a** Middle-aged male found in his bedroom with incised wounds to his neck. The room is tidy and no evidence of forced entry: (a) Male lying on his back opposite a dressing table with a mirror (arrow) and a knife to his right side.

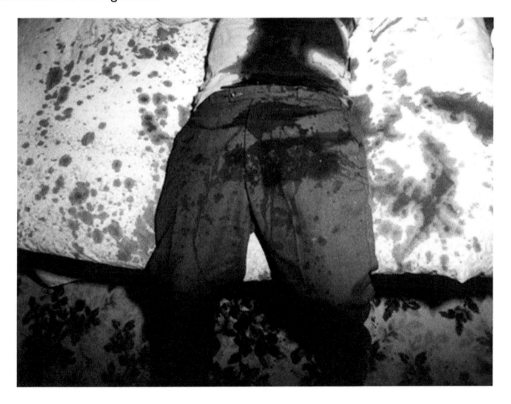

▲ **Figure 10.14b** Pattern of blood staining indicating that he had been sitting on the edge of the bed prior to collapsing on to his back.

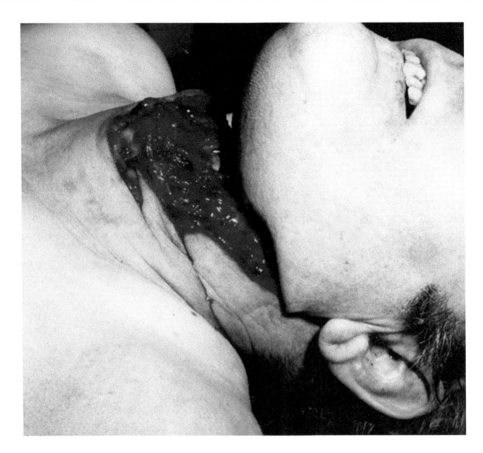

▲ **Figure 10.14c** Self-inflicted parallel incised wounds of the neck.

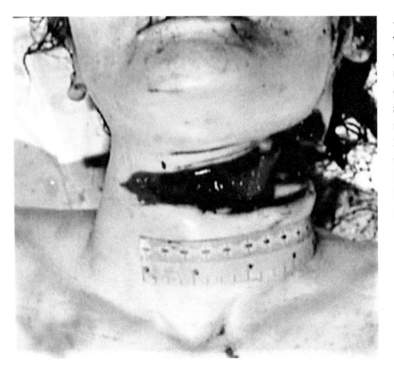

◀ **Figure 10.15** Homicide: Young woman with deep incised wounds to the neck. The wounds have exposed underlying vasculature of the left carotid sheath. There are two parallel linear injuries which might be misinterpreted as being self-inflicted. Small puncture wounds are also seen to the left of the suprasternal notch. Fingernail marks are also seen on her lower face where she had been held down.

# Complex (Combination) Suicides

Complex suicides which involve more than one method of injury are very uncommon but when they occur they can present a real challenge to investigators in differentiating between homicide and suicide (Simonit et al. 2018). The term was first used by Marcinkowski et al. (1974) when reporting the case of a 23-year-old man who simultaneously hanged and electrocuted himself. Letters at the scene showed that the complex suicide had been previously planned. Complex suicides may be classed as planned (primary) or unplanned (secondary). A primary or planned complex suicide is recognised as a combination of more than one previously planned method in order to prevent the first method from failing. Conversely, in secondary or unplanned complex suicide, the victim employs an alternative second method only after the first method failed, was too slow or proved to be painful.

In relation to cases of sharp force trauma where other methods are also employed, Peyron et al. (2018) report a suicide by self-stabbing and drowning. The case is of a young man found submerged in a river, stabbed nine times with two wounds that had penetrated the thorax and had caused lung injuries and a haemo-pneumothorax. This was a challenging case for the police to differentiate between homicide and suicide. The post-mortem and histological examinations were consistent with a death caused by drowning, but the manner of death, whether homicide or suicide, still remained undetermined. The police investigation finally concluded that it was a suicide, although no suicide note had been left and the victim had no underlying diagnosed mental disorder. Furthermore, the authors were of the view that it was an unplanned complex suicide because the intrathoracic stab wounds were not immediately life threatening thus allowing the victim to remain conscious and able to undertake physical activity for a few minutes. The submersion was considered to have occurred as a backup method, after self-stabbing had initially failed to cause death. A further complex unplanned suicide is described by Kulkarni et al. (2020), in which a middle-aged male used a knife to stab himself seven times and also produce other incised wounds. As this did not appear to be immediately effective, he

then walked in front of a train and died as a result of crushing head injuries.

A complex suicide classified as planned after a police investigation, was reported by Christin et al. (2018), of a 27-year-old man, working as a butcher, who was found dead in his crashed car. Although, initially it was thought that it was an uncomplicated road traffic collision, a knife was discovered penetrating the driver's chest. The cause of death was exsanguination from vascular thoracic lesions and internal blood loss.

The author of this book encountered a case of a 45-year-old male who lived in a fourth-floor apartment (Figures 10.16, 10.17 and 10.18 Figures 10.16–10.20). He was suffering from depression and had expressed suicidal thoughts to his family. He was found lying with a severe head injury on the ground, below his apartment. It was thought that he had jumped to his death from the balcony opposite his apartment. It was also noticed that he had sustained a large number of incised and stab wounds of varying sizes. His left hand appeared to have been severed and was not present on the ground. He was not under the influence of alcohol or drugs at the time of his death. Examination of his apartment which was directly above where he lay, revealed a broken Swiss Army Knife, a substantial amount of blood spattering and an amputated left hand.

## Complicated Suicide

A complex suicide, whether planned or unplanned, should not be confused with a "complicated suicide" – a term that was first used by Töro and Pollak (2009). These authors in their investigation of 1217 suicides at the Budapest Institute of Forensic Medicine from 2004 to 2006 found six cases which they described as "complicated suicides." These involved a situation where a suicide attempt was made and failed but during the course of the suicide attempt, there is an unforeseen event (presumed accidental), which caused death. They give as one example: the case of a 38-year-old man who attempted to hang himself from a tree, during which the rope broke and he died as a result of a fall from a height.

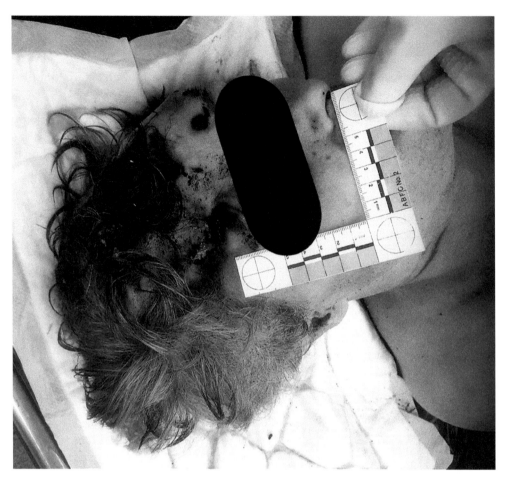

▲ **Figure 10.16** Head of the deceased, which has impacted on hard ground as a result of falling from a height. There is an indentation of the right frontal region, beneath which are substantial cranial injuries. (Source: Author)

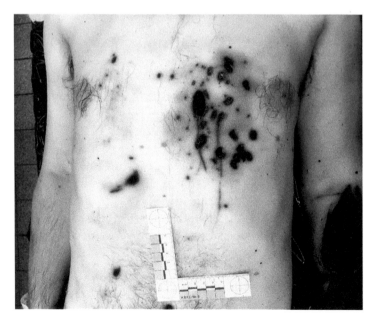

◀ **Figure 10.17a** There are multiple stab and incised wounds mostly situated on the left mid and lower chest. The smaller pinpoint wounds among the larger ones can be described as hesitation marks.

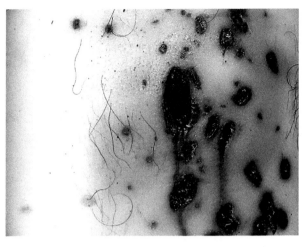

◄ **Figure 10.17b** Close up of wounds.(Source: Author)

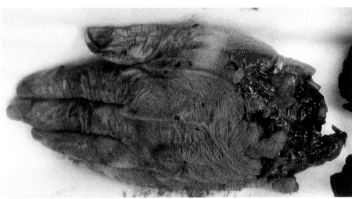

◄ **Figure 10.18a** Self-amputated severed left hand.

**221**

◄ **Figure 10.18b** Forearm (Source: Author)

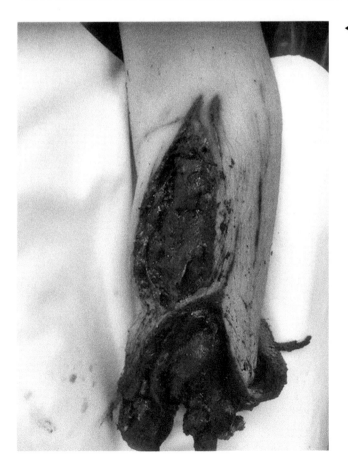

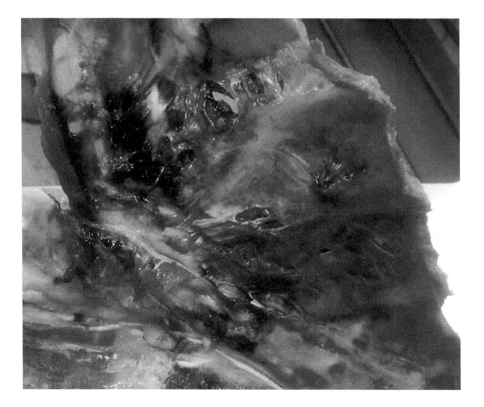

▲ **Figure 10.19** Multiple stab wounds seen to the inside of the rib cage. (Source: Author)

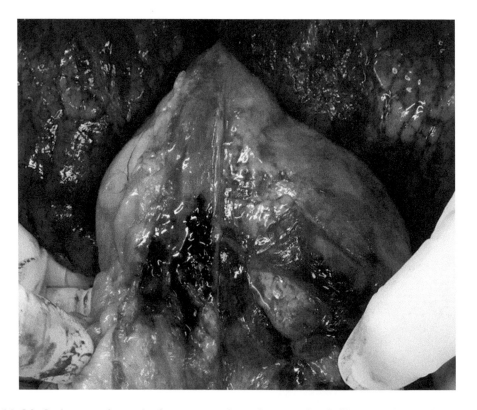

▲ **Figure 10.20** Stab wounds to the heart are relatively superficial. (Source: Author)

# Sharp Force Wounds to the Extremities and Elsewhere on the Body with Non-suicidal Intention

A substantial number of cases of self-wounding including mutilation of the body are seen by forensic pathologists and in living subjects which have not been caused with a suicidal intention (Eckert 1977). The motives may be complex and it is important wherever possible to assess the pattern and distribution of injuries in the context of the lifestyle history of the individual. One commonly finds self-harm injuries in persons abusing drugs and in others who are suffering with various mental health problems. Veeder and Leo (2017) discussed different types of male genital mutilation in 173 cases. The psychiatric disorders in their patient data included the schizophrenia spectrum (49%), substance use (18.5%), personality (15.9%) and gender dysphoric disorders (15.3%).

Self-inflicted wounds are seen in accessible regions, most commonly to the trunk and upper limbs on exposed regions and to the opposite side of the dominant hand. The face, eyes and mouth are usually – though not exclusively – avoided, being more commonly seen where severe mental issues predominate (Figure 10.12).

The vast majority of self-inflicted injuries clearly predominate at the extremities, most commonly at the wrists and forearms, more typically on the ventral aspect and occasionally on the back of the hands. They are usually superficial and occasionally slightly deeper at the start than when tailing off (Figure 10.21). They are frequently multiple, orientated transversely, arranged in parallel, show symmetry and may be present up to the elbow. They are occasionally seen to run in the long axis of the arm. They frequently accompany other self-inflicted cutting wounds to other parts of the body. Occasionally, death may supervene if for example, blood loss is extensive, although in most cases, they are seen as older healing wounds or scars accompanying a different manner/cause of death (Figure 10.22). Where suicide had been intended, the individual may, in

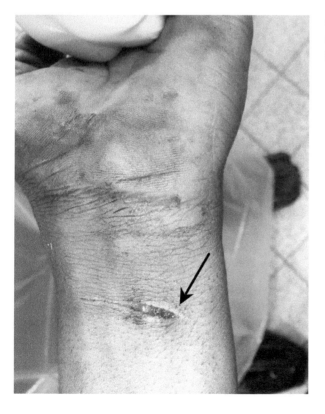

◀ **Figure 10.21** Wound on the right wrist, slightly deeper at the end where the cut began (arrow) then decreasing in depth. (Source: Author)

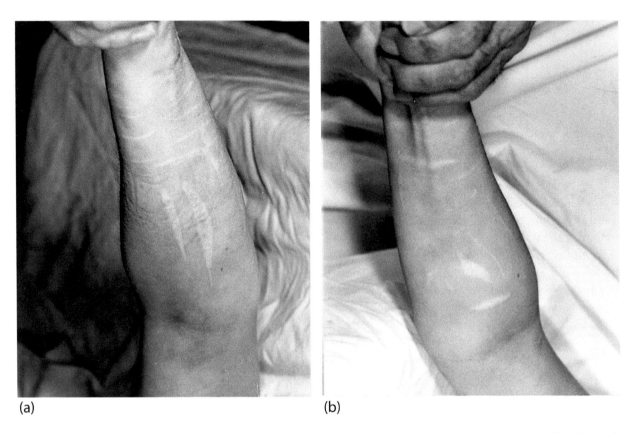

(a)  (b)

▲ **Figure 10.22** Multiple old scars from self-inflicted wounds on the ventral aspects of the left (a) and right arm (b). Some wounds on the left arm are along the longitudinal axis, although most are transverse. (Source: Author)

addition, use another more effective method, such as stabbing a vital organ or hanging.

Occasionally self-inflicted wounds may be seen which are produced by an individual with the intension of simulating an attack by an imagined assailant, in order to appear to be the victim rather than the aggressor to gain sympathy, avoid arrest or incriminate another person. Injuries may also be produced to defraud for the purpose of financial gain or to draw attention to oneself for some other reason. Karger et al. (1997) reported on 14 cases with self-inflicted injuries intended to simulate a criminal offence. One of their cases involved a 20-year-old woman, who had previously attempted suicide. She informed the police that a man who had raped her weeks before had raped her again and injured her with a knife ("not a kitchen knife"). Her injuries: comprised multiple superficial scratches (depth increasing towards the centre of the body) sparing the head, genitals and breasts. There were scars from scratches at

the back of the hands. It was thought that the possible motivation was related to her being sexually abused as a child. The weapon used was a kitchen knife.

In one case seen by the author, the subject – a young adult male – could not face sitting his final university examinations; therefore when he missed his sitting, he invented a story that he had been assaulted and knifed. The casualty surgeon suspected that this was not the case and a forensic opinion was sought (Figure 10.23).

A further case of self-inflicted injury used to simulate a crime and attract attention was reported by Doberentz et al. (2013). A young male student of Asian origin pretended to have been assaulted to force him to convert to Islam. He claimed that he had been beaten and his tongue had been cut with a knife. The clinical and medico-legal examination did not show any signs of blunt force, but only sharp force injuries in the form of superficial scratches and cuts on the forehead and tongue.

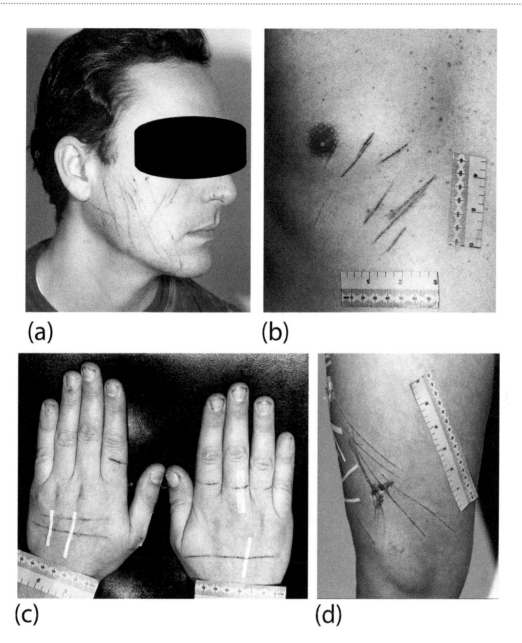

(a)

(b)

(c)

(d)

▲ **Figure 10.23** Young male with multiple self-inflicted incised wounds. The wounds are all superficial, have a regular parallel distribution and are on accessible parts of his body. (a) Right side of face. (b) Right side of chest. (c) Back of both hands. (d) Right upper leg. (Source: Author)

# References

Atreya A, Rijal D, Kanchan T, Shekhawat RS. (2017). Abdominal self-stabbing: a case report. *Med Leg J* 85, 97–99.

Bhattacharjee N, Arefin SM, Mazumder SM, Khan MK. (1997). Cut throat injury: a retrospective study of 26 cases. *Bangladesh Medical Research Council Bulletin*, 23, 87–90.

Byard RW, Klitte A, Gilbert JD, James RA. (2002). Clinicopathologic features of fatal self-inflicted incised and stab wounds: a 20-year study. *Am J Forensic Med Pathol*, 23, 15–18.

Christin E, Hiquet J, Fougas J, Dubourg O, Gromb-Monnoyeur S. (2018). A planned complex suicide by self-stabbing and vehicular crash: an original case and review of the literature. *Forensic Sci Int* 285, e13–e16.

Di Paolo M, Guidi B, Vergaro G, Emdin M. (2015). Self-inserted needles in the heart. *Am J Cardiol* 116, 1315–1317.

Dickson ED. (1876). Report on the death of the ex-sultan Abdul Aziz Khan. *Br Med J*, 2, 41–42.

Doberentz E, Albalooshi Y, Madea B. (2013). An unusual case of a self-inflicted injury to the tongue to simulate a criminal offence. *Arch Kriminol* 232, 201–207.

Durmić T, Atanasijević T, Bogdanović M. (2018). Circumferential suicidal cutting of the lower legs. *Forensic Sci Med Pathol* 14, 561–563.

Eckert WG. (1977). The pathology of self-mutilation and destructive acts: a forensic study and review. *J Forensic Sci* 22, 242–250.

Fukube S, Hayashi T, Ishida Y, Kamon H, Kawaguchi M, Kimura A, Kondo T. (2008). Retrospective study on suicidal cases by sharp force injuries. *J Forensic Leg Med* 15, 163–167.

Giles C. (1956). Suicidal laryngectomy. *J Forensic Med*, 3, 91–93.

Gill JR, Catanese C. (2002). Sharp injury fatalities in New York City. *J Forensic Sci*, 47, 554–557.

Janík M, Straka Ľ, Novomeský F, Krajčovič J, Hejna P. (2016). Circular saw-related fatalities: a rare case report, review of the literature, and forensic implications. *Leg Med (Tokyo)* 18, 52–57.

Jo YM, Lee SH. (2015). Case report of suicide by cutting the tongue with a pair of scissors. *Korean J Leg Med* 39, 132–135.

Karakasi MV, Nastoulis E, Kapetanakis S, Vasilikos E, Kyropoulos G, Pavlidis P. (2016). Hesitation wounds and sharp force injuries in forensic pathology and psychiatry: multidisciplinary review of the literature and study of two cases. *J Forensic Sci.*, 61, 1515–1523.

Karger B, DuChesne A, Ortmann C, Brinkmann B. (1997). Unusual self-inflicted injuries simulating a criminal offence. *Int J Legal Med* 110, 267–272.

Karger B, Niemeyer J, Brinkmann B. (2000). Suicides by sharp force: typical and atypical features. *Int J Legal Med* 113, 259–262.

Karlsson T. (1998). Homicidal and suicidal sharp force fatalities in Stockholm, Sweden. Orientation of entrance wounds in stabs gives information in the classification. *Forensic Sci Int* 93, 21–32.

Karlsson T, Ormstad K, Rajs J. (1988). Patterns in sharp force fatalities—a comprehensive forensic medical study: Part 2. Suicidal sharp force injury in the Stockholm area 1972–1984. *J Forensic Sci* 33, 448–461.

Kato K, Kimoto K, Kimoto K, Takahashi Y, Sato R, Matsumoto H. (2014). Frequency and clinical features of patients who attempted suicide by Hara-Kiri in Japan. *J Forensic Sci* 59 1303–1306.

Kemal CJ, Patterson T, Molina DK. (2013). Deaths due to sharp force injuries in Bexar County, Texas, with respect to manner of death. *Am J Forensic Med Pathol.* 34, 253–259.

Kharbach Y, Tenkorang S, Ahsaini M, Mellas S, El Ammari J, Tazi MF, Khallouk A, El Fassi MJ, Farih MH. (2014). Suicide attempt by self-stabbing of the bladder: a case report. *J. Med. Case Reports*, 8, 391.

Kranioti EF, Kastanaki AE, Nathena D, Papadomanolakis A. (2017). Suicidal self-stabbing: A report of 12 cases from Crete, Greece. *Med Sci Law*, 57, 124–129.

Kulkarni C, Mohite S, Meshram V. (2020). Unplanned complex suicide by self-stabbing and rail suicide: a case report and review of literature. *Am J Forensic Med Pathol* 41, 78–80.

Marcinkowski T, Pukacka-Sokolowska L, Wojciechowski T. (1974). Planned complex suicide. *Forensic Sci* 3, 95–100.

Ozdemir B, Celbis O, Kaya A. (2013). Cut throat injuries and honor killings: review of 15 cases in eastern Turkey. *J Forensic Leg Med* 20, 198–203.

Peyron PA, Casper T, Mathieu O, Musizzano Y, Baccino E. (2018). Complex suicide by self-stabbing and drowning: a case report and a review of literature. *J Forensic Sci* 63, 598–601.

Racette S, Sauvageau A. (2007). Planned and unplanned complex suicides: a 5-year retrospective study. *J. Forensic Sci*, 52, 449–452.

Rautji R, Behera C, Kulshrestha P, Agnihotri A, Bhardwaj DN, Dogra TD. (2004). An unusual suicide with a safety razor blade—a case report. *Forensic Sci Int* 142, 33–35.

Rouse DA (1994). Patterns of stab wounds: a six year study. *Med Sci Law*, 34, 67–71.

Schuessler WW. (1944). Self-inflicted excision of the larynx and thyroid and division of trachea and oesophagus with recovery. *J Am Med Association*, 125, 551–552.

Schyma C, Albalooshi Y, Madea B. (2013). Extended suicide by use of a chain saw. *Forensic Sci Int* 228, e16–e19.

Simonit F, Bassan F, Scorretti C, Desinan L. (2018). Complex suicides: a review of the literature with considerations on a single case of abdominal self stabbing and plastic bag suffocation. *Forensic Sci Int* 290, 297–302.

Start RD, Milroy CM, Green MA. (1992). Suicide by self-stabbing. *Forensic Sci Int* 56, 89–94.

The death of the Sultan Abdul Aziz. ( no authors) (1876). *Br Med J* 1, 740.

Töro K, Pollak S. (2009) Complex suicide versus complicated suicide. *Forensic Sci Int* 184, 6–9.

Vanezis P, West IE. (1983). Tentative injuries in self stabbing. *Forensic Sci Int* 21, 65–70.

Veeder TA, Leo RJ. (2017). Male genital self-mutilation: a systematic review of psychiatric disorders and psychosocial factors. *Gen Hosp Psychiatry* 44, 43–50.

Watanabe T, Kobayashi Y, Hata S. (1973). Harakiri and suicide by sharp instruments in Japan. *Forensic Sci*, 2, 191–199.

World Health Organisation. (2019). Latest data on suicide. www.who.int/mental_health/suicide-prevention/en/.

# Chapter 11
# Accidental Injuries Including Injuries from Animals

## Introduction

The use of the term "accident" in a forensic sense requires careful consideration and differentiation from other manners of death. Keywords which define an accidental event are "unexpected" and "unintentional". Furthermore, accidents may be due to the influence of external and/or internal factors in an environment.

Animal-related injuries are included in this chapter because the manner of death caused by animals (except in circumstances where there is deliberate involvement of a person with the intention of causing harm to another or to themselves with the use of an animal) should be regarded as accidental.

An accident, it has to be said, can occur in a number of different situations and as a result of a number of factors acting together which may include the actions of the victim, or circumstances outside the control of the injured person These in general terms include:

- The dynamics or motion of the victim to increase the risk of an accidental injury to occur, for example, falling on to a glass door, possibly when inebriated.

- The non-deliberate action of a third party holding or throwing a sharp object.

- Working in an environment where sharp implements are regularly used and where the risk of accidental injury may be high.

- Transportation accidents where the collision causes impact against glass or other sharp surfaces.

- Explosions, of accidental non-intentional origin, with a risk of injury from flying glass or other sharp fragments.

## Demographics

In accidental deaths from sharp force trauma, it is well recognised that the majority in most series involve impact against a glass surface, whereas fewer by comparison are due to wounding from knives or other sharp implements (Karger et al., 2001).

### Incidence

Fatalities from accidental stab or incised wounds, from whatever sharp object, are very unusual or rare. In two large studies (Karger et al., 2001; Prahlow et al., 2001) the incidence was 2.3% and 3.5%, respectively. Their findings are mirrored by other published literature I have found and from my own experience of 44 years of examining sharp force trauma deaths in the United Kingdom.

### Type of Sharp Object, Victim and Circumstances

*Glass*

Karger op. cit., in their retrospective evaluation of 799 consecutive autopsies of victims of sharp force trauma, performed between 1967 and 1996 in Münster and Berlin, found 18 cases classified as accidents. There was a typical pattern in 15 of their cases: They were adults who were inebriated (1.4–3.6g/l BAC) and had fallen into an architectural glass surface in the form of a door or window (12 cases), an aquarium, a mirrored wardrobe or a telephone kiosk. Another man fell into a large drinking glass! The other two victims were not injured with glass. One was a farmer who suffered a head injury from a fall onto the long prong of a pitch fork, and in the other case, the victim fell onto a knife in his hand and his death was complicated by pneumonia following inadequate medical therapy.

In the other large series Prahlow op. cit., reviewed all accidental sharp force injury deaths investigated at the Southwestern Institute of Forensic Sciences, Indiana, USA, from 1990 to 1999 and found 22 cases of accidental sharp force injury from 630 cases of all sharp force deaths. The victims' ages ranged from 2 to 71, with most deaths occurring in older teenagers and younger adults. Male subjects (17) were involved much more frequently than female subjects (5). In 50% of the cases, ethanol or other drug use was a possible underlying contributing factor in the accident. Their series included 5 incised wounds, 11 stab wounds, four chop wounds, and 2 deaths caused by dog attacks. About half of the cases involved some type of motorised machinery. As with other studies, broken glass was a major cause of injury occurring in the five cases in which incised wounds were described.

Glass was also involved in the two cases categorised as accidents by Mazzolo and Desinan (2005) in their series of 21 cases. Case 1 was a 56-year-old female, found at home in a large pool of blood, with an incised-stab wound in the left arm, caused by broken glass from a nearby glass showcase. The cause of death was exsanguination. Case 2 was a 55-year-old male, found in a coma in a garden and later pronounced dead in hospital, with an incised wound in his right forearm.

In Vassalini et al.'s (2014), series of 11 cases of accidental deaths from sharp force trauma, five were injured in their own home by splinters of glass (46%); three others at work using chain saws (27%) and two others from metal chips (18%). Six cases (54.5%) had a single sharp force injury. Where there was more than one injury, they were mostly superficial, incised wounds distributed in a random manner: they were due to the breaking of the glass surface and the consequent production of more fragments with sharp edges and pointed tip. They found that the number of fatal injuries was distributed as follows: two on the head, three on the neck, one on the right anterior chest, one on the epigastrium, two on the left upper limb and two on the left lower limb.

Accidental glass injuries may be mistaken for assaults with knives and if there is no evidence of glass in the wound, it may be extremely difficult or impossible to differentiate between the two from the

autopsy alone. Rothschild et al., 2001 reported on three cases with fatal puncture wounds caused by broken glass which resembled stab wounds from a knife with a single edge blade. All were initially the subject of a murder investigation. Stab injuries from glass are rare but in the authors' three cases, the glass shards were very much shaped like a knife and could easily be mistaken as such. Radiographic examination in such cases may be useful if the tip of a shard or fragments of glass are found within a wound or elsewhere on the body, as glass appears opaque and can be easily identified.

*Road Traffic Collisions*

In road traffic collisions, over the last few decades there has been a dramatic drop in serious glass injuries, whereas, 50 years ago the number of persons with such injuries was much more prevalent. This is mainly due to the use of shatterproof glass windscreens which have a laminated coating preventing the escape of numerous glass fragments. However, laminated glass can shatter and penetrate the skin and can be missed both on clinical examination and on a radiograph. Ahmad et al. (2009) reported the case of a 38-year-old man who presented to casualty, having been involved in a road traffic collision three hours earlier in which his small family car had collided at 50 mph with the back of a truck. He had been wearing his seat belt at the time. His car's front windscreen and passenger side window were smashed. He suffered multiple injuries and radiographs a month later revealed that he had glass fragments in the back of his right hand which were subsequently surgically removed.

Although toughened glass has a different configuration to laminated glass – typically breaking into small cubic fragments rather than slithers – both can produce a similar radiographic appearance and it is not always possible to be certain of the source, i.e. toughened side windows or a laminated windscreen. Contrary to common belief, laminated safety glass can shatter and produce foreign bodies of glass density following penetration.

Swain et al. (2018) reported two unusual deaths of two auto-rickshaw drivers where the broken windshield of the auto-rickshaw was responsible for the wounds. Although the wounds on the neck initially suggested homicide, they were found to have occurred accidentally as a result of a road traffic accident involving a head-on collision of the two rickshaws. The injuries were inflicted by the shattered glass of the windshield.

## Machine-operated Saws

Accidental injuries may very occasionally occur from the use of machine operated saws. Such injuries can be caused by a number of types of saws including table or portable circular, band and chainsaws. They often occur in an environment where wood is being cut and in particular if the appropriate safety procedures are not followed with such equipment. The mechanisms which result in injury include direct contact by the saw, or by fragments from the machinery. The most commonly reported regions injured are the head, neck, and limbs, especially the hands.

Sidlo and Sidlova (2018) reported the case of an accidental fatal penetrating craniocerebral injury to a 26-year-old man at work cutting wood. An angle grinder with an accessory for cutting, similar to a chainsaw, was used to shorten some wooden boards. He did not put a steel protective cover on the cutting blade or made use of the required personal protective equipment, particularly a plexiglass shield protector. During the work, the chain broke, and a loose chain fragment caused a penetrating head and brain injury with bleeding. Resuscitation was unsuccessful and death occurred shortly after injury. The chain fragment broke through the facial part of the head to the left and penetrated the brain in the region of the left parietal bone of the cranial vault. The death occurred as a result of a violation of safety precautions.

A further case is reported by Demirci et al. (2008) of a 30-year-old man, in a workshop operating a cutting machine, where a spinning circular saw from the machine came off its place and cut his throat.

There was an incision (15 cm × 5 cm) that began in the middle of the neck down the thyroid cartilage, extended horizontally to the left of the neck and ended on the outer part of the neck in the outer left side of the trapezius muscle. Death occurred because of exsanguination caused by the cutting of the carotid artery and jugular vein.

# Movement Between Object and Victim

## Sharp Object Moving Towards the Victim

Hirt and Karger (1999) describe a fatal brain injury caused by the free-flying blade of a knife while handling a special type of knife. A spring in the shaft of the knife accelerated the blade, which perforated the orbital cavity and the frontal lobe at the right side. The initial velocity of the blade was measured to be 15 m/s. The authors carried out some experimental work on pig cadaver skin and found that the skin and 5–10 cm of soft tissue were penetrated as long as the distance of the blade from the skin did not exceed 1 m. For distances longer than 1 m, the free flight of the blade did not remain stable and resulted only in superficial wounds.

With explosions there is a high risk of injury from flying glass or other fragments with a sharp surface. Indeed, impact from surrounding objects and debris produces a "peppering" effect with discolouration from dust blasting (Figure 11.1). The peppering effect described by Marshall is caused by bruising,

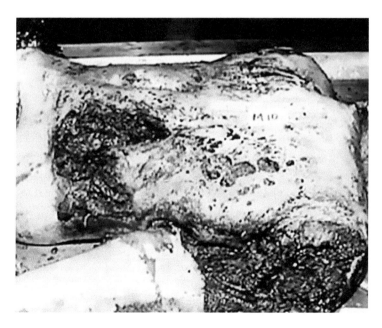

◀ **Figure 11.1** Explosion injuries. Peppering, and multiple lacerations are present.

lacerations and punctate wounds and is well known as Marshall's triad (Marshall 1976).

*Victim Moving Towards the Sharp Object*

Motion of the victim in relation to glass injuries has been alluded to above. In addition, these further cases are examples of rare accidents occurring as a result of movement of the victim.

Marecová et al. (2018) presented the case of a young man with stab and cut injuries due to a duralumin rod embedded in his chest. Examination of the body revealed that death was due to penetration of the thoracic aorta by a duralumin rod. Careful investigation of the circumstances surrounding the death was able to confirm a case of accidental death due to falling from a ladder onto tomato seedlings that were supported by duralumin rods.

In one of the cases described by Ormstad et al. (1986), accidental stab and incised wounds were sustained by a female alcoholic, causing transection of the right femoral artery, resulting in a fatal haemorrhage. The injuries were caused by a beer bottle that was carried in the right trouser pocket which shattered as she fell down a staircase during and epileptic seizure.

Irandoust et al. (2013) report the unusual case of a fatal accidental wound to the neck seen in a 29-year-old employee on a sheep farm. The injury occurred whilst a sheep that was being sheared suddenly moved unexpectedly causing the victim to lose control of the electric shears and inflict an incised wound to his neck, cutting the left internal jugular vein and common carotid artery. He was found to be dead on arrival at hospital.

Park et al. (2015) report a case of a 42-year-old woman who developed Brown-Sequard syndrome caused by an accidental stab injury of the cervical spine at C6-C7 level. The stab wound was on the right side of the posterior neck. She had apparently slipped and fallen onto a knife that was lying in a fruit basket. The clinical aspects of this case are well described. However, there has been no consideration of the position of the knife in the fruit basket and whether the injury could have been the result of an assault rather than an accident. The former, in my view, seems more plausible.

Having regard to possibly other contents of a fruit basket being associated with injury, it has been shown that accidental hand injuries may occur whilst cutting an avocado pear. The first such case

to be reported in the literature was by Rahmani et al. in 2017. Their patient was a 32-year-old woman who accidentally stabbed her left ring finger. On arrival to the emergency department, the knife was still impaled through patient's finger with the attached avocado. The severed digital radial nerve was repaired (Figure 11.2). According to the authors, there has been an apparent increase in avocado-related hand injuries because of the increase in popularity of avocado and its recognition as a highly beneficial health food. The fruit is typically held in the non-dominant hand and knife in the dominant hand to cut or peel it. The mechanism of injury is usually a stabbing action, with the knife slipping past the stone and through the soft flesh.

Following this first publication, Farley et al. (2019) carried out a national survey in the United States of avocado-related knife injuries from 1998 to 2017. They estimated that there were 50,413 (95%) of such injuries and the incidence had increased significantly over this period (1998–2002=3143; 2013–2017=27,059). This increase correlated closely with a rise in avocado consumption. Women comprised 80.1% of injuries seen and much more common on the left (and likely non-dominant) hand.

# Accidental Auto-erotic Deaths from Sharp Force Trauma

Auto-erotic deaths are uncommon and even more so where the mechanism of death involves sharp force trauma as in the two cases described below.

Schmeling et al. (2001) describe a fatal autoerotic accident of a 23-year-old man who derived sexual pleasure from painful irritation of the peritoneum by sharp force. For this purpose, he clamped two knife blades into a vice suspended from a rope-pulley construction so that he could lower it to pierce the abdominal skin with the tips of the knives. When one of the ropes broke, the vice with the knives fell onto the man's abdomen piercing the inferior vena cava and leading to death by exsanguination.

The other case reported by the author of this book was of an elderly male found dead in his living room with two horseshoe nails hammered into the soles of his shoes (Figure 11.3). Nearby were electric cables with clips prepared for attachment to the nails. The cables were attached to a transformer which was plugged in the electricity supply so as to deliver a low voltage. When the shoes were removed

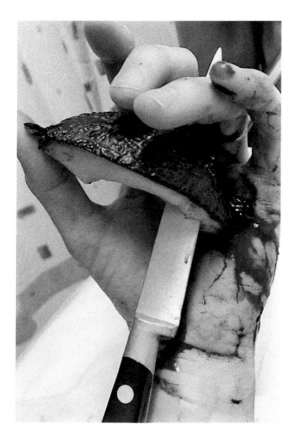

◀ **Figure 11.2a** Hand with knife in the left ring finger with avocado attached.

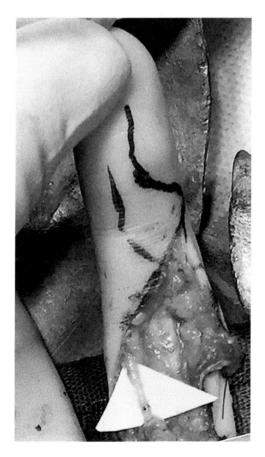

◀ **Figure 11.2b** Ring finger during repair of digital radial nerve branch. (Courtesy Rahmani, Martin-Smith and Sullivan, 2017. The Avocado Hand. *Ir Med J* 110, 658 (Source Figures 1 and 2).)

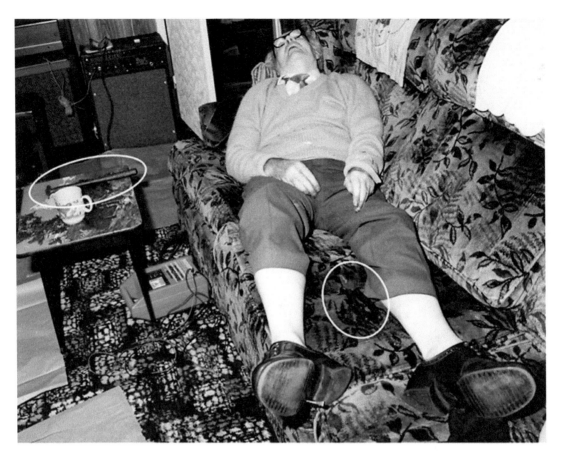

234

▲ **Figure 11.3a** The deceased is seen lying on the couch in his living room. The transformer with cables are nearby and on the coffee table a hammer is seen and a pair of pliers to remove the nails, between his legs (both circled).

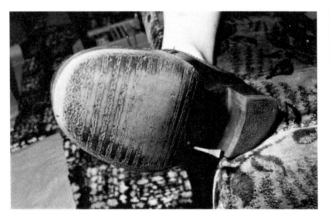 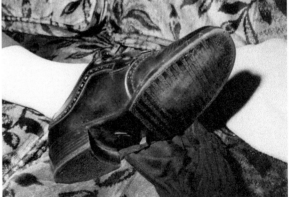

▲ **Figure 11.3b and c** Both soles of shoes have nails driven into them.

at autopsy, it was found that the nail on the left shoe had been hammered beyond its intended depth (apparently, the depth to which he normally hammered the nails was so that they were just touching the soles of his feet and thus able to convey a mild electric shock). In fact, he had hammered the nail with enough force for it to go through the sole of his foot and appear on the dorsal surface. He apparently died soon after this act as there were no signs of him attempting to remove the nail. The cause of death was cardiac failure from ischaemic heart disease and from the timing of his death very likely to have been contributed to by the pain and stress caused by the nail.

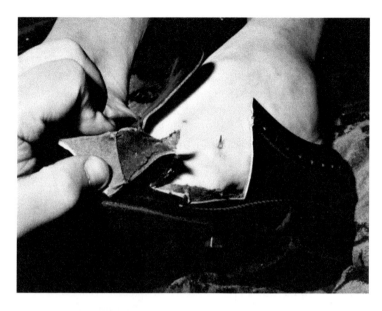

◀ **Figure 11.3d** Part of the left shoe has been cut away to reveal the underlying injury to the left side of the dorsum of the foot with the impaled nail in situ.

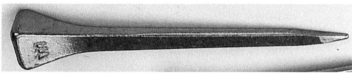

◀ **Figure 11.3e** Horse shoe nail of the type seen in this case.

# Animal-related Sharp Force Trauma

235

Animals have always interacted with humans and been exploited by them in many ways and for different reasons. From time to time such a relationship results in injury to humans, not forgetting that there are also many circumstances in which people abuse and neglect animals both in domestic situations and in the wild.

Animals may cause injury to humans which can range from minor wounding to fatal trauma. The extent and type of injury will depend on the circumstances in which the animal is encountered, the class and species as well as anatomical characteristics. Essentially injuries result from blunt or sharp forces and frequently a combination of both. Other fatalities may occur from envenomation from many types of creatures, including mammals, reptiles, spiders, wasps and some fish. The type of injuries seen will also, to a great extent, be associated with the make-up of the animal population, both in the wild and in captivity, in different geographical regions.

## Incidence of Fatal Animal-related Injuries

In the USA, there were 1943 human fatalities caused by animals between 1991 and 2001 (Langley 2005).

Comparing the venomous to the nonvenomous categories, venomous animals caused 39.1% of the fatalities and 60.9% resulted from the nonvenomous category. In the nonvenomous category, dogs caused the majority of fatalities (about 19 per year).

## Dog Attack Fatalities

Deaths from dog attacks appear to be increasing as the population of both humans and dogs continues to increase (Langley 2009). Of the 504 victims between 1991 and 2001, 58.1% were males and 41.9% females. Children are at the greatest risk of death. Victims less than one year of age accounted for 10.9% of deaths and under the age of 10 fatalities accounted for 55.6% of the cases. The highest number of deaths occurred in children aged one to four, accounting for 29.9% of the total deaths. Infants less than oneyear-old had the highest age-specific death rate. The next most vulnerable group were elderly individuals aged 65 or older, accounting for 24.0% of fatalities.

In the United Kingdom, dog bites, including the number of fatalities, continue to increase. The Office for National Statistics (2016) reported 72 fatal cases between 1981 and 2015 (50 of them were from 2001 to 2015).

The Dangerous Dogs Act 1991 (section 3) stated that it is a criminal offence (for the owner and/or the person in charge of the dog) to allow a dog to be "dangerously out of control." A "dangerously out of control" dog can be defined as a dog that has injured someone or a dog that a person has grounds for reasonable apprehension that it may do so. In addition, the 1991 Act recognised that some breeds were particularly aggressive and the following breeds were banned under the Act: The Pit Bull Terrier; Fila Brasiliero; Dogo Argentino and the Japanese Tosa.

The Act was amended in 1997 (Dangerous Dogs (Amendment) Act 1997) which allowed removal of the mandatory destruction order provisions on banned breeds and re-opened the Index of Exempted Dogs for dogs which the courts consider would not pose a risk to the public. The courts were given discretion on sentencing, with only courts able to direct that a dog be placed on the list of exempted dogs. It should be borne in mind however, that amongst the banned dogs, seven pit bull terriers since 2005 in the United Kingdom have been involved in six fatalities, more than any other breed.

The Government recently introduced legislative changes to the Dangerous Dogs Act 1991 and introduced the Anti-Social Behaviour, Crime and Policing Act 2014 to extend section 3 of the Dangerous Dogs Act 1991 in order that it covers incidents that take place on private property (as well as in public places). This is a welcome change and accounts for the fact that most bites occur from a familiar dog in familiar surroundings. In addition, they removed the mandatory requirement for police to seize and kennel prohibited dogs which they do not consider to be of risk to the public. The Act further introduced Control Orders to prevent incidences of dog aggression.

With around 35 fatal UK dog attacks occurring within 10 years (between 2006 and 2015, [ONS 2016]), pressure has been put on the government to enact more control measures and protect the public. There appears to be a lack of understanding between victim/owner behaviour and the dog's motive and signs it gives out prior to an attack (Westgarth et al. 2018). The dog may be provoked in a number of ways causing it distress and become aggressive, as well as the possibility of being unrestrained in its owner's property and have easy access to young children who are particularly vulnerable.

A dog attacks and bites the region of the head, neck and face and these areas are where most of the fatal injuries occur. They first produce penetrating wounds with their teeth (Figure 11.4) and then tear at the tissue described as the "hole and tear" pattern. Death commonly occurs from exsanguination and/or air embolism. Fractures and penetration of the skull may also be seen particularly in children. In addition to the findings on the victim, when the dog is examined, the victim's blood and hair may be

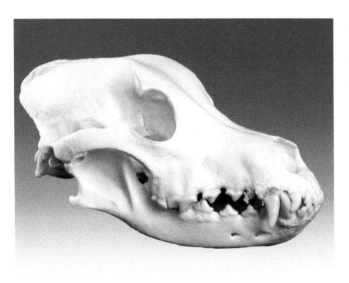

◄ **Figure 11.4** Canine skull. The animal's dentition can be compared with bite marks on victim. Note prominent canine tooth used for tearing and locking on to tissue.

found around or in the mouth. The gastro-intestinal system should be examined by radiography as well as by dissection to look for any of the victim's tissues.

In the case reported by Oshima et al. (2008), a Japanese Tosa attacked a frail elderly woman who died from a vertebral arterial laceration with the C5 vertebral fracture. The detection of the offending dog was made by comparisons of the dental casts of the dog with the victim's wounds. The woman was found dead lying face down on the street. Her body was covered extensively with blood. When an ambulance team arrived at the scene, she was in a state of cardiopulmonary arrest and was bleeding profusely from her right neck. She was confirmed dead at an emergency hospital about one hour later. In relation to the attack, apparently the dog owner who usually kept the dog in a cage on this occasion failed to lock the door of the cage and let his dog run loose out of the cage. The autopsy revealed deep lacerations over both sides and on the back side of the neck. She also had other injuries to her chest and left leg. Internally, it was found that the right internal jugular vein was lacerated, C5 vertebral transverse process fractured and there was about an 0.3 cm long laceration of the right vertebral artery at the level of C5. Death was attributed to exsanguinations due to neck blood vessels' laceration subsequent to dog bite.

## Large Cats

Like dogs, they attack the neck region and shake their prey causing cervical spine injury. They also produce penetrating injuries to the neck and nearby areas from teeth. Death may result from exsanguination and/or air embolism. Deaths from large cats are rare and mostly occur in relation to captive animals in zoos attacking either keepers or members of the public who climb into the cat enclosures. Wolf and Harding (2014) reported on seven deaths in Florida. One case involved a 49-year-old experienced male volunteer worker employed in a private compound, which bred animals for zoos. The victim was mauled by a Siberian tiger weighing 550 lbs (249 kg) which was shot to death by the owner of the park so paramedics could enter the enclosure. The victim was dead at the scene. The autopsy revealed five puncture wounds of the neck, multiple superficial puncture wounds and abrasions/superficial sharp force injuries to the torso typical of claw marks. There were also incised wounds to the arms and hands. The largest of the wounds to the neck,

perforated the left sternocleidomastoid muscle and the left external jugular vein, dislocated the first cervical vertebra, and lacerated the upper cervical spinal cord. There were also left-sided rib fractures.

## Alligators and Crocodiles

Alligator and crocodile attacks on humans are rare with 376 reported attacks in the United States between 1948 and 2006 resulting in only 15 fatalities (Harding and Wolf 2006). Deaths result from exsanguination and drowning, with a combination of blunt and sharp force trauma.

## Aquatic Animals

### Sharks

Great white sharks are responsible for the most unprovoked attacks against humans. The other two common varieties that are also involved in unprovoked attacks are the Bull shark and Tiger shark. There are only approximately six fatal shark attacks a year worldwide (Byard et al. 2006). Injuries are usually caused by rows of triangular sharp teeth moving in a saw-like motion leaving deep wounds (Figure 11.5).

In South Australia, there have been 15 deaths attributed to sharks since 1926, with two patterns of injury being identified: those with bites to the limbs who often exsanguinate and/or drown after removal from the water (Bury et al. 2012), and those where the body is either never found or only small fragments of tissue and organs, such as the lung, are identified (Byard et al. op. cit.). Comparison of serrations of bite marks to the teeth of a shark may enable the identification of the species of the attacker (Nambiar et al. 1996). In Australia, divers and fishermen are most at risk from shark attack with between 4 and 6% of deaths in fisherman between 1982 and 1984 being attributed to sharks. Over the same time period, 68% of deaths were caused by drowning (Driscoll et al. 1994).

### Stingrays

Stingrays have a tail and within it is the sharp stinger, a blade with barbed edges which can also release venom (Figure 11.6). The type of injuries they cause are from the effects of venom and also from the puncture wounds caused by the blade. These fish will only attack if provoked and rarely cause serious

237

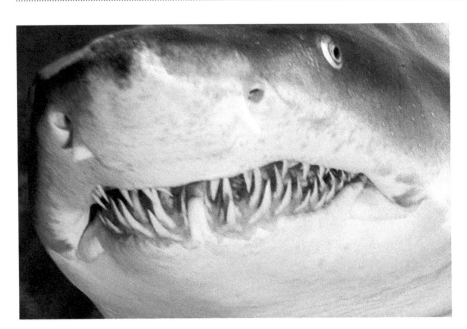

◀ **Figure 11.5a** Mouth of great white shark showing rows of sharp teeth.

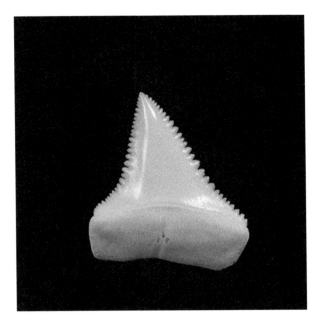

◀ **Figure 11.5b** Close-up of triangular-shaped tooth; note serrated margins.

injury. Fatalities are rare and have been reported from Australia, New Zealand, Columbia, Mexico, Texas, and Fiji (Meyer 1997). Fatalities typically result from penetration of the heart and abdomen. Fenner et al. (1989) reported the case of a 12-year-old boy who died six days after chest penetration and the effects of venom causing myocardial necrosis followed by tamponade. A further case is reported of a fisherman who pulled up a stingray in a fishing net. He attempted to remove the large bull ray, estimated to be 250 k, from the nets, when the stingray flicked its tail, which led to a 12-inch barb piercing his chest. The barb which struck just above his heart, was removed when the stingray pulled away, but left the fisherman in immense pain, before being taken to hospital (Vercoe 2016, Coffs Coast Advocate) (Figure 11.7).

*Catfish*

Catfish have sharp prominent barbels resembling cat's whiskers. They possess a strong, hollow, bony leading spine-like ray on their dorsal and pectoral fins. As a defence, these spines may be locked into place so that they stick outwards and can inflict severe wounds. In several species catfish can use these fin rays to deliver a stinging protein if the fish is irritated. This venom is produced by glandular cells in the epidermal tissue covering the spines and is strong enough that it may hospitalise humans who are unfortunate enough to receive a sting. While

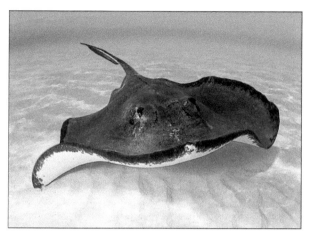

◀ **Figure 11.6a** Stingray.

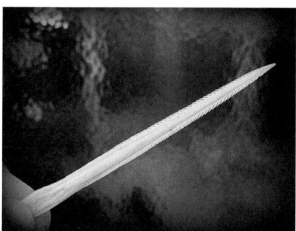

◀ **Figure 11.6b** Stingray barb.

**239**

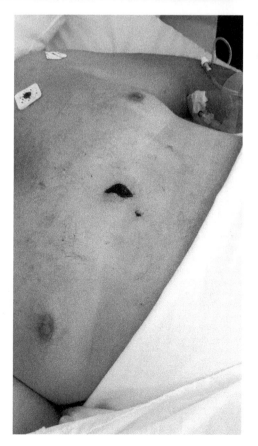

◀ **Figure 11.7** Stab wound produced by stingray barb on lower chest. (Courtesy, Vercoe 2016. Coffs Coast Advocate).

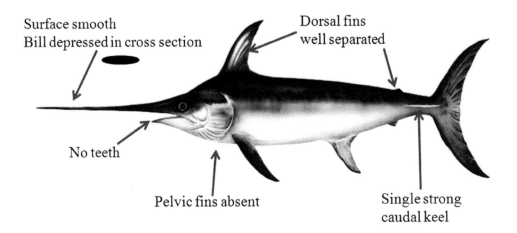

Surface smooth
Bill depressed in cross section

Dorsal fins
well separated

No teeth

Pelvic fins absent

Single strong
caudal keel

No scales on body

▲ **Figure 11.8** Swordfish (Xiphias gladius).

most human encounters are nonlethal, involving lacerations and envenomation, the stings in some species are sufficiently long and sharp to cause severe penetrating trauma. Haddad et al. (2008) reported the case of a fisherman who died after penetration from a catfish sting that perforated his left ventricle.

*Swordfish*

There have been very few attacks from swordfish that have been unprovoked.

Swordfish have long flat pointed bills which are very sharp. The upper jaw measures at least one-third the length of the body. They are large fish that can grow to over three metres in length and the average fish caught commercially weighs between 90 and 150 kg (Figure 11.8).

Their habitat is near the surface of water rather than on the bottom or in coastal areas and they are well known for their powerful jumping. They have been observed moving through schools of fish, thrashing their swords to kill quickly, turning to consume their catch. When provoked they can jump and use

their swords to pierce their target. Gooi et al. (2007) reported a case where it was that thought that the swordfish was attracted by the fisherman's flashing lights mistaking it for food. The unfortunate victim was a 39-year-old fisherman who was attacked by a swordfish which jumped towards him and pierced his right eye when he flashed a torch light at the water from his fishing boat. He was immediately rushed to the nearby hospital by his companion. Clinical examination revealed a penetrating wound at the upper eyelid. About 20 hours after the incident, he became unconscious with a Glasgow Coma Scale score 7. He was intubated and the computed tomography scan showed proptosis of the right eye with subarachnoid haemorrhage and cerebral oedema at the right frontal region. Pneumocranium was also noted. Despite all support, he deteriorated and died one day after admission. The autopsy demonstrated that he had a penetrating injury of his head. The bill had penetrated through the right upper eyelid and traversed through the right orbit, with subsequent penetration into the third ventricle and cavernous sinus through the right optic canal and the right superior orbital fissure.

# References

Ahmad Z, Devaraj VS, Jenkins JP, Silver DA. (2009). Penetrating injury from laminated glass—a trap for the unwary. *Br J Radiol* 82, e114–e116.

Bury D, Langlois N, Byard RW. (2012). Animal-related fatalities—part I: characteristic autopsy findings and variable causes of death associated with blunt and sharp trauma. *J Forensic Sci* 57, 370–374.

Byard RW, James RA, Heath KJ. (2006). Recovery of human remains after shark attack. *Am J Forensic Med Pathol* 27, 256–259.

Dangerous Dogs Act 1991. www.legislation.gov.uk/ukpga/1991/65/contents.

Dangerous Dogs (Amendment) Act 1997. www.legislation.gov.uk/ukpga/1997/53/contents.

Demirci S, Dogan KH, Gunaydin G. (2008). Throat-cutting of accidental origin. *J Forensic Sci*, 53, 965–967.

Driscoll TR, Ansari G, Harrison JE, Frommer MS, Ruck EA. (1994). Traumatic work related fatalities in commercial fishermen in Australia. *Occup Environ Med* 51, 612–616.

Farley KX, Aizpuru M, Boden SH, Wagner ER, Gottschalk MB, Daly CA. (2019). Avocado-related knife injuries: describing an epidemic of hand injury. *Am J Emerg Med* 2019 Jul 2. [Epub ahead of print].

Fenner P, Williamson J, Skinner R. (1989). Fatal and non-fatal stingray envenomation. *Med J Aust* 151, 621–625.

Gooi BH, Khamizar W, Suhani MN. (2007). Swordfish attack—death by penetrating head injury. *Asian J Surg* 30, 158–159.

Haddad V, de Souza RA, Auerbach PS. (2008). Marine catfish sting causing fatal heart perforation in a fisherman. *Wilderness Environ Med* 19, 114–118.

Harding BE, Wolf BC. (2006). Alligator attacks in southwest Florida. *J Forensic Sci* 51, 674–677.

Hirt M, Karger B. (1999). Fatal brain injury caused by the free-flying blade of a knife—case report and evaluation of the unusual weapon. *Int J Legal Med* 112, 313–314.

Irandoust S, Heath K, Byard RW. (2013). Sheep shearing and sudden death. *J Forensic Leg Med* 20, 944–946.

Karger B, Rothschild MA, Pfeiffer H. (2001). Accidental sharp force fatalities—beware of architectural glass, not knives. *Forensic Sci Int* 123, 135–139.

Langley RL. (2005). Animal-related fatalities in the United States—an update. *Wilderness Environ Med* 16, 67–74.

Langley RL. (2009). Human fatalities resulting from dog attacks in the United States, 1979–2005. *Wilderness Environ Med* 20, 19–25.

Marecová K, Uvíra M, Dokoupil M, Handlos P. (2018). Stab wounds of the chest caused by penetration of duralumin rods. *Forensic Sci Med Pathol* 14, 558–560.

Marshall TK. (1976). Death from explosive devices. *Med Sci Law* 16, 235–239.

Mazzolo GM, Desinan L. (2005). Sharp force fatalities: suicide, homicide or accident? A series of 21 cases. *Forensic Sci Int* 147(Suppl.), S33–35.

Meyer PK. (1997). Stingray injuries. *Wilderness Environ Med* 8, 24–28.

Nambiar P, Brown KA, Bridges TE. (1996). Forensic implications of the variation.in morphology of marginal serrations on the teeth of the great white shark. *J Forensic Odontostomatol* 14, 2–8.

Office for National Statistics. (2016). Deaths from dog bites, England and Wales, 1981 to 2015. www.ons.gov.uk/peoplepopulationandcommunity/birthsdeathsandmarriages/deaths/adhocs/006077deathsfromdogbitesengland1981to2015.

Ormstad, K, Karlsson T, Enkler L, Law B, Rajs J. (1986). Patterns in sharp force fatalities—a comprehensive forensic medical study. *J Forensic Sci* 31, 529–542.

Oshima T, Mimasaka S, Yonemitsu K, Kita K, Tsunenari S. (2008). Vertebral arterial injury due to fatal dog bites. *J Forensic Leg Med* 15, 529–532.

Park SD, Kim SW, Jeon I. (2015). Brown-sequard syndrome after an accidental stab injury of cervical spine: a case report. *Korean J Neurotrauma* 11, 180–182.

Prahlow JA, Ross KF, Lene WJ, Kirby DB. (2001). Accidental sharp force injury fatalities. *Am J Forensic Med Pathol* 22, 358–366.

Rahmani G, Martin-Smith J, Sullivan P. (2017). The avocado hand. *Ir Med J* 110, 658.

Rothschild MA, Karger B, Schneider V. (2001). Puncture wounds caused by glass mistaken for stab wounds with a knife. *Forensic Sci Int* 121, 161–165.

Schmeling A, Correns A, Geserick G. (2001). An unusual autoerotic accident: sexual pleasure from peritoneal pain. *Arch Kriminol* 207, 148–153.

Sidlo J, Sidlova H. (2018). Accidental fatal craniocerebral injury caused by broken chain of sawing tool. *Forensic Sci Int* 289, e15–e17.

Swain R, Dhaka S, Sharma M, Bakshi MS, Murty OP, Sikary AK. (2018). Accidental cut-throat injuries from the broken windshield of an auto rickshaw: two unusual cases. *Med Sci Law* 58, 183–185.

Vassalini M, Verzeletti A, De Ferrari F. (2014). Sharp force injury fatalities: a retrospective study (1982-2012) in Brescia (Italy). *J Forensic Sci*, 59, 1568–1574.

Vercoe R. (2016). Man survives barb through chest from 250kg stingray the Coffs coast advocate. https://www.coffscoastadvocate.com.au/videos/fisherman-survives-sting-ray-barb-chest/45322/ (accessed April 2020).

Westgarth CJ, Brooke M, Christley RM. (2018). How many people have been bitten by dogs? A cross sectional survey of prevalence, incidence and factors associated with dog bites in a UK community. *Epidemiol Community Health* 72, 331–336.

Wolf BC, Harding BE. (2014). Fatalities due to indigenous and exotic species in Florida. *J Forensic Sci* 59, 155–160.

# ■ Chapter 12

# Post-Mortem Injuries, the Effects of Putrefaction and Artefacts

## Introduction

Post-mortem changes to the body for whatever reason may well be challenging to the pathologist in their investigation of the cause of death and reconstruction of an assault. The changes that one sees include the natural changes that occur after death in the different stages of decomposition until and including skeletonisation. There may also be deliberate interference with the body after death by destroying or disposing of it in some way in order to prevent its discovery and identification. In some circumstances in order to make disposal easier and prevent identification, the deceased is dismembered and/or mutilated, particularly with the removal of hands and head which are frequently either destroyed or found in separate locations to other parts of the body. In sharp force trauma as in other forms of injury, wounds may be modified by the effects of post-mortem change and in addition there may be further wounds, caused deliberately or accidentally after death, and these need to be thoroughly examined to assess how they were caused, and whether they are ante- or post-mortem injuries. Artefactual features resembling injuries are not unusual findings when there has been some form of post-mortem mutilation including from the effects of burns.

## Ante-mortem or Post-mortem Injury?

One of the problems frequently faced by pathologists is the assessment of whether injuries were caused before or after death or during the process of dying. In situations where there are multiple stab wounds to the body, it is not unusual to find that the victim, has at some stage, stopped moving and was lying still whilst the assailant continued the attack. The pathologist will be required, as in all cases, to advise on the possible sequence of injuries, length of survival, type of weapon, whether more than one weapon had been involved, and in particular which injuries were most likely to have occurred whilst the victim was still alive and which had been inflicted after death. It is in fact a very difficult assessment for the pathologist to make, within such short periods and indeed, may not be possible to do so as there is considerable overlap between the gross and microscopical tissue findings in wounds sustained just before death (late agonal phase) or just after death (early supravital period (Grellner and Madea 2007).

Differentiation between ante-mortem and post-mortem injury relies on whether there is evidence of a circulation having been present giving a vital reaction to the injury, i.e. bleeding from damaged blood vessels around a wound giving the appearance of a bruise within the wound and frequently surrounding it, or no obvious loss of blood from the wound, giving it a yellow/orange appearance. Edges of the wound may have a dry brown appearance and there is no evidence of bruising in the skin surrounding the wound (Figures 12.1 and 12.2). As mentioned above, there may be a considerable overlap between the appearance of ante-mortem or post-mortem injuries on gross appearance as well as at the microscopical level. When there have been multiple wounds inflicted and the wounding is continued when the circulation ceases, then one might expect a combination of wounds with a vital reaction with the later wounds showing a brown/yellow bloodless appearance. In situations where there has been rapid exsanguination leading to death from large wounds, there may be no obvious vital appearance to the surface injuries on gross inspection when compared to a more prolonged period before death ensues (Figures 12.3).

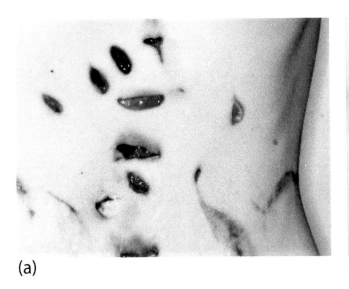
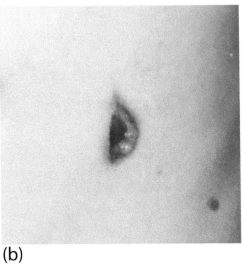

(a)                                       (b)

▲ **Figure 12.1** (a) Victim with multiple stab wounds. The assailant continued stabbing after she had died. A combination of wounds with bruising and a dark appearance can be seen as well as some with a yellow/brown bloodless appearance which appears to have been caused after death (one such wound is magnified and shown in (b).

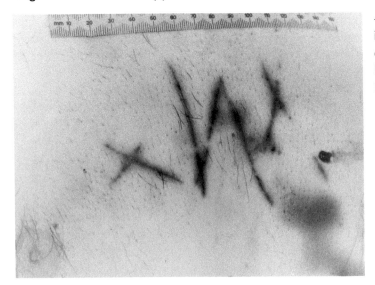

◀ **Figure 12.2** Peri-mortem superficial incised wounds depicting the letter "W" carved on the victim's chest following fatal head injuries from kicking. Slight bruising is noted in part of the wound.

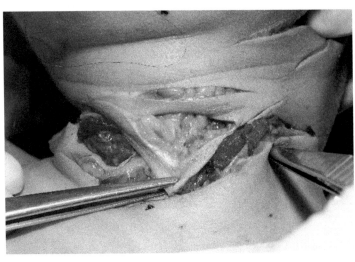

◀ **Figure 12.3** Multiple incised wounds to the neck which were caused just prior to death. There is no bruising associated with these wounds as a result of rapid exsanguination and death occurring rapidly.

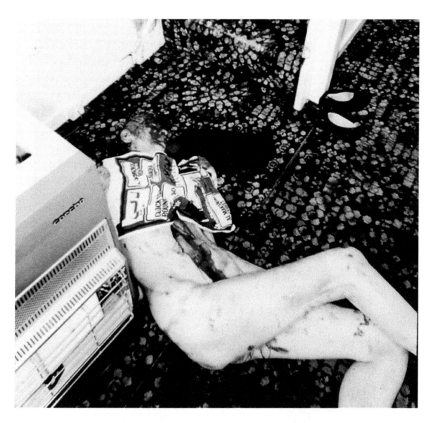

◀ **Figure 12.4a** Elderly woman seen at the bottom of a flight of stairs.

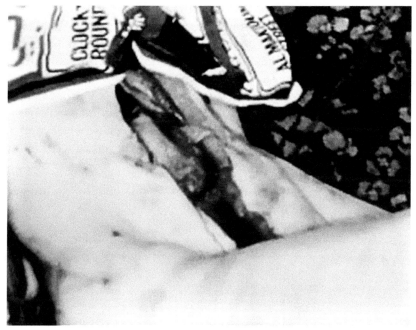

◀ **Figure 12.4b** There is a longitudinal post-mortem wound produced using an electric carving knife, by the assailant who suffered from schizophrenia.

**245**

A further case seen by the author of this book involved an elderly woman who was bludgeoned to death. An electric carving knife was attached to an electrical socket on the wall by her head and used by the assailant, who was suffering from paranoid schizophrenia, to incise her abdomen to reveal the internal organs (Figure 12.4).

## Histological and Immune-histochemical, Biochemical and Molecular Techniques

These techniques have been used or are in the developmental stage in the assessment of the timing of injury and vitality. The subject has been widely studied in the forensic pathology field and more recently in veterinary forensic pathology, with timing and vitality of injuries becoming increasingly important in animals as well (Barington and Jensen 2017).

Wound healing occurs through the following broad successive phases with overlap between them and subject to large intra- and inter-individual variations:

- Inflammatory phase (1–3 days after injury): vascular, haemostatic and cellular response. During the inflammatory phase, platelet aggregation at the injury site is followed by the infiltration of leukocytes such as neutrophils, macrophages, and T-lymphocytes into the wound site.

- Proliferative phase (up to 10–14 days after injury): epithelial and connective tissue regeneration. In the proliferative phase, re-epithelialisation and newly formed granulation tissue begin to cover the wound area to complete tissue repair. Angiogenesis is indispensable for sustaining granulation tissue

- Reorganisation or remodelling phase (several months after injury). Advanced cell biological studies have demonstrated that many cytokines, growth factors, proteases, and so on are closely involved in the wound healing process to complete normal tissue repair after damage (Singer and Clark 1999; Martin 1997).

Biochemical changes may also be attempted in determining vital reaction by testing skin wound edges for serotonin and histamine (Raekallio 1972; Vaněrková et al., 1997).

A particular issue which needs careful interpretation in order to avoid making an incorrect assessment of the timing of a wound relates to the migration of leukocytes. Saukko and Knight (2004) stated that, despite cardiac arrest and circulatory failure, leukocytes can survive and may be motile for more than 12 hours after death. However, only leukocytes outside an area of bleeding can be regarded as a reactive vital change, since cells present in the blood may drift passively into tissue and give a false impression of a vital reaction (Betz 1994; Kondo 2007; Oehmichen 2004; Raekallio 1973).

More recently, many bioactive substances have been found to be involved in skin wound healing to assist in timing of injury and whether caused before or after death. These include collagens, growth factors and cytokines. Of the cytokines, Interleukin-6 and tumour necrosis factor-alpha (TNF-a) were found to be the most useful in the early phase of injury showing a statistically significant increase in the first 30 minutes in the study carried out by Birincioglu et al., 2016). A good review of the subject is provided by Kondo (op. cit.) who also discusses the application of gene expression to wound age determination and emphasises that although still in the experimental stage, it appears that in future determination of wound vitality or wound age will be established at the molecular as well as the protein level. MiRNA expression data from the study by Neri et al. (2019) confirmed the relevance of miRNA expression in traumatic skin lesions bearing in mind its role in the regulation of the inflammatory phase which aims at inhibiting the intracellular signals that occur in the first few minutes of injury.

Further detailed discussion on the techniques employed in the timing of injuries is beyond the scope of this textbook.

# Dismemberment[1]

Dismemberment refers to the removal of major parts of a body such as the limbs, trunk, head or parts of the upper and lower limbs such as the hands or feet. It may be carried out after death or, very rarely, whilst the individual is alive. During life it may result accidentally from road traffic or mass transportation accidents; explosions; accidents with heavy sharp implements such as from mechanised saws, propeller blades from vessels; as part of an execution (usually decapitation), punishment or torture.

## "Hanged, Drawn and Quartered"

In medieval England and beyond up to 1790, one could be subjected to execution by being hanged, drawn and quartered for the crime of high treason. A convicted traitor was taken to the gallows, then hanged until nearly dead, then disembowelled, beheaded, and chopped into four pieces. The four quarters were then exhibited at well-known landmarks throughout the country. London Bridge was such a popular location.

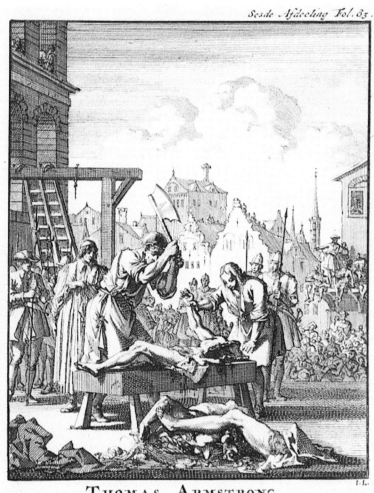

*Sesde Afdeeling Fol. 83.*

THOMAS ARMSTRONG,

*Binnen Londen, gehangen en geviererdeele.*

247

Such was the fate of Sir Thomas Armstrong, who was convicted of high treason against King Charles II. He was Member of Parliament for Stafford and was implicated in the Rye House Plot. This was an alleged Whig conspiracy to rebel against Charles II because of his Roman Catholic sympathies. The ill-fated Sir Thomas was dragged to Tower Hill, where he was hanged, drawn and quartered, on 20 June 1684. His head was displayed at Westminster Hall and three of his quarters in London, and the fourth at Stafford (source: Encyclopaedia Britannica 2019) (Figure 12.5).

A few years earlier, Samuel Pepys – the celebrated medieval diarist https://www.pepysdiary.com/ who lived in seventeenth-century London – wrote of the execution of Major General Thomas Harrison[2], which he had witnessed and is seen from his entry for Saturday 13 October 1660:

*To my Lord's in the morning, where I met with Captain Cuttance, but my Lord not being up I went out to Charing Cross, to see Major-general Harrison hanged, drawn, and quartered; which was done there, he looking as cheerful as any man could do in that condition. He was presently cut down, and his head and heart shown to the people, at which there was great shouts of joy. It is said, that he said that he was sure to come shortly at the right hand of Christ to judge them that now had judged him; and that his wife do expect his coming again.*

*Thus it was my chance to see the King beheaded at White Hall, and to see the first blood shed in revenge for the blood of the King [Charles I] at Charing Cross. From thence to my Lord's, and took Captain Cuttance and*

*Mr. Sheply to the Sun Tavern, and did give them some oysters. After that I went by water home, where I was angry with my wife for her things lying about, and in my passion kicked the little fine basket, which I bought her in Holland, and broke it, which troubled me after I had done it.*

*Within all the afternoon setting up shelves in my study. At night to bed.*

## Dismemberment After Death

In cases involving homicide, nearly all cases of dismemberment occur after death apart from specific instances such as decapitation or amputation of limbs, which may be carried out whilst the person is still alive (as we have seen above), with dismemberment continued after death. The killer uses a very sharp cutting weapon or weapons such as a saw, knife, axe, etc., to sever the limbs and cut the body into small pieces. The dismemberment is usually carried out very quickly after the death or in some cases after a delay of some time.

Dismemberment after death is not always deliberate at the hands of another person. Predation of a body causing dismemberment may occur from animals either on land or at sea. Furthermore, a deceased person in water may suffer post-mortem wounds of various types including from the propeller blades of sea craft, which may result in dismemberment or mutilation

## Dismemberment Categories

There are a number of reasons why dismemberment is carried out after death. Indeed, it has been categorised into different types to reflect the motive of the perpetrator (Rajs et al., 1998; DiNunno et al., 2006).

### Defensive Dismemberment

The vast majority of cases fall into the category of *"defensive dismemberment,"* where the aim is to reduce the body to smaller parts to facilitate transportation from the scene rather than moving the whole intact victim and also by doing so delay investigations until a body is found. Prevention of identification is another reason high in the killer's mind. Many bodies that are dismembered have their head and hands removed and disposed of in different locations to make identification more difficult.

### Aggressive Dismemberment or Mutilation

This is another category where there is an element of hate and aggression in the perpetrator towards the victim. In such cases the dismemberment may begin before death has supervened and continue afterwards. Disfigurement or mutilation of the face or genital area may be present. Together with this category there is sometimes an overlap which is more sexually motivated, often referred to as *offensive dismemberment* and is combined with sadistic pleasure in dehumanising the victim in this way.

### Necromantic Dismemberment

Yet a further type, which relates to performing sexual acts on an inanimate body following its mutilation and may also include bizarre ritualistic practices, fetishes, including the retention of pieces of the body as trophies or even for cannibalism (Pettigrew 2019).

For the investigators, therefore, a dismembered corpse may provide significant challenges in the investigation. Firstly, in addition to evidence lost from the scene or difficulty in identification, to ascertain the cause and circumstance in which the person was killed may be very difficult to achieve, particularly if the killer has deliberately, by dismembering the body, attempted to cover or destroy wounds or other evidence related to the deceased.

## Pattern of Dismemberment

Most victims, particularly in the defensive type of dismemberment are divided into six or eight sections, comprising the head, trunk, upper limbs and lower limbs (on many occasions the thighs and lower legs are separated further). There are of course variations to this common pattern. For example, the person many only be decapitated or just have the hands removed or both head and hands and the rest of the body left intact, to conceal identification.

## Examination of Cut Marks on Soft Tissue and Bone

The different implements that are used in dismemberment leave characteristic marks on soft tissue and in bone which can be examined morphologically both naked eye and at the microscopic level including with the use of the scanning electron microscope (SEM) particularly with energy dispersive

X-ray analysis as well as micro CT (Rutty et al., 2013) (see also Chapter 7). The combination with Energy Dispersive X-ray Analysis (EDX) allows for the assessment of the chemical composition of metallic residues detected on the surveyed sample together with evaluations of the morphological features (Porta et al., 2016).

The killer frequently uses a combination of a knife and a saw, either a mechanised type, e.g. chain saw, a non-mechanised variety such as a hacksaw or a chopping implement such as an axe; in fact, whatever is available that is suitable for dismembering the victim. In a planned dismemberment, where it is intended to kill the victim and then dismember their body, such implements would have most likely been gathered beforehand. It would not be the case when such an act was not planned which is in fact the more common practice, but thought of only after the death of the victim. In such cases there may be a delay for a number of reasons. The perpetrator, may not immediately think of dismembering the victim until it is realised that in order to dispose of the body and cover up the crime, he/she will need to find a way of facilitating its removal from the scene. Occasionally the perpetrator may have to procure the required cutting

implements and any other equipment necessary for the task to ensure the body can be moved easily and safely from the scene and also to attempt to clean up the area where the dismemberment occurred, where it will inevitably be heavily blood stained. It should be appreciated that the place where the dismemberment occurs is in most instances, where the victim was killed therefore the scene of death may well be in disarray and heavily contaminated with blood and other material of evidential value.

Some examples of the type of marks left on the body (skin, underlying soft tissue and bone) from dismemberment/mutilation are shown below.

*Skin Marks*

Beginning with the skin, the killer would in most instances use a knife, which may of course vary in size and shape but one that is sharp and has the ability to cut down into the soft tissue until bone or cartilage is reached. The appearance of the cuts that are made on the skin, since they are after death, will have a bloodless appearance. There may be nearby superficial cuts which may well reflect the killer gauging the most suitable place to make incisions (Figure 12.6). Although it is understood that dismemberment

**249**

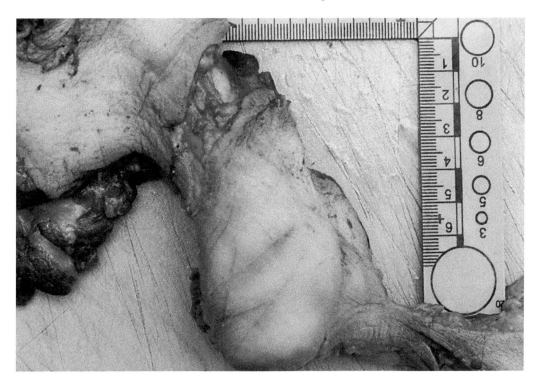

▲ **Figure 12.6** Skin cuts showing bloodless appearance. Superficial post-mortem incised wounds are also seen. The victim was dismembered within a few minutes of death (from last victim in Crossbow cannibal cases).

involves removal of major body parts, many killers also remove and flay bodies removing much smaller pieces of tissue thus presenting a much more complex task for the pathologists and other scientists.

If the body parts are found after some time has elapsed, then the appearance of the cuts may be modified and be more difficult to assess as to whether they were caused prior to or after death as in Figure 12.7.

One further aspect relating to the use of knives was explored in the Buck Ruxton case (see also below). This issue related to blunting of a sharp knife during the dismemberment process and the use of more than one implement. As was stated by Professor John Glaister, Regius Professor of Forensic Medicine at the University of Glasgow, during Ruxton's trial at Manchester Assizes in March 1936 – when he was examined by the prosecution – a knife is likely to become blunt during the process and might require the use of a second sharp knife, unless the initial implement is sharpened (Blundell and Wilson 1950).

Cuts in the skin which are made as part of the dismembering/mutilating process may be deliberately employed to destroy, mutilate or modify any fatal ante-mortem wounds.

### Marks Found in Bone and Cartilage

Marks found in bone are mostly produced by saws (either manual or mechanised) and very occasionally, by axes or hatchets. Where a body is dismembered by disarticulation, knives, particularly small knives which are easier to hold and manipulate within joints, are preferred. The marks they make on bones are smaller than saws and leave a sharper notch on the bone (see Figure 12.13 in the section on the Buck Ruxton case).

As stated, in various published series of cases and in my own experience, most dismemberments are achieved by sawing through bone. Porta et al. (2016) reported their findings in six dismemberment cases, including well-preserved cadavers and skeletal remains. They found that two of their cases had their forearms and limbs disarticulated from the rest of the body rather than sawn through bone at any point. They stressed the point that the method used by a killer in dismembering their victim may assist, if there is likely to be more than one victim, in linking findings between victims and building a profile of the killer and his/her modus operandi.

When a saw cuts into a bone it leaves a kerf mark or groove (Symes 1992; Symes et al., 1998). Saw

250

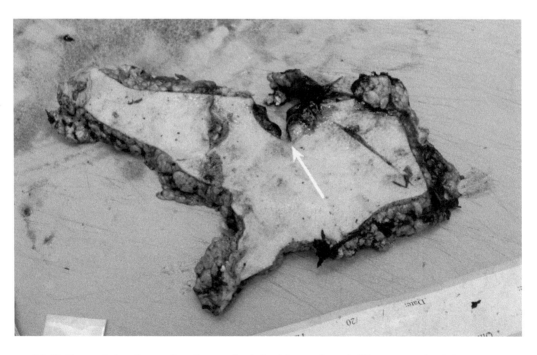

▲ **Figure 12.7** Part of skin from the chest which had been flayed. The victim had disappeared about a month prior to discovery of her remains. Incised wounds can also be seen within the cut margins (arrow). The sharpness of the knife used is evident from the production of such well demarcated and neat cuts in the skin. (from second victim in Crossbow Cannibal cases)

mark analysis involves examination of saw cut kerf floors and walls. Floor contour includes false starts (Figure 12.8) and, occasionally, breakaway spurs. Kerf floors offer the most information about saw class by revealing the relationship of saw teeth to each other. The information includes set and number of teeth per inch.

The characteristics of the kerf walls and floors are used to assist in the identification of the class of saw. The arrangement of the ridges or striations (edges of the kerf walls) will indicate the direction that the bone has been sawn and towards the end of one edge of each will be seen where the bone may have chipped off depending on how the saw has been used (Figure 12.9). It should be appreciated that the width of each ridge edge does not necessarily indicate the distance between the teeth on the saw but could well be more in keeping with the force applied (Symes et al., 2010). The latter authors give a detailed analysis of and guidance on how the various characteristics that are found in cut bone that can assist in the diagnosis of saw class.

## Case Studies

There are numerous examples of homicide cases involving dismemberment, some of which have become notorious in the annals of crime. An example of one such case from the first half of the twentieth century is given below together with some cases from my own files.

### The Buck Ruxton Case

Undoubtedly this case is one of the first to demonstrate the close cooperation and team work, between different scientific experts and the police in bringing together all the necessary evidence to bring the perpetrator to justice. The case is also remembered for the use of forensic techniques, fledgling or innovative at that time, to assist with identification.

The case involved the Parsi doctor Dr Bukhtyar Rustomji Ratanji Hakim who changed his name to Buck Ruxton by deed poll when he settled in the United Kingdom. He was born in Mumbai on 21 March 1899 and executed by hanging in Strangeways Prison Manchester on 12 May 1936, for the murder

251

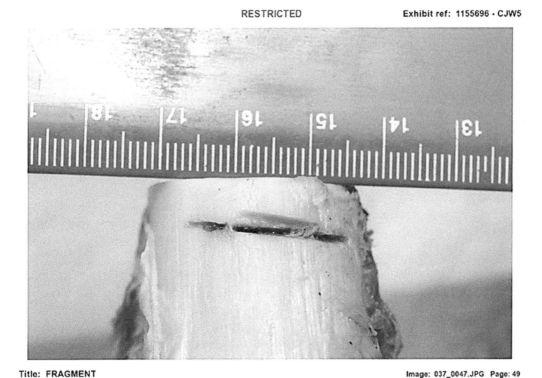

Title: FRAGMENT

**▲ Figure 12.8** Marks on the bone known as "false starts." These are preliminary attempts at sawing through bone. Note the square kerf walls and flat floor, compared to a knife which causes a "v"-shaped mark because of its sharp surface.

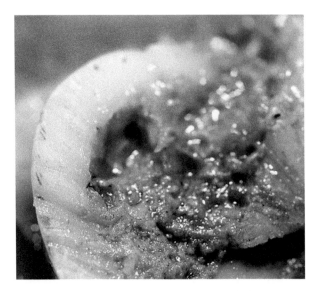

◄ **Figure 12.9a** Hand saw marks. Sawn proximal end of radius showing broad and flat kerf floors. The use of a hand operated saw is in keeping with the unevenness in the striations. One can also see that where the saw has cut through most of the bone, at the exit path of the saw on the bone the remaining uncut bone has chipped off.

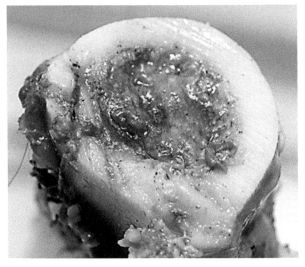

◄ **Figure 12.9b** The striations in this image show a change of direction and fracture of bone at the exit side.

252

of his common-law wife, Isabella Ruxton, and their housemaid Mary Jane Rogerson.

He moved to Lancaster, England, in 1930 and lived at 2 Dalton Square with his wife and their three children. He opened a general practitioner surgery there and was well respected and popular with his patients.

Dr Ruxton and his wife appeared to have a love-hate relationship and had regular rows. He was said to be morbidly jealous and was convinced that she was having an affair although there was no evidence of this.

Eventually his jealousy overwhelmed him and on 15 September 1935 he manually strangled Isabella. In order to prevent their housemaid, Mary Jane Rogerson, from discovering his crime before he could dispose of the body, he also killed her. He then dismembered and mutilated both bodies to hide their identities.

On 29 September 1935 various human body parts in four bundles and others scattered separately were found dumped in the bed of Gardenholme Linn, below the bridge where the stream runs into the River Annan, crossed by the Edinburgh–Carlisle road, two miles to the north of the town of Moffat in Dumfriesshire, Scotland (Figure 12.10). A total of 70 separate body parts were discovered and sent for examination. Some of the human remains were wrapped in newspapers and unfortunately for Ruxton, one of the newspapers he had chosen for this purpose was a special "slip" edition of the Sunday Graphic that was sold only in the Morecambe and Lancaster areas. The date shown on the paper coincided with the day the two women disappeared and proved a crucial piece of evidence in tracking its origin back to Ruxton's neighbourhood.

The bodies were examined by John Glaister, Regius Professor of Forensic Medicine at Glasgow University and James Couper Brash, Professor of Anatomy at Edinburgh University together with the cooperation

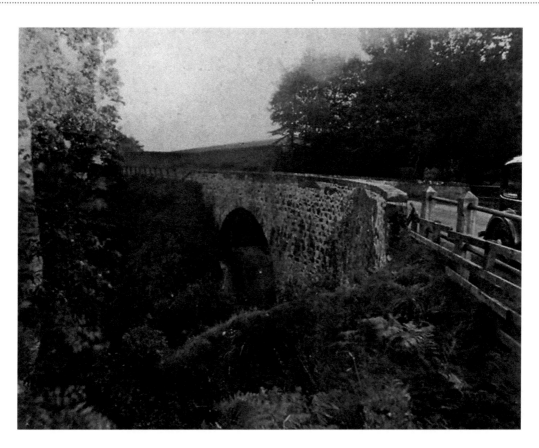

▲ **Figure 12.10** Gardenholme Bridge on the Moffat-Edinburgh Road from the North where the human remains were found (Glaister J and Brash JC (1937). Medico-legal aspects of the Ruxton case. Livingstone, Edinburgh)

of the police. The remains, which were initially separated by Glaister and Brash into two individuals known as body 1 and body 2, were later identified as Mary Rogerson and Isabella Ruxton, respectively (Figure 12.11), by comparing them with ante-mortem information, employing fingerprints and forensic anthropology including superimposing a photograph over the X-ray of a victim's skull. Forensic entomology by identifying the age of maggots, assisted in estimating the approximate date of death.

It will be noted that the technique used by Ruxton to dismember his victims was essentially disarticulation (Figures 12.12 and 12.13) using one or more sharp knives (or by knife called a "slip knife" which has more than one blade), as remarked by the Judge in his summing up. Ruxton also removed the fingertips of one of the victim's (Isabella) in order to prevent identification.

Ruxton was arrested on 13 October 1935 and charged with the murder of Mary Rogerson; he was subsequently charged on 5 November with the murder of his wife, Isabella. His trial started on 2 March 1936 and lasted for 11 days, ending on 13 March 1936 when the jury returned a verdict of "guilty,"

and Mr Justice Singleton sentenced him to death. An appeal for clemency was dismissed and he was hanged at Strangeways prison, Manchester, on the morning of 12 May 1936 (Blundell and Wilson 1950; Glaister and Brash 1937).

*Body Parts at Women's Refuge in East London*
Six black plastic bin liners neatly wrapped with sealing tape to conceal their contents were discovered within bins outside a "battered women's refuge" in East London (Figure 12.14). When they were examined in the mortuary they were found to contain six limb parts. These were one each of a left and right lower leg, thighs and arms. The torso and head were never found. The method of dismemberment appeared to be with the use of a knife, with the limbs all having been disarticulated at the joints (Figure 12.15).

Forensic tests revealed that the remains were those of a female in her twenties, about 1.65 m (5' 6"), not pregnant, with traces of diazepam in her tissues. From her feet, she showed all the signs of having led a fairly active life (examined by a chiropodist). She had multiple old linear scars on both wrists

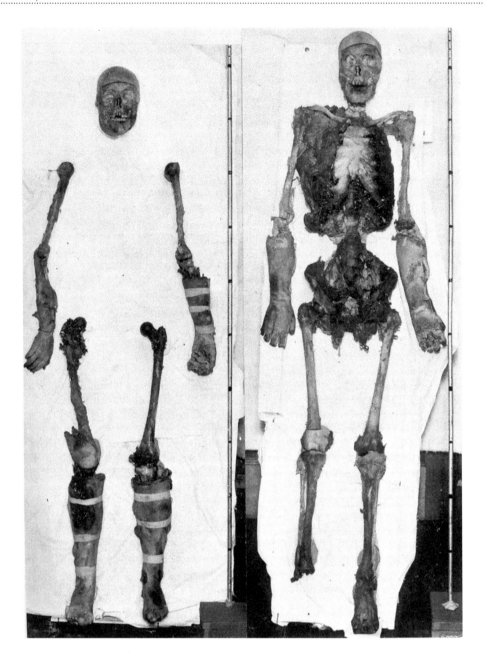

▲ **Figure 12.11** Skeletons of both sets of human remains reassembled as Body No.1 (left) and Body No. 2 (right). (Glaister J and Brash JC (1937). Medico-legal aspects of the Ruxton case. Livingstone, Edinburgh)

and forearms (Figure 12.16) indicating that she had self-harmed in the past. Furthermore, the scene was misleading and hindered the correct avenue of investigation, as she had no connection with the "battered women's refuge." Her body parts, as discovered later, were placed there by chance. Identification remained unknown for 5 years after their discovery.

Five years later, a young man, recently settled in North West London and living in the same block of flats as the victim, walked into a Police station and confessed to killing and dismembering a young woman. He apparently met his victim, a young woman in her early twenties, by chance when she knocked on his door in error, looking for a friend. He struck up a conversation with her then, after inviting her into his flat, tried to have sexual intercourse with her. She refused and then he strangled her. He hid her under his bed, went to sleep and woke up the next morning incredulous at what he had done. He eventually removed her from under the bed and placed her near a radiator where she sustained some post-mortem burns (Figure 12.17). The

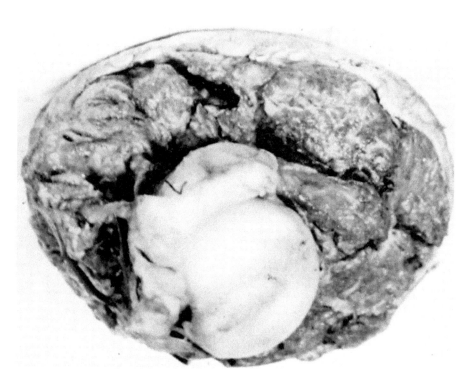

▲ **Figure 12.12** Upper end of right arm of Body 1 showing the head of the humerus which articulates with the shoulder joint. The cartilage was slightly scratched only (Glaister J and Brash JC (1937). Medico-legal aspects of the Ruxton case. Livingstone, Edinburgh)

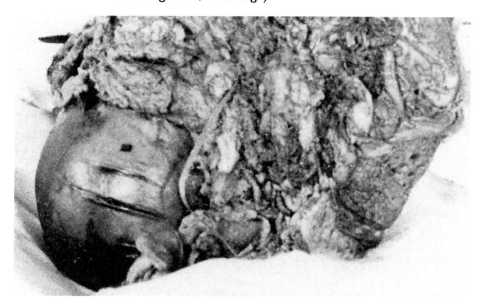

▲ **Figure 12.13** Head of right femur of Body 1, which articulates with the hip joint, showing several cuts on the articular cartilage. This was the worst damage of the articular aspect of any bone of either body (Glaister J and Brash JC (1937). Medico-legal aspects of the Ruxton case. Livingstone, Edinburgh).

same day he dismembered her with a carving knife. He placed her head and trunk into two bin liners in bins outside the flats and they were taken away by refuse collectors, disposed of in the usual way and have remained undiscovered to this day. The rest of the remains, as there was no more room in the bins outside the flats, were placed into two heavy-duty carrier bags. He then took a London Underground train and crossed over to the East side of London to the only other location in London that he knew.

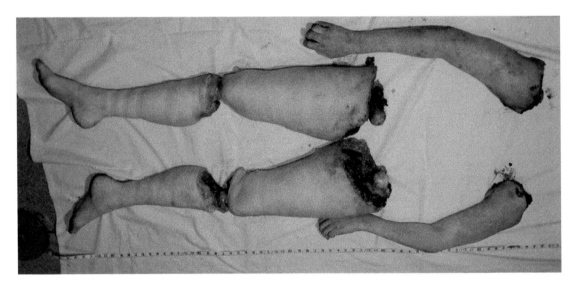

▲ **Figure 12.14** Dismembered limbs wrapped up in bin liners secured with white adhesive tape. They were found stacked by some bins outside a terrace house used as a "battered women's refuge."

▲ **Figure 12.15** All limb parts have been disarticulated with very little damage at the articular surfaces.

He then walked about half a mile and placed them, purely by chance, in the location where they were found the day after they had been deposited.

The dismemberment was carried out using only a carving knife. The offender was not known to have any skills in anatomical dissection, or had any medical training or connection with the butchery trade.

*The "Crossbow Cannibal"*

Stephen Griffiths, self-styled as the "crossbow cannibal" lived in Bradford for over a decade before beginning his short but notorious criminal career. He was enrolled part-time in a PhD programme in criminology at Bradford University. Bradford is the city where the infamous Yorkshire Ripper Peter Sutcliffe committed a series of murders against

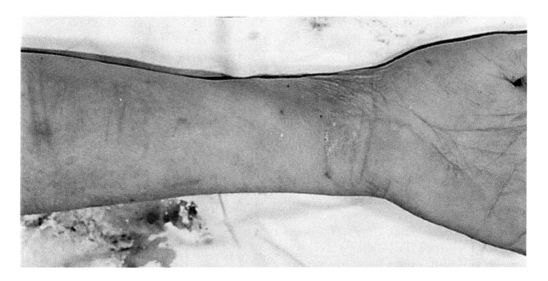

▲ **Figure 12.16** Left forearm showing multiple linear scars from self-inflicted wounds.

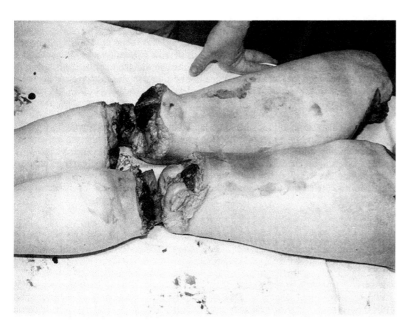

◀ **Figure 12.17** View of the back of the legs. Note the post-mortem burning on the backs of both thighs and right lower leg near the back of the knee. These had been caused by placing the body close to a radiator with the legs straightened before they were dismembered.

257

women, mostly prostitutes, in the 1970s. Griffiths lived on the top floor of Holmfield Court, a building that had once been a Victorian textile factory.

Griffiths befriended the neighbourhood's sex workers. He would cook for them, wash their clothes and let them stay with him if they needed to. Many of them later reported that he had seemed harmless and even clueless, and a couple have admitted that they stole from him.

Griffith's first victim was a 43-year-old female whose body was never found, and, while investigators believed that Griffiths had beaten her to death with a hammer, the only physical evidence tying him to her

death was a trace amount of her blood in the bathroom of his apartment.

The second victim was a female, aged 31, who was supporting her boyfriend by working the streets. However, it took the boyfriend a few days to contact authorities when she disappeared in April 2010. Investigators would find only parts of her shoulders, vertebrae and some connective tissue. When Griffith's cell phone was found, it still had video footage on it, showing his victim in a bathtub, hog-tied and splayed on a bed, with the words "My Sex Slave" spray-painted on her bare back.

The following month the third female, aged 36, disappeared. She had walked out on her boyfriend the night before after an argument; and did not return by the next night. He searched for her, then phoned her mother, who called the police. His third victim, in common with the other two women, had been a prostitute. Police recovered 81 body parts from the river Aire, later identified as belonging to the third victim. A security camera, that Griffith was aware of, captured her trying to run away from him and then he holding her and then murdering her. He was also captured on camera as he was leaving his flat holding a number of bags some time later. When security personnel returned the following weekend, the security cameras were routinely checked. What they witnessed caused alarm and the police were informed.

The scene of discovery of the remains was attended by the pathologist the evening following information received from the security personnel on discovery of a plastic bag which was at first thought to contain a football, but in fact was the head of his third victim. There followed further discoveries of human remains in bags in the following week.

The post-mortem examination was carried out the following day using disaster victim identification (DVI) protocol, bearing in mind that it was uncertain as to whether parts from other individuals might be found. Prior to examining the body parts all were labelled, photographed and those containing bones were radiographed. The post-mortem examination was carried out over a period of days. Example of the remains found from one bag is shown in Figure 12.18.

There were a number of features on the body parts that clearly demonstrated that the type of dismemberment carried out followed the pattern of the aggressive offensive type, with cannibalistic elements. She had been killed by the use of a crossbow and stabbed with a knife, both to the chest and to the head. The knife tip had broken off in the skull and he had broken part of the shaft of the crossbow bolt (Figures 12.19 and 12.20). Much of the bony skeleton was defleshed with a knife. It was noted that her face was stripped and her nose separated (Figure 12.21). All internal organs were missing apart from the brain and internal genitalia. It was also found that he had stabbed her prior to death on

258

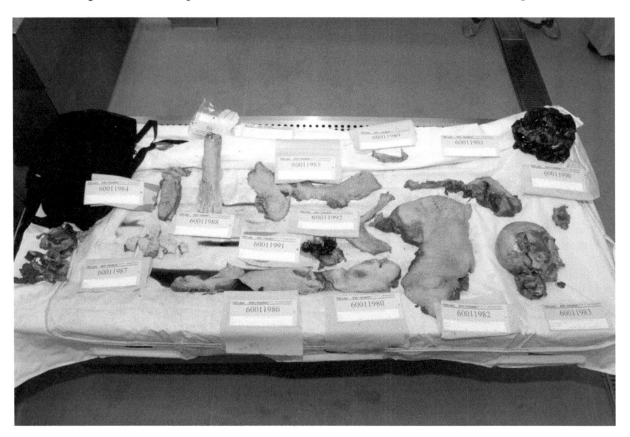

▲ **Figure 12.18** Dismembered remains labelled and displayed with the bag in which they were found.

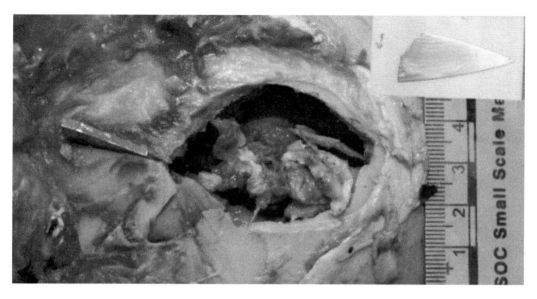

▲ **Figure 12.19** Broken knife tip embedded in skull. Inset: tip of knife blade

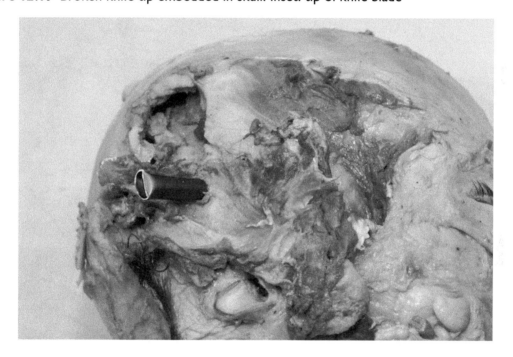

▲ **Figure 12.20** Broken shaft of crossbow bolt embedded in the skull.

the areolar region of the left breast (Figure 12.22). A hand saw was also used to saw through some of the bones (Figure 12.23). All body parts of the third victim were approximately matched visually and by CT scans, although definitive association was through DNA analysis.

Griffiths was convicted of murder at Bradford Crown Court and given three life sentences with a recommendation to remain in prison with a life order.

*Paralysed Victim and Use of Chainsaw*

In a further case seen by the author, the perpetrator was thought to have stabbed his paralysed victim, who was unable to defend himself, in the lower half of the chest and then proceeded to dismember his body using a chainsaw which included division of his torso at the site of the stab wound which coincided with cuts seen on the heart and left lung. After his body had been dismembered he stored him in two freezers (Figure 12.24).

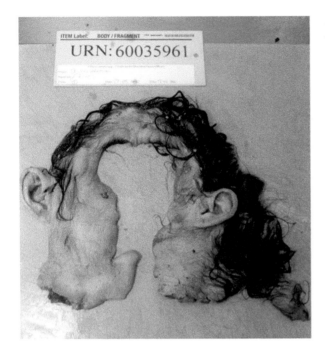

◀ **Figure. 12.21a** Face cut away (stripped) from the skull by a knife.

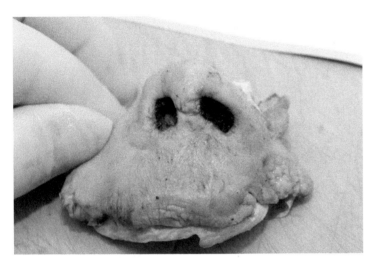

◀ **Figure. 12.21b** Tip of nose cut off.

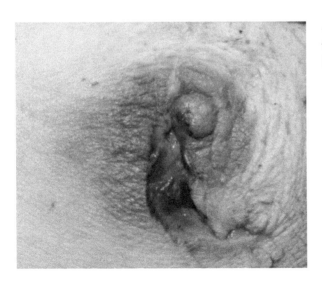

◀ **Figure 12.22** Stab wound before death on the areola of the left breast. Note the associated bruising.

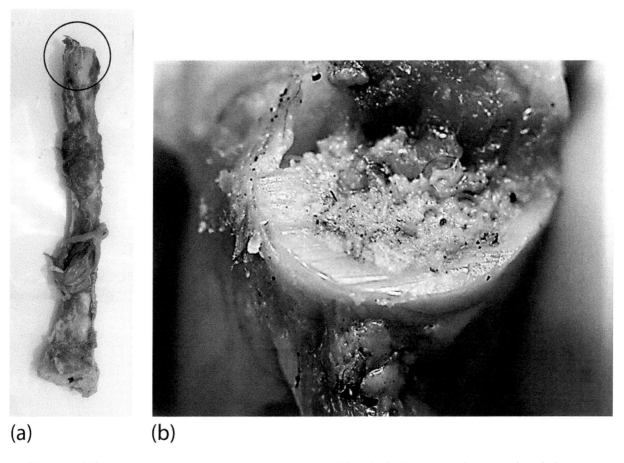

(a)          (b)

▲ **Figure 12.23** Left radius with proximal end sawn off (circled). Close up of proximal end showing saw marks.

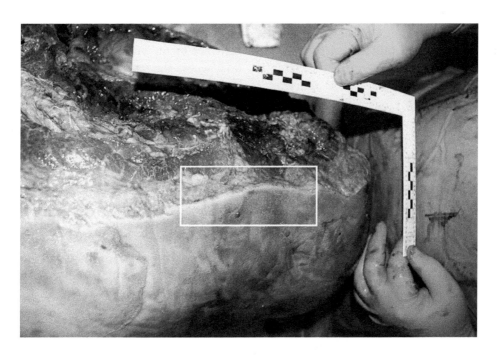

▲ **Figure 12.24a** Border of cut skin from part of dismembered torso.

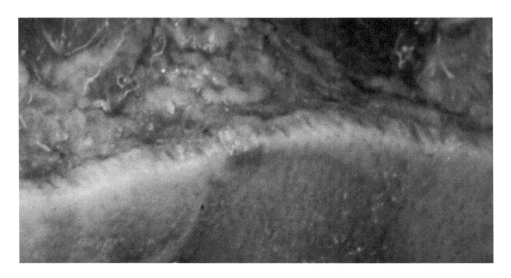

▲ **Figure 12.24b** The area within the white rectangle is magnified to show the serrations produced by a chain saw at the skin margin.

# Post-mortem Changes with Putrefaction and Associated Artefacts

After death, if the body is not preserved in some way, either artificially such as embalming, or in very cold environment from around freezing and below, one will see post-mortem deterioration (decomposition). This is a continuous process once cellular death has occurred. The rate at which such changes occur will depend on climatic conditions, the environment and the effects of predation. Occasionally changes are seen in such circumstances which resemble ante-mortem injury and it is essential to differentiate between the two (see section on "ante-mortem or post-mortem injury").

## Surgical Incisions and Post-mortem Injuries

Surgical incisions may be modified or dehiscence may occur with putrefaction due to the action of underlying gases causing bloating of the body and have an appearance similar to incised wounds (McGee and Coe 1981; Byard et al., 2006; Gill et al., 2009). The latter authors describe the case of a 53-year-old male with a history of colon cancer who had advanced putrefactive changes and multiple defects of the anterior torso that resembled stab wounds. It was found that he had had a transection of his colon about a year earlier.

The following case seen by the author of this text of a woman in her late 70s, demonstrates the difficulty faced by the police and the pathologist with decomposing cadavers, in assessing the status of some defects to ascertain whether they are ante-mortem wounds or caused after death. The deceased had lived alone and had not been seen for three weeks prior to discovery. Her apartment was secure and there was no disturbance in any of the rooms. She was found on the floor where she had apparently fallen from her bed. She was only wearing a pair of knickers. The police deemed the death to be non-suspicious and requested a routine coroner's autopsy. Once in the mortuary, the deceased was examined and found to have a vertical wound in the midline of the back of her neck. Her hands showed some loss of skin giving the appearance of wounds, which may have been defensive injuries, modified by decomposition and the widespread maggot infestation (Figure 12.25). Further questioning by the police of the undertakers who removed the body from the scene confirmed that the body was difficult to remove from the scene and they believed that they knocked her head and back against some objects as the body was being extracted. The autopsy did not confirm any deep injury to underlying muscle and no mark to the skull or cervical spine was found. She had died from ischaemic heart disease.

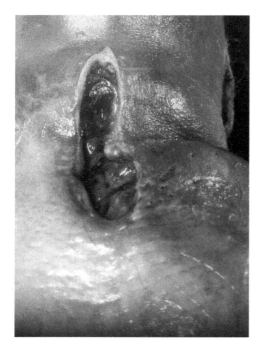

◀ **Figure 12.25a** Vertical wound at the back of the neck which has a central notch, a sharp pointed end uppermost and a blunted end lowermost. The dark discolouration around the wound could be misinterpreted as bruising.

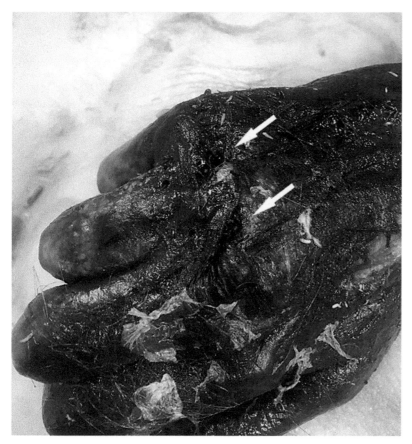

◀ **Figure 12.25b** Defects on the knuckles of the right hand (arrows).

263

In addition to artefacts produced in decomposing bodies, where ante-mortem sharp force wounds are present, these may be modified in shape, and any accompanying bruising may become diffuse or dissipated so that they are not visible (Figure 12.26).

## Insect and Larger Animal Predation

Insects and larger animals may alter ante-mortem wounds or produce artefacts resembling injuries. Careful evaluation is essential in such cases

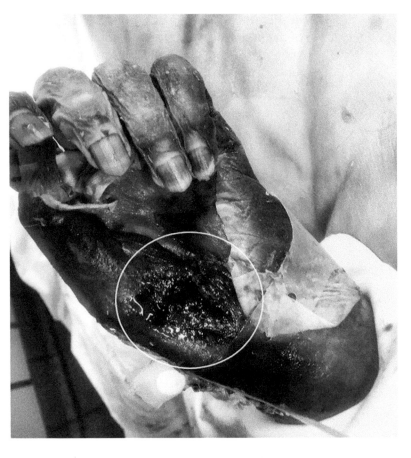

◀ **Figure 12.25c** Palm of left hand (circled) could be interpreted as defence injuries.

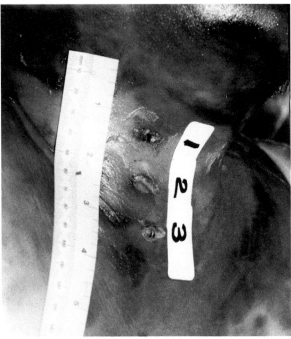

◀ **Figure 12.26a** Three stab wounds on the right side of the neck. They appear rounded and slightly modified by the effects of tissue autolysis during putrefaction.

(Viero et al., 2019) (Figure 12.27). It is particularly important to consider the opportunity for household pets in particular to gain access to the scene where the body is located. Other animals such as rodents may also access the body. Furthermore, if the body is easily accessible to the external environment other animals such as foxes may gain access. The teeth marks of animals need to be carefully examined and it may be appropriate to involve a dental specialist or veterinarian to assist if there is any doubt.

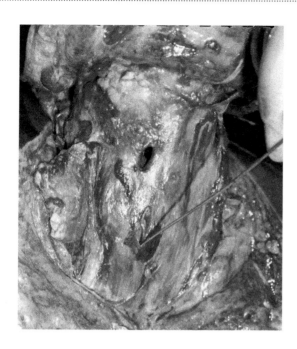

◀ **Figure 12.26b** Dissection of the neck shows three wounds which have become partly autolysed and any blood in the region has dispersed.

Rossi et al. (1994) reported four cases of wounds caused by pets (three by dogs and one by cats). There were a number of important common factors between these cases which included free movement of pets within the home, no available source of food within the home, social isolation of the deceased and having a predisposing condition causing sudden death.

A further case encountered by the author of the text (Figure 12.28) is of an elderly lady found deceased alone in her home. She lived on her own and had not been seen by her neighbours for three days. They called the police who gained entry and found her dead, sitting in an armchair in the lounge with her knickers torn and a small pool of blood under the chair. Although there was no sign of a disturbance in the room and the house was locked from the inside, the police were concerned at the fact that there were a number of injuries around her genitalia. Closer examination of the injuries confirmed that they were of animal origin rather than caused by human hand. The culprit appeared to be her pet cat that was discovered alive in the same room. Post-mortem examination revealed that she had died from the effects of ischaemic heart disease.

## Sharp Force Trauma in Burnt Victims

Disposal of a body by burning following homicide is not uncommon and the forensic pathologist should therefore take great care when conducting an autopsy in which the body has been burnt (Tümer et al., 2012). Wounds on the surface of the body may be difficult to see or may have been modified (Figure 12.29) and where charring has occurred may have been destroyed. Nevertheless, careful dissection of the body may reveal evidence of sharp force trauma, in bone and soft tissue and internal organs, which in most cases found in such circumstances are reasonably well preserved.

Modification of the appearance of sharp force trauma on bone after burning has been examined by Macoveciuc et al. (2017). They carried out experiments on burnt sheep radii and concluded that marks associated with sharp and blunt force trauma could be recognised and were not masked or destroyed by heat exposure. Their work demonstrates the need for careful analysis of burnt remains, particularly in scenarios where there has been an attempt to conceal trauma by burning.

## Embalmed Bodies

Pathologists should be aware that the post-mortem examination of an embalmed body may present difficulties in interpretation of findings because of the artefacts caused by the embalming procedure. Such a situation may occur in a number of different circumstance and in all manner of deaths where embalming has taken place prior to or after a post-mortem examination. Some deceased may have

265

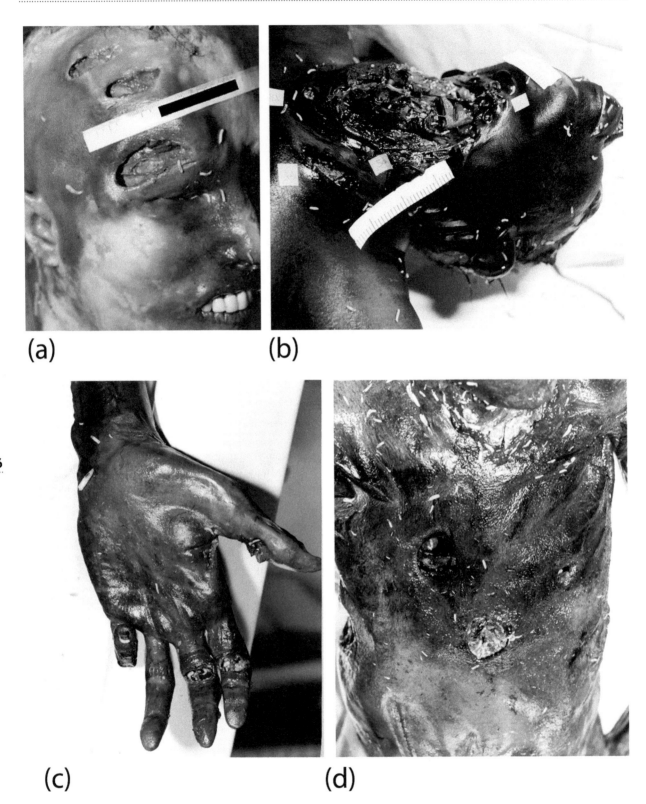

(a)

(b)

(c)

(d)

▲ **Figure 12.27** Examples of incised wounds showing rounding and enlarging of wounds with some loss of original features caused by larval action (fly maggot). (a) Stab wounds to head. (b) Incised neck wounds. (c) Defence wounds on left hand. (d) Trunk.

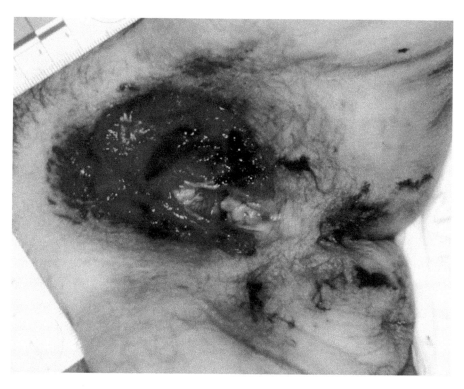

▲ **Figure 12.28** Genitalia showing large lacerated wound caused by the pet cat. Scratches are noted at the edge of the wounded area.

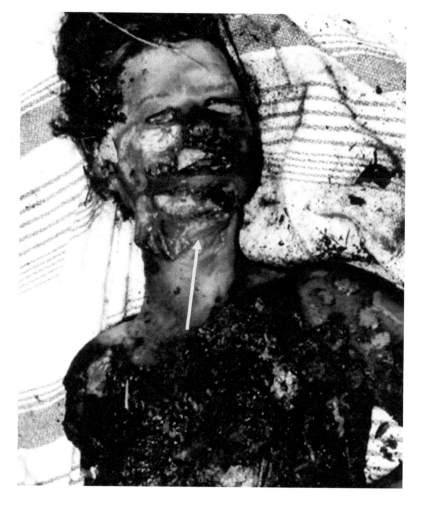

**Figure 12.29** Severely burnt young adult female who had been killed with incised wounds to her neck (arrow). The area where the wound was seen had been partially spared from burning because of flexion of the neck during the conflagration. There were no signs that she had been alive prior to the fire.

267

been repatriated from abroad and it should be borne in mind that embalming practices may vary in different countries.

In relation to cases where stab wounds are suspected or present, it is essential to take into account that cavity embalming involving the use of a trochar to produce numerous incisions in the thoracic and abdominal organs, may resemble wounds caused during life. Stab wounds on the skin surface may be obscured or modified by the application of cosmetics and their tracks altered and artificial ones produced (Opeskin 1992).

# Notes

1. For a detailed description of various aspects of dismemberment, including tool mark analysis, that are beyond the scope of this text, the reader is recommended to the following text: *Criminal Dismemberment—Forensic and Investigative Analysis* edited by Sue Black et al. CRC Press, Taylor and Francis Group, 2017.

2. He was an extreme puritan who was one of the Fifth Monarchists. He was also one of the signatories to Charles I death warrant in 1649. Shortly after the Restoration, he was found guilty of regicide and hanged, drawn and quartered in October 1660.

# References

Barington K, Jensen HE. (2017). Forensic aspects of incised wounds and bruises in pigs established post-mortem. *Res Vet Sci* 112, 42–45.

Betz P. (1994). Histological and enzyme histochemical parameters for the age estimation of human skin wounds. *Int J Legal Med* 107, 60–68.

Birincioğlu I, Akbaba M, Alver A, Kul S, Ozer E, Turan N, Sentürk A, Ince I. (2016). Determination of skin wound age by using cytokines as potential markers. *J Forensic Leg Med* 44, 14–19.

Blundell RH, Wilson GH (Eds.). (1950). *Trial of Buck Ruxton. Notable British Trials.* 2nd ed. London: William Hodge and Company. pp 155–156.

Byard RW, Gehl A, Anders S, Tsokos M. (2006). Putrefaction and wound dehiscence: a potentially confusing postmortem phenomenon. *Am J Forensic Med Pathol* 27, 61–63.

DiNunno N, Costantinides F, Vacca M, DiNunno C. (2006) Dismemberment: a review of the literature and description of 3 cases. *Am J Forensic Med Pathol* 27, 307–312.

Encyclopaedia Britannica. (2019). https://www.britannica.com/event/Rye-House-Plot (accessed 2019).

Gill JR, Cavalli DP, Ely SF. (2009). Pseudo-stab wounds: putrefactive dehiscence of remote surgical incisions masquerading as stab wounds *J Forensic Sci* 54, 1152–1154.

Glaister J, Brash JC. (1937). *Medico-legal aspects of the Ruxton case.* Livingstone: Edinburgh.

Grellner W, Madea B. (2007). Demands on scientific studies: vitality of wounds and wound age estimation. *Forensic Sci Int* 165, 150–154.

Kondo T. (2007). Timing of skin wounds. *Leg Med* 9, 109–114.

Macoveciuc I, Márquez-Grant N, Horsfall I, Zioupos P. (2017). Sharp and blunt force trauma concealment by thermal alteration in homicides: An in-vitro experiment for methodology and protocol development in forensic anthropological analysis of burnt bones. *Forensic Sci Intern*, 275, 260–271.

Martin P. (1997). Wound healing—aiming for perfect skin regeneration. *Science* 276, 75–81.

McGee MB, Coe JI. (1981). Postmortem wound dehiscence: a medicolegal masquerade. *J Forensic Sci* 26, 216–219.

Neri M, Fabbri M, D'Errico S, Di Paolo M, Frati P, Gaudio RM, La Russa R, Maiese A, Marti M, Pinchi E, Turillazzi E, Fineschi V. (2019). Regulation of miR-NAs as new tool for cutaneous vitality lesions demonstration in ligature marks in deaths by hanging. *Sci Rep* 9, 20011.

Oehmichen M. (2004). Vitality and time course of wounds. *Forensic Sci Int* 144, 221–231.

Opeskin K. (1992). An unusual injury. *Med Sci Law* 32, 58–60.

Pettigrew M. (2019). Corpse dismemberment and a necrofetishist. *J Forensic Sci* 64, 934–937.

Porta D, Amadasi A, Cappella A, Mazzarelli D, Magli F, Daniele Gibelli D, Rizzi A, Picozzi M, Gentilomo A, Cattaneo C. (2016). Dismemberment and disarticulation: a forensic anthropological approach. *J Forensic Leg Med* 38, 50–57.

Raekallio J. (1972). Determination of age of wounds by histochemical and biochemical methods. *Forensic Sci* 1, 3–7.

Raekallio J. (1973). Estimation of the age of injuries by histochemical and biochemical methods. *Z. Rechtsmed* 73, 83–102.

Rajs J, Lundstrom M, Broberg M, Lidberg L, Lindquist O. (1998). Criminal mutilation of the human body in Sweden—a thirty year medico-legal and forensic psychiatric study. *J Forensic Sci* 43, 563–580.

Rossi ML, Shahrom AW, Chapman RC, Vanezis P. (1994). Postmortem injuries by indoor pets. *Am J Forensic Med Pathol* 15, 105–109.

Rutty GN, Brough A, Biggs MJ, Robinson C, Lawes SD, Hainsworth SV. (2013). The role of micro-computed tomography in forensic investigations. *Forensic Sci Int* 225, 60–66.

Singer AJ, Clark RA. (1999). Cutaneous wound healing. *N Engl J Med* 341, 738–746.

Saukko P, Knight B. (2004). The pathology of wounds. In: P Saukko, B Knight (Eds.), *Knights forensic pathology*. London: Arnold. pp 136–173.

Symes, SA. (1992). Morphology of saw marks in human bone: identification of class. characteristics. Ph.D. Dissertation, Department of Anthropology, University of Tennessee, Knoxville, TN.

Symes, SA, Berryman HE, Smith OC. (1998) Saw marks in bone: introduction and examination of residual Kerf Contour. In: KJ Reichs (Ed.), *Forensic Osteology II, advances in the identification of human remains*. Springfield, IL: Charles C. Thomas. pp 333–352.

Symes SA, Chapman EN, Rainwater CW, Cabo LL, Myster SMT. (2010). Knife and saw toolmark analysis in bone: a manual designed for the examination of criminal mutilation and dismemberment. U.S. Department of Justice.

Tümer AR, Akçan R, Karacaoğlu E, Balseven-Odabaşı A, Keten A, Kanburoğlu C, Unal M, Dinç AH. (2012). Postmortem burning of the corpses following homicide. *J Forensic Leg Med* 19, 223–228.

Vaněrková H, Klír P, Jezková J, Fedorowiczová A. (1997). Detection of free histamine and serotonin in the evaluation of the vital reaction in injuries. *Soud Lek* 42, 39–42.

Viero A, Montisci M, Pelletti G, Vanin S. (2019). Crime scene and body alterations caused by arthropods: implications in death investigation. *Int J Legal Med* 133, 307–316.

**269**

# Chapter 13

# Iatrogenic, Needlestick and Other Related Sharp Force Trauma

## Introduction

In this chapter, we will focus on the mechanical and technical misadventures that can occur with any device or intervention that requires penetration into the patient via a needle or other sharpened implement, be it related directly to the sharp force trauma that can occur or from the sequelae of the use of the related device or procedure. The chapter will also deal with sharp force trauma from medical devices out with the healthcare setting i.e. in the instance of intravenous drug abuse, as well as discussing the exposure of healthcare providers to the occupation hazards of working with needles and other sharp implements.

## Therapeutic Misadventure – General Considerations

The range of therapeutic options available to modern-day clinicians to treat their patients is ever expanding. Despite the advances in sophisticated imaging modalities and non-invasive treatment options, the administration of therapeutic agents and the performance of diagnostic investigations in a number of medical and surgical specialties is still heavily reliant on gaining access to the vascular tree or viscera. Iatrogenic complications can occur both as a direct result of the insertion of sharpened instruments or as a result of the subsequent use and management of products after the initial access has been gained.

Langford defines therapeutic misadventure as an "adverse event caused by medical management rather than by an underlying disease" (Langford, 2010) The term in itself does not directly imply negligence on the part of the healthcare provider (although certainly negligence does play a role in some cases) but rather more the term encompasses the broader spectrum of harm that can be inadvertently caused to patients through their interaction with healthcare services, be they human or system error. On a broad level, errors can be subdivided into the following categories:

- *System errors* i.e. an error caused by poor infrastructure, communication channels, staffing levels or any other environmental and/or cultural factors in the workplace that make human error likely or even inevitable.

- *Mistakes* i.e. a failure to adequately plan for a particular situation, or an action or procedure that is undertaken without the necessary requisite knowledge.

- *Slips* i.e. an unobserved or unnoticed unintended action or error.

- *Lapses* i.e. an observed unintended action or error.

- *Lack of skill or technical error* i.e. an error occurring when a procedure or action is performed in the absence of adequate experience or training.

- *Violation of standard practise* i.e. deviating from best practise, usually to save time or due to convenience.

Iatrogenic therapeutic misadventure, in the absence of overt negligence or maleficence, can be caused by any of the error types described.

# Scope of the Problem

Medical misadventure as a whole has been well publicised to be the third leading cause of death per year in the USA (Heron, 2019; Makary and Daniel, 2016). Similarly, data from other developed Western countries including European Union member states, Canada and Australia estimates that hospital adverse events caused by medical misadventure occur in around 7.5–13.5% of all hospital admission and around 12% of all intensive care unit admissions (Aranaz et al., 2006; Baker et al., 2004; Darchy et al., 1999; Jackson et al., 2006; Levinson, 2010; Perla et al., 2013). The way these figures are collected and reported have been recently brought under sharp scrutiny (Shojania and Dixon-Woods, 2017); nevertheless, the problem remains real and ever present. With regard to the data pertaining specifically to procedures, investigations or treatments which require the insertion of an intravascular or other intra-visceral devices, the data is less robust but data available from Sweden and the USA pertaining to iatrogenic vascular injuries suggests it is a growing problem (Giswold et al., 2004; Rudström et al., 2008).

# Complications from Inserting Intravascular Lines or Sheaths

## Indication for Intravenous Access

Intravenous access is the cornerstone for a myriad diagnostic and treatment options in both the outpatient and inpatient hospital setting. The vast majority of intravenous access devices are smaller bore peripheral cannulas, usually sited in the upper limbs and ranging from 14 to 26 gauge. The cannulas are usually self-contained proprietary products that are inserted over a needle. Once access is obtained into the vein, the needle introducer is removed and the plastic catheter remains indwelling. These catheters allow for the administration of fluids, medications, nutrition, blood products and diagnostic contrast or stress agents (e.g. for use in magnetic resonance imaging [MRI], computed tomography [CT] and nuclear imaging) as well as allowing for intermittent and regular blood sampling.

Larger bore or central venous access become necessary in some cases, usually in the inpatient setting however some exceptions occur (for example patients with end-stage renal failure with long-term central access in situ). Access can be gained via the Seldinger technique (described later) or via surgical cut-down. The most common sites for central venous access include the internal jugular veins, subclavian veins, axillary veins and common femoral veins. The author observed, as a coincidental finding unrelated to the patient's death, a broken needle in an elderly person from attempted access into the left femoral vein (Figure 13.1).

Depending on the indication for access, cannulas can range from 2.7 French (F) in paediatrics to greater than 25 F for some venous sheaths in adults. Large-bore intravenous access can be gained for short or longer-term indwelling central catheters or as a conduit to perform certain procedures.

Typical short-term indwelling catheters are used for the administration of inotropic or vasopressor agents or certain therapeutics that can be necrotoxic or caustic in the case of extravasation (e.g. amiodarone), when emergency intravenous access is required, for nutritional support, to perform haemodialysis, to monitor central venous pressure, to allow regular blood sampling or to allow the passage of a temporary pacing wire to the right ventricle or a pulmonary artery catheter to monitor pulmonary arterial or wedge pressures. Larger bore access to the venous system is also required in some forms of mechanical circulatory support such as venous to venous (VV) or venous to arterial (VA) extracorporeal membrane oxygenation (ECMO) as well as cardiopulmonary bypass during cardiac surgery.

Typical longer-term indwelling catheters are often tunnelled under the skin to reduce the risk of infection and for greater comfort to the patient and are used for regular haemodialysis, the administration of long-term therapeutic agents such as antibiotics or chemotherapy agents, bone marrow transplantation and long-term nutritional support.

Temporary venous access (via venous sheaths) is also gained for a number of procedures including right heart catheterisation, placement of right heart

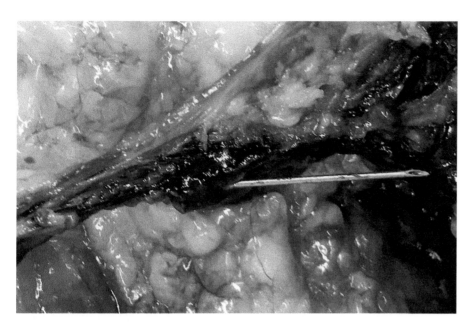

◀ **Figure 13.1** Broken needle (gauge 20) in an elderly female who had died from an unrelated cause. The vein has been lacerated and there is extensive surrounding soft tissue haemorrhage. (Source: Author)

support devices such as the Impella RP® and insertion of leadless pacemakers in the right ventricle.

## Indication for Intra-arterial Access

Intra-arterial access has a more limited indication than intra-venous access. Smaller sized indwelling cannulas can provide continuous arterial pressure monitoring as well as frequent arterial blood sampling and are commonly cited in the radial or femoral arteries. Furthermore, a number of procedures are carried out via sheath insertion with sheath sizes varying from 4 F to over 20 F.

Commonly performed procedures performed via smaller bore access sites such as the radial and ulnar artery include coronary catheterisation and coronary angioplasty and via larger bore access sites such as the femoral, iliac, subclavian or axillary arteries include transcatheter aortic valve implantation (TAVI), the placement of certain circulatory support devices such as intra-aortic balloon pumps (IABP), left-sided Impella support devices, complex coronary angioplasty procedures and endovascular arterial repair procedures. In some settings, intra-arterial access can also be used to administer certain pharmacotherapies.

## Seldinger Technique

Surgical cut-down to gain access to the vascular tree allows for direct visualisation of the vessel and was the predominant method of vascular access in the first half of the twentieth century. Despite this invasive technique having been superseded in many

areas in favour of the Seldinger technique (original and modified), it is still the preferred method of vascular of visceral access in some settings, for example for central arterial and venous access in VA-ECMO, after failed peripheral access attempts to the vasculature or the insertion of large-bore chest drains into the pleural cavity using blunt dissection. The Seldinger technique can also be used to gain access to the thoracic and abdominal cavities in a similar fashion to that described for vascular access.

The Seldinger technique, as first described by Sven-Ivar Seldinger in 1953, allows the insertion of a wire through a hollow needle which has punctured the vessel or cavity space (Figure 13.2). The needle is removed and over the wire within the desired space, a catheter or sheath is introduced and then the wire removed (Higgs et al., 2005). The modified Seldinger technique, which applies more specially to vascular access, has adapted the original principle but avoids the back wall puncture of the vessel with the puncture needle (so-called through and through) and has been shown in a number of arenas to be non-inferior to the original Seldinger technique in terms of procedural success rates with reduced vascular complication rates such as bleeding and vascular injury (Lee et al., 2015; Song et al., 2018; Warrington et al., 2012).

One of the major drawbacks of the Seldinger technique is the lack of direct visualisation of the vessel or cavity space to which access is being obtained. The use of adjunctive ultrasound has greatly mitigated this problem; however, various complications can

273

## SVEN IVAR SELDINGER

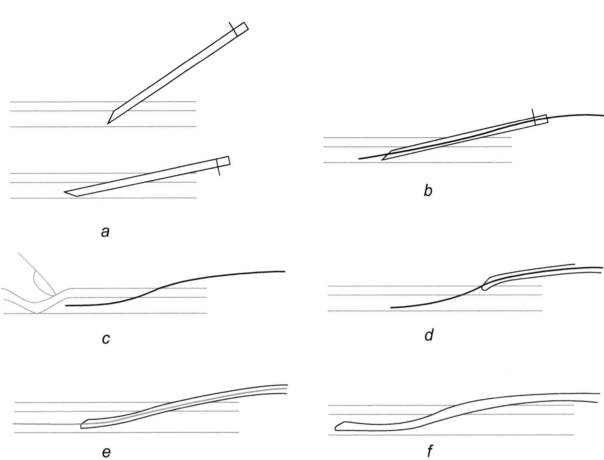

▲ **Figure 13.2** Original technique described by Seldinger. (a) Arterial puncture with needle. (b) Wire insertion. (c) Needle removal and compression over puncture site. (d) Catheter threaded onto wire. (e) Catheter placed into vessel over the wire. (f) Wire removed (Adapted from Seldinger, S. I. (1953). Catheter Replacement of the Needle in Percutaneous Arteriography: A new technique. Acta Radiologica, 39(5), 368–376.).

occur at multiple stages of the procedure (Moore, 2014). The first and most obvious complication is failed access to the desired site. If this goes unnoticed, the introduction of catheters and sheaths can cause significant damage to surrounding structures. The puncture needle itself can inadvertently puncture surrounding structures; however, recognition of the fact before insertion of catheters and sheaths greatly reduces the potential for harm. In the case of attempted vascular access, puncture of both vein and artery can cause a tract between the two structures which can lead to the development of arterio-venous malformations. If care is not taken, access to the venous rather than the arterial space or vice-versa can occur if imaging, pressure waveform testing or blood gas sampling is not performed, leading to a potential number of misadventures, the most

serious being inadvertent drug or fluid administration into the arterial system after attempted venous cannulation. Guide wire embolisation is also a serious complication of the Seldinger technique and care must be taken by the operator at all times to ensure control of the wire to avoid embolisation as such an event usually requires surgical intervention to remove the embolised wire (Figure 13.3) (Schummer et al., 2002).

Delayed complications included pseudoaneurysm formation, which can also occur after arterial access is gained, especially in patients with larger body mass indices who are heavily anticoagulated during the procedure and require larger sheath insertion sizes. The management of pseudoaneurysms vary greatly depending on the site and size and

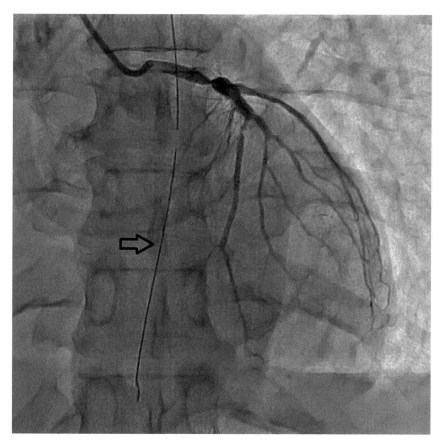

▲ **Figure 13.3** Guidewire embolisation after femoral central venous line insertion. Fluoroscopic images performed during subsequent coronary angiography in this patient demonstrated a free floating central line insertion wire in the super vena cava, highlighted by the arrow. This required surgical removal. Courtesy of Dr Neil Brass, CK Hui Heart Centre.

management includes a conservative approach with manual compression to seal the neck of the

pseudoaneurysm, thrombin injection or interventional or surgical repair(Stone et al., 2014).

# Air Embolisation

When air is introduced into the circulatory system, it forms bubbles in the liquid blood due to surface tension. The accidental introduction of a small volume of air into the venous system after access has been obtained i.e. approximately less than 3–5ml/kg in adults (Mirski et al., 2007), usually has minimal or no serious sequelae. Larger volumes of air in the venous system can lead to pulmonary obstruction and ventilation/perfusion mismatch and respiratory collapse. Furthermore only air bubbles less than ~20μm are able to cross capillary membranes in the lungs into the arterial system. Larger bubbles eventually dissipate in the venous circulation. However, a passage can be gained to the arterial system in the presence of a shunt allowing for paradoxical embolisation of air.

More prevalent shunts include arteriovenous malformation in the lungs or liver or a patent foramen ovale (PFO) or atrial septal defect (ASD) in the heart.

When air bubbles are introduced into the arterial system, either directly through arterial access or indirectly through venous access and across a venous to arterial shunt, the bubbles can quickly become lodged in organ capillary networks leading to end-organ ischaemia if there is inadequate collateral blood supply to that organ. The clinical manifestations of arterial air embolisation clearly are related to the organ(s) affected, for example cerebral embolisation can lead to stroke symptoms and/or seizures whereas coronary embolisation can lead to chest pain and/or cardiac arrest. As well as mechanically induced end-organ dysfunction, air bubbles can also stimulate a cytokine-mediated systemic inflammatory response (Kapoor et al., 2003).

In a case series of 67 patients where air embolisation was identified by searching through the hospital records of a single US centre over 25 years, the most common causes identified for this event included

central venous line placement and removal, cardiac surgery, neurosurgery and bronchoscopic Nd:YAG laser procedures (McCarthy et al., 2017). As the size of the air bubbles is inversely proportional to the higher the atmospheric pressure, the mainstay of treatment includes the use of hyperbaric oxygen therapy to reduce the size of the bubbles in the circulation and attempt to relieve any mechanical obstructions in the vasculature (Leach et al., 1998).

# Iatrogenic Perforation

Perforation is a broad term and in this section is used to mean the creation of a hole or communication through the walls of viscera in the body. Whilst it commonly used to describe perforations of the gastrointestinal tract caused by surgery, iatrogenic induced perforations can also be encountered in the vasculature and thoracic cavities, each of which will be dealt with separately in the following sections.

## Gastrointestinal Tract Perforations

One of the main arenas in which inadvertent iatrogenic perforation is a major cause of morbidity and mortality is surgery or instrumentation of the gastrointestinal tract, in which perforation can lead to bleeding, infection and subsequent sepsis, shock, delayed wound healing, fistula formations or hernias. Procedures that may cause iatrogenic perforation include open or laparoscopic abdominal surgery, upper gastrointestinal endoscopy (including transoesophageal echocardiography), colonoscopy, sigmoidoscopy, stent placement within the gastrointestinal tract, sclerotherapy, oesophageal dilatation, nasogastric tube insertion, abdominal drain insertion, peritoneal dialysis and the insertion of percutaneous feeding tubes (Covarrubias et al., 2013; Ghahremani et al., 1980; Nassour and Fang, 2015; Schmitz et al., 2001).

Anastomotic leaks after intestinal anastomosis are a particular fear for surgeons in the post-operative period (Hyman et al., 2007). After closure of the surgical wound, the manifestation of an intra-abdominal perforation can often times be delayed with non-specific presentation hence vigilance is required after surgery to monitor for the first signs of a complication. Hecker et al. (2015) suggested in a small randomised trial that identification of intestinal

perforation and early intervention to avoid sepsis decreases mortality.

Another site of perforation with a high incidence of mortality is the oesophagus. Pooled data suggests a mortality rate of between 12 and 19% (Paspatis et al., 2014; Tullavardhana, 2015) as well as an associated increase in hospital stay. Treatment options include surgical exclusion and diversion, oesophagectomy or endoscopic approaches such as clips or stents (Figure 13.4).

The management of iatrogenic gastrointestinal perforation relies on prompt diagnosis and is based on the detection of free gas (pneumoperitoneum or pneumomediastinum), gastrointestinal fluids or faeces within the abdominal or thoracic cavity or the mediastinum, depending on the section of the tract involved. Common diagnostic tests include erect chest X-ray and abdominal CT scanning (Figure 13.5). In some situations, specific organ imaging is required, e.g. water-soluble contrast studies to detect oesophageal perforation. On occasions, exploratory laparoscopic or open surgery is required to identify the site of the perforation and facilitate repair. Depending on the site and severity of the perforation, management approaches can vary from conservative (including nutritional support and fluid management), medical (including the use of antibiotics), percutaneous drainage and open surgical repair.

## Tracheal and Airway Perforations

Iatrogenic perforation of the trachea can occur as a consequence of endotracheal intubation or bronchoscopy. It is more common in women, people over the age of 50 and of short stature (Minambres et al., 2009) and can lead to surgical emphysema, respiratory distress and haemoptysis, although the

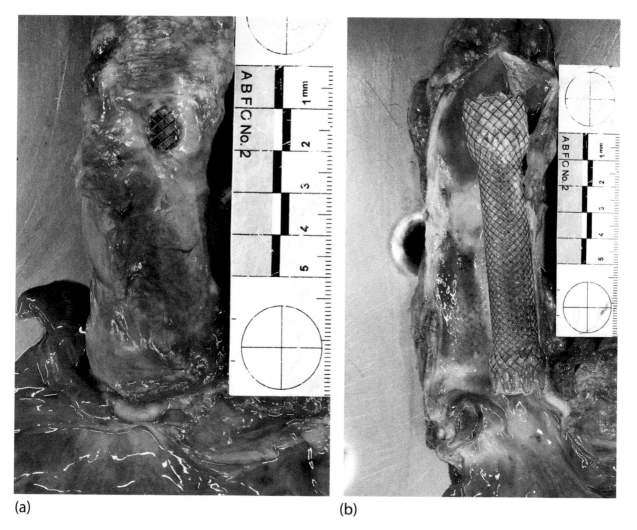

(a)                         (b)

▲ **Figure 13.4** Oesophageal perforation in an elderly patient which occurred during oesophagoscopy to investigate a stricture. (a) External view of perforation which has been stented. (b) Oesophagus opened showing stent.

overall pooled mortality rates are low at around 0.005% (Borasio et al., 1997). With regard to endo-tracheal intubation, perforation can occur directly from blunt tip trauma, over inflation of the balloon cuff or by vigorous movement of an already placed tube whilst in situ (Jougon et al., 2000). In addition, adjuncts used to aid in airway intubation such as introducers, gum-elastic bougies and stylets can also directly cause perforation (Evans et al., 2015). Iatrogenic perforation from endotracheal tubes typically occurs from blunt trauma which causes longitudinal tears to the posterior part of the trachea as it lacks cartilaginous support (Figure 13.6) (Lobato et al., 1997).

Fibre-optic bronchoscopy is regarded as the gold standard for the diagnosis of suspected tracheal or upper airway perforations and can pinpoint the exact location of the lesion. Depending on the size and location of the lesion, treatment can be conservative or may require surgical repair (Minambres et al., 2009). Bronchoscopy itself can result in perforations below the level of the main bronchi and can lead to pneumomediastinum and/or pneumothorax. The incidence is significantly increased with transbronchial biopsy with a reported incidence of perforation of 4% in a large retrospective study (Pue and Pacht, 1995).

## Vascular Perforations

The indications for vascular access and more general complications that can ensue with these procedures have been described in an earlier section. This

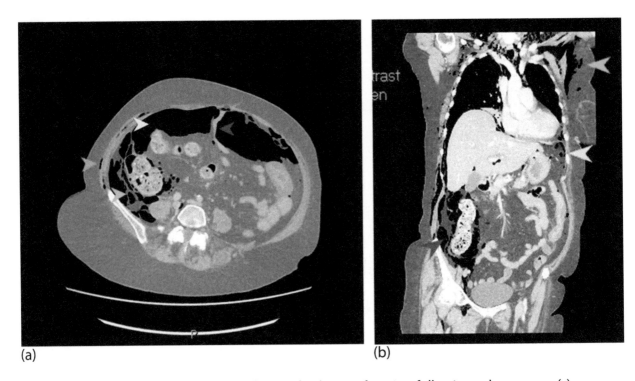

(a)                                                              (b)

▲ **Figure 13.5** CT scans showing evidence of colon perforation following colonoscopy. (a) Cross-sectional slice of abdominal CT. Intraperitoneal free air (pneumoperitoneum) is visible (yellow arrow), delineating the inferior aspect of the falciform ligament at its attachment to anterior abdominal wall (red arrow). Locules of gas are seen surrounding the ascending colon and extending into both the retroperitoneum and the mesentery (green arrow). Subcutaneous gas (surgical emphysema) is also visible superficial to and within the muscles of anterior abdominal wall (blue arrow). (b) Coronal view of thoraco-abdominal CT showing intraperitoneal free air (pneumoperitoneum, yellow arrow), retroperitoneal free air (red arrow) and subcutaneous gas (surgical emphysema) extending into the upper chest wall (green arrow) is evident. (Courtesy of Mr James Park, University of Glasgow).

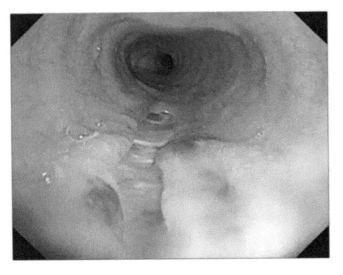

◀ **Figure 13.6** Diagnostic bronchoscopy demonstrating an iatrogenic posterior membranous wall laceration of the trachea. (Lim, H., Kim, J. H., Kim, D., Lee, J., Son, J. S., Kim, D. C., & Ko, S. (2012). Tracheal rupture after endotracheal intubation - A report of three cases. Korean journal of anesthesiology, 62(3), 277–280; used with permission and courtesy of the *Korean Journal of Anesthesiology*)

section will focus specifically on the perforating vascular injuries that can occur. Rather than serving as a panacea for all the perforating injuries described in the literature, we have concentrated on some of the more commonly performed procedures with well-described incidence of such complications and discuss any specific nuances to diagnosis and management for each procedure.

*Femoral Arterial Access and Retroperitoneal Haemorrhage*

Femoral arterial access is used for a number of cardiac, coronary, vascular and neuro-interventional procedures. Anatomical land marks and the use of fluoroscopy and ultrasound are commonly used to aim for a puncture above the bifurcation of the profunda and superficialis branches of the common femoral artery and below the inferior border of the inferior epigastric artery (Feldman, 2014).

High puncture sticks with back wall puncture run the risk of a retroperitoneal haemorrhage as the common femoral artery dives deep into the pelvis above the level of the inferior epigastric artery. The rates of retroperitoneal haemorrhage have fallen in the United Kingdom during percutaneous coronary interventional (PCI) procedures from 0.09% to 0.03% between 2007 and 2014, but this is mainly driven by a significant shift in performing PCI procedures via the radial artery (Kwok et al., 2018). Nevertheless the authors of this review demonstrated a three-fold increase in mortality and a five-fold increase in adverse cardiovascular outcomes with retroperitoneal haemorrhage and this is relevant to procedures where femoral access remains the norm, such as TAVI. Compression of the bleeding in high punctures is not possible due to the location in the pelvis and hence management involves fluid and/or blood resuscitation and often requires vascular or interventional techniques, such as covered stents, to stop the bleeding.

*Coronary Artery Perforation during Percutaneous Coronary Intervention (PCI)*

Coronary artery perforation (CAP) can occur during diagnostic coronary angiography but more frequently during PCI. The overall rates of CAP have previously been reported to be as high as 1% in PCI procedures but more recently data from the UK analysing 28,537 PCI procedures demonstrated a perforation rate of 0.36% (Guttmann et al., 2016). The risk of perforation is greater in more complex procedures, especially in chronic total occlusion PCI where perforation rates have been reported at 2.9% (Patel et al., 2013). CAP is also associated with female sex, complex and tortuous coronary anatomy, increasing age and aggressive sizing and dilatation of coronary balloons and stents, as well as the use of adjunctive devices such as rotational and orbital atherectomy (Shimony et al., 2011). Coronary perforation can be categorised into three classes according to severity (Ellis et al., 1994) (Figures 13.7 and 13.8). In a large cohort analysis by Lemmert et al. (2017) the 30-day mortality following CAP was 10.7%.

Cardiac tamponade is the most feared consequence of CAP and can rapidly lead to cardiac arrest. The focus on treatment in this setting is sealing the perforation with the use of prolonged balloon inflations, the placement of covered stents or the deployment of vascular coils, embolisation of fat or the injection of thrombin. The rapid insertion of a pericardial drain is also often required. In some situation, emergency surgery may be needed to alleviate the tamponade. Previous conventional wisdom dictated that CAP in the context of previous coronary artery bypass surgery (CABG) was relatively benign as much of the pericardium is stripped away during the operation. In fact, recent data has shown that CAP after previous CABG can present significant problems due to pericardial adhesions formed in much of the pericardium that was left behind after CABG which can lead to loculated effusions which can be challenging to detect using transthoracic echocardiography and difficult to drain percutaneously. In such patients, Kinnaird et al. (2017) demonstrated a one-year post-event -dds ratio of excess mortality of 1.35 in the CAP after CABG group compared with matched survivors without a CAP.

*Pulmonary Artery Perforation during Right Heart Catheterisation*

Pulmonary artery catheterisation has a number of indications including the diagnosis and characterisation of pulmonary hypertension, shunt assessment, the provision of pre-surgical assessment information to calculate valve disease severity and for the continuous monitoring of critically ill patients with cardiogenic shock. Typically, a Swan-Ganz catheter is placed (varying from 4-8F) via the femoral vein or large vein in the antecubital fossa (typically the medical cubital vein) and advanced across the tricuspid valve into

279

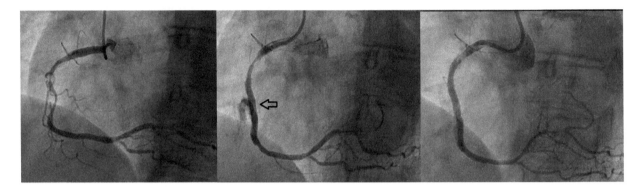

▲ **Figure 13.7** Ellis classification of coronary perforations. Grade I. No extravasation but extra-luminal, usually indicative of a contained dissection. Grade II. Blush of contrast into the pericardium or myocardium without an overt jet. Grade III. Frank perforation with extravasation of contrast, usually through a hole ≥ 1mm. Adapted from Rogers and Lassa (2004)

▲ **Figure 13.8** Grade 2 perforation of the proximal right coronary artery in a patient after insertion of a drug-eluting stent. Left panel shows the pre-PCI angiogram. Middle panel shows the perforation and extravasation of contrast immediately after stent insertion where contrast can be seen in the myocardium (arrow). This was treated with two covered stents to seal the perforation with the final angiogram shown in the right panel. Courtesy of Dr Andrew Vanezis, Trent Cardiac Centre, Nottingham.

the right ventricle and up into one of the pulmonary arteries. Many catheters have a balloon tip to allow access across the tricuspid valve and also facilitate obtaining a pulmonary capillary wedge pressure when placed deep into the pulmonary arterial system. It is at this juncture that the risk of pulmonary arterial haemorrhage can take place. Whilst a rare complication with an incidence of up to 0.2% of all cases, the mortality has been reported to be as high as 70% in the literature (Schramm et al., 2009). Associated risk factors include chronic obstructive pulmonary disease (COPD), pre-existing pulmonary hypertension, the use of anticoagulation, female sex and advancing age (Hoeper et al., 2006; Kearney and Shabot, 1995).

The mechanism of pulmonary haemorrhage during right heart catheterisation is usually either by over advancement of the catheter too distally with significant manipulation whilst trying to obtain a wedge pressure or by over inflation of the balloon tip of the catheter whilst in the end arteriolar space. Typically, patients present with haemoptysis, a decline in

oxygen saturations and rapid circulatory collapse. Emergent treatment includes the reversal of heparin and replacement of blood loss with blood products and fluids followed by attempts to stop the bleeding, either by percutaneous embolisation of the affected pulmonary arteriole or stent graft placement. Surgical intervention may be required if massive haemothorax has developed. A pulmonary artery false aneurysm (PAFA) has been reported to occur in around 25% of survivors of pulmonary arterial rupture and haemorrhage which can lead to subsequently fatal bleeding in the future and usually mandates closure (Boyd et al., 1983; Sirivella et al., 2001).

*Transcatheter Aortic Valve Implantation (TAVI)*
The indications and role for TAVI are evolving and with the recent publication of two large non-inferiority trials of TAVI compared to surgical aortic valve replacements in low-risk patient groups with severe aortic stenosis, the number of TAVI procedures is likely to increase dramatically worldwide over

the next few years (Mack et al., 2019; Popma et al., 2019). The majority of TAVI procedures are now performed via the femoral artery using 14F sheaths. As well as the traditional complication associated with femoral arterial access as described earlier in this chapter, there are some vascular complications that can occur more readily in this procedure due to the patient demographic, size of sheath involved and arterial site closure techniques. The use of stiff 0.035" diameter guidewires to aid valve deployment can lead to left ventricular (LV) perforation or damage of the mitral valve or subvalvular apparatus causing mitral regurgitation. The likelihood of LV perforation increases with a smaller cavity size, when the LV is hypercontractile with a thin muscular wall and if there is a narrow angle between the aortic and mitral valve (Owais et al., 2017). The advent of specialised guidewire with coiled tips and protocols to minimise the time the guidewire spends in the LV cavity has helped reduce the incidence of this complication (Nielsen et al., 2019).

Dissection of the aorta during valve or sheath manipulation can occur throughout any part of the aorta and is often fatal. The incidence has been up to 1.9% in some series (Thomas et al., 2010). Concurrent transoesophageal echocardiography can aid in the diagnosis but a high index of suspicion is required in the context of chest or abdominal pain and an unexplained drop in blood pressure during the procedure. Treatment includes strict blood pressure control and in the context of Type A dissections, prompt surgical or endovascular repair. Another vascular complication feared by TAVI operators is that of ileal-femoral dissection when attempting to pass the initial delivery system or when attempting to withdraw the sheath. The incidence of this complication has been reported as high as 7% and can lead to significant dissection or perforation which can compromise lower limb vascular run-off directly or lead to thrombus formation and vessel closure sub-acutely (Chaudhry and Sardar, 2017). Depending on the degree and nature of the vascular injury, treatment can vary from medical management with anticoagulation, endovascular repair with ballooning +/- stenting or open surgical repair. Sudden haemodynamic compromise during TAVI may suggest ileal-femoral rupture and if prompt endovascular techniques fail (often from the contralateral femoral artery), emergent surgical repair is required (Mussardo et al., 2011).

Finally, at the end of the TAVI procedure, the removal of the large femoral sheath has the potential to cause significant haematoma and vascular compromise, even with prolonged manual pressure. Contemporary practice is to close the larger arteriotomy site with either two Perclose ProGlide® (Abbott Laboratories, Chicago, IL, USA) suture-based closure devices or one Manta (Essential Medical Inc., USA) collagen-based vascular plug (Figure 13.9). The use of these devices has significantly reduced the rates of haematomas and vascular bleeding complications. There is conflicting data as to which device is the safest but it is clear that their safety profile is in part reliant on operator experience and patient selection (Biancari et al., 2018; Hoffmann et al., 2018).

## Chest Drain Insertion and Thoracic Injury

There are numerous clinical scenarios that necessitate the insertion of an intercostal drain into the thoracic cavity including for the treatment of pneumothoraces or haemothoraces, large or loculated pleural effusions and empyemas. It can also be inserted to perform pleurodesis, alleviate surgical emphysema and is placed routinely following thoracic surgery. Larger bore traditional drains are placed using either blunt dissection or with the aid of a trocar. The trocar technique is associated with a higher rate of complications (John et al., 2014). Some of the more common injuries associated with larger chest drain insertion include intercostal arterial injury, insertion of the tube or trocar into the lung parenchyma (Figure 13.10) or a misdirection of the tube into other mediastinal structures such as heart or diaphragm or extrathoracic structures such as abdominal organs. A Canadian analysis of residents placing large bore chest drains in trauma patients demonstrated an overall complication rate of 16%, of which 7% involves an intercostal arterial laceration and 3% involved a lung parenchymal placement (Ball et al., 2007).

More recently (except in cases of trauma) there has been a move from a larger surgical style chest drain to smaller 10–12F Seldinger drains. This removes the need for the trocar and penetrating injuries that can occur as a result of its use. However, some studies suggest that the risks of iatrogenic injuries remain high in the hands of inexperienced operators. Indeed, damage to the intercostal artery, puncture

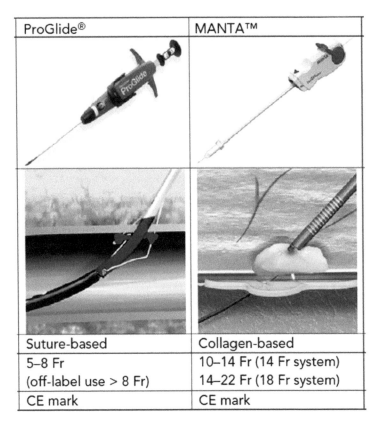

| ProGlide® | MANTA™ |
|---|---|
| Suture-based | Collagen-based |
| 5–8 Fr | 10–14 Fr (14 Fr system) |
| (off-label use > 8 Fr) | 14–22 Fr (18 Fr system) |
| CE mark | CE mark |

◀ **Figure 13.9** New Large-bore Vascular Closure devices and techniques. a. Perclose Proglide® device. b. Manta™ closure device. (Source Abbott Medical and Teleflex.)

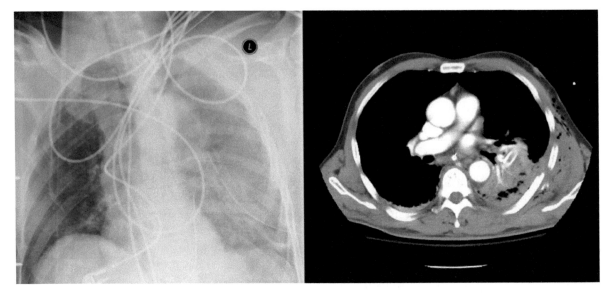

▲ **Figure 13.10** Chest drain insertion into the lung parenchyma. Left panel shows a chest x-ray after attempted drain insertion in the left thoracic space. The right panel shows the tube in the lung parenchyma with associated haemorrhage. (Ball, C. G., Lord, J., Laupland, K. B., Gmora, S., Mulloy, R. H., Ng, A. K., Schieman, C., Kirkpatrick, A. W. (2007). Chest tube complications: how well are we training our residents? *Canadian Journal of Surgery. Journal Canadien de Chirurgie*, 50(6), 450–458; used with permission and courtesy the *Canadian Journal of Surgery*)

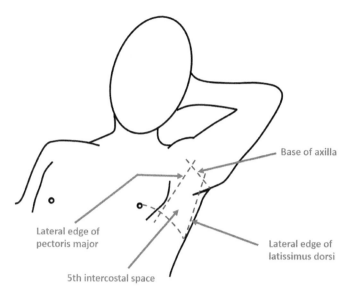

◀ **Figure 13.11** Safe triangle for insertion of chest drains to minimise the possibility of iatrogenic injury. The drain should be inserted above the rib with the use of ultrasound if available. Adapted from the British Thoracic Society pleural diseases guidelines (Davies et al., 2010)

Base of axilla

Lateral edge of pectoris major

Lateral edge of latissimus dorsi

5th intercostal space

of major vessel or instrumentation of parenchyma of the lung or other thoracic or abdominal organs can still occur (Maskell et al., 2010). Many of these issues can be mitigated by the use of ultrasound to guide equipment insertion as well as locating the insertion site for the chest drain (if feasible) in the so-called safe triangle (Figure 13.11). The introduction of kits with shorter dilators and adequate training for those inserting the drains have also reduced the rates of complications (Laws et al., 2003).

# Needle Stick Injuries

Needle stick injuries (NSIs) are an ever-present occupational hazard for healthcare workers. The World Health Organisation (WHO) Report in 2007 estimated that each year 2 million healthcare workers experience a NSI from a sharp object such as a needle, scalpel or broken glass vial that has been contaminated with the patient's blood or other bodily fluid that could expose them to infectious diseases (Pruss-Ustun et al., 2005).

The most commonly transmitted blood borne virus is hepatitis B (HBV), for which an immunisation exists and is routinely recommended (if not mandated) for healthcare workers at risk of NSIs (Lewis et al., 2015). However, a number of other serious diseases can be transmitted for which no vaccine exists including human immunodeficiency virus (HIV), hepatitis C (HCV), malaria and syphilis. It is for these reasons that healthcare systems must ensure rigorous procedures are in place to minimise the likelihood of NSIs as well as making sure that if an NSI does occur, the healthcare worker has access to prompt and effective post-exposure prophylaxis (PEP) to minimise the risk of the disease developing. The risks of infection

to the healthcare worker after an NSI with a contaminated sharp is ~0.3% for HIV, 3% for HCV and up to 10% for HBV if not vaccinated (Pruss-Ustun et al., op .cit.). The risk of HIV transmission can be as high as 5% if the healthcare worker sustains a deep wound, the patient has a high viral load or a device has been used to access the vasculature directly (Ippolito et al., 1999). Healthcare workers who have particular risk of NSIs, such as surgeons, can reduce the chance of disease transmission by other simple measures such as double gloving or using tools that are not blunted or overly re-used (Hasak et al., 2018).

Factors that increase the risk of NSIs occurring including a lack of specific training pertaining to the correct handling of sharps and needles, re-sheathing needles into their original plastic housing, needles without engineered safety containment devices including retractable needles and auto disposable syringes (Figure 13.12), a lack of sharps disposable bins or containers and poor practice between healthcare workers including passing needles or sharps and picking up suture sharps with fingers rather than instruments.

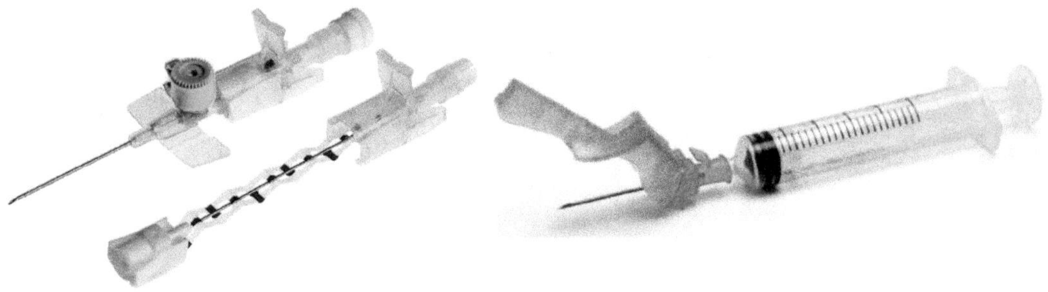

▲ **Figure 13.12** On the left is the BD Vacutainer®, an example of a propriety IV cannula with a lock mechanism that encapsulates the needle tip after the cannula has been placed. On the right is an example of an injection needle the BD Eclipse™ with a lock mechanism attached to the needle itself (used with permission and courtesy of BD Medical UK).

NSIs also pose a significant risk to some non-healthcare workers. One significant source of NSI in the community come about through home administered needle-based therapies, both through mishandling of the syringes by the user or care giver and subsequently by inappropriate disposal. In the United States, the Coalition for Safe Community Needle Disposal estimated that there were more than 7.5 billion medical syringes in the community in the country (Gold, 2011).

# Recreational Intravenous Drug Use

Intravenous recreational drug use is associated with significant morbidity and mortality. This is in a large part related to high rates of drug overdose, serious psychiatric disorders and homelessness, but is also heavily influenced by increased rates of blood-borne viruses such as HIV and HCV from risk-tolerant behaviours such as needle sharing and multiple injections as well as increased rates of bacterial and fungal infections and thromboembolic events (Bruneau, et al., 2012). This section will discuss the scope of the problem and focus on the more frequent as well as rarer but more serious medical sequelae that can ensue from this behaviour.

## Scope of the Problem

Current research suggests that in the Western world at least, the use of recreational intravenous drug use had declined over the last 2 decades, although the numbers have plateaued in recent years and indeed there has been an increase in those aged 15–29 (Kraus et al., 2003; Mathers et al., 2008). Mathers et al., who performed a systematic review of intravenous drug use from all available literature around the world in 2008, estimated that there were between 11 and 21 million intravenous drug users at that time, of which they estimated approximately 3 million are HIV positive. This review does not take into account sub-Saharan Africa and a number of other developing world countries where economic and social conditions may point towards even higher rates of intravenous drug use (Figure 13.13).

## Soft Tissue and Dermatological Infections

IV drug abuse is frequently associated with local complications around the site of injection. Predisposing factors to the development of such sequelae include poor self-hygiene, needle reuse, the sharing of needles and accessory equipment such as cooking devices or cotton filters, the repeated use of the same injection site and poor injection technique with injections into the subcutaneous tissue or muscle (Ebright and Pieper, 2002). Local site complications remain the commonest reason for hospitalisation in this group and at any one time it is estimated that around a third of IV drug users are affected by some form of soft tissue infection (Binswanger et al., 2000).

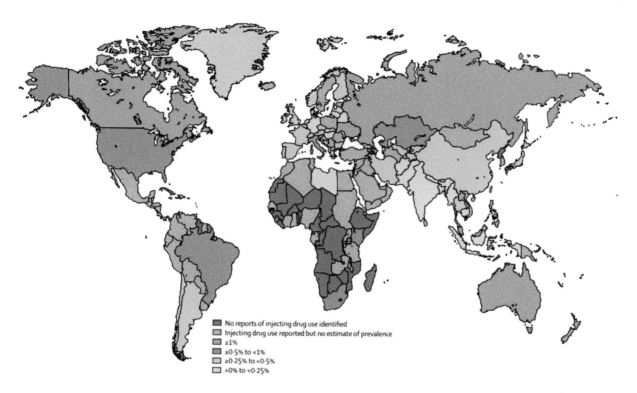

No reports of injecting drug use identified
Injecting drug use reported but no estimate of prevalence
≥1%
≥0·5% to <1%
≥0·25% to <0·5%
>0% to <0·25%

▲ **Figure 13.13** Prevalence of intravenous drug use. (Courtesy Mathers et al., 2008)

Some of the specific site issues that can occur include abscess formation, cellulitis (which can be mild or limb and life threatening and include necrotising fasciitis within this spectrum), mycotic aneurysm formation, compartment syndromes and gas gangrene. Broken needle tips are commonly encountered in such patients and whilst commonly can cause abscess formation or localised soft tissue infection, these events can often cause no ill effect to the patient (Figure 13.14). The most common causative organisms for infection are the local skin commensal *Staphylococcus* aureus or *Staphylococcus* epidermidis, streptococci as well as gram-negative bacilli such as Pseudomonas species. Depending on the nature of the condition, soft tissue and local sites infections may be treated with targeted antimicrobial therapy or may require incision and drainage in the case of abscess formation, surgical repair of mycotic aneurysms or in extreme cases of infection or gangrene, amputation of limbs to preserve life.

## Blood-Borne Infections

Local injection site infections can lead to sepsis and a systemic inflammatory response syndrome (SIRS). Some of the more common and widely recognised blood-borne infective sequelae of IV drug abuse includes bacterial and fungal infective endocarditis, viral illnesses such as HIV and hepatitis B and C, pneumonias often caused by septic embolisation or opportunistic infections as well as mycotic abscesses in the brain, spinal and endovascular system. However this list is not exhaustive as the infectious sequelae from illicit IV drug use is vast. This is reflected by the evolving pattern of drug use and the products being abused over time which can lead to users presenting with rare infections such as clostridial and anthrax derived skin-infections as well as systemic infections caused by lactobacillus and cornyebacetria species (Wurcel et al., 2015).

Infective endocarditis remains a particularly problematic clinical condition as it has a high morbidity and mortality associated with it (Colville et al., 2016). In this group, *staphylococcus aureus* predominates making up around 70% or all causative organisms, followed by streptococci and enterococci species (Murdoch et al., 2009). IV drug users also show higher rates of fungal and pseudomonal endocarditis (Ellis et al., 2001). Most endocarditis in this group affect the right heart (namely the tricuspid and pulmonary valves). Treatment is based around prolonged antimicrobial therapy with directed surgical

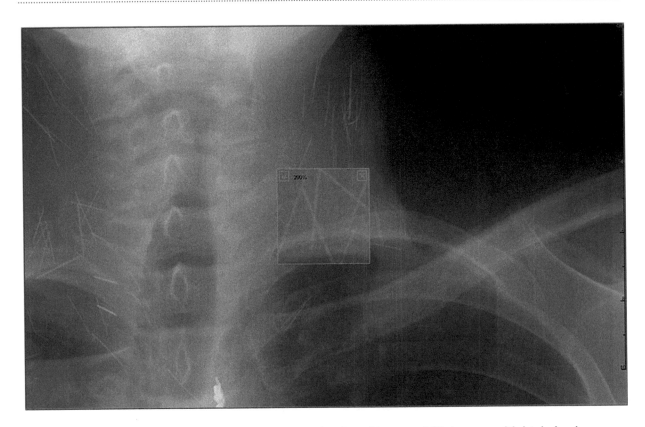

▲ **Figure 13.14** X-ray of the neck in a patient with a long history of IV drug use. Multiple broken needle fragments can be seen bilaterally. On visual examination the patient had some mild scarring in the neck but was otherwise asymptomatic (Petrovic, M., M.D., Berkow, L., M.D., & Merritt, W., M.D. (2011). Needles, Needles, Everywhere! Anesthesiology: The Journal of the American Society of Anesthesiologists, 114(3), 681–681; used with permission and courtesy Wolters Kluwer).

intervention in selected instances where there is either severe right heart failure despite good diuretic therapy, the presence of particularly difficult-to-eradicate organisms such as fungi, abscess formation or persisting fever or large vegetations >20mm on the tricuspid valve which persist or embolise to the lung (Habib et al., 2015).

## Venous Thromboembolic Phenomena

Thromboembolic phenomena related to IV drug injection are common with a study of patients in England treated for opioid abuse showing a deep vein thrombosis (DVT) prevalence of 14%, over 100 times higher than in non-IV drug users (Cornford et al., 2011). DVTs are more likely to occur in the femoral veins at the site of injections in IV drug users and the risk of pulmonary embolism in this group is around 7% overall and 10% for DVTs situated more proximally in the leg (Syed and Beeching, 2005). Long-term sequelae including recurrent pain syndromes, the need for long-term anticoagulation in this high-risk group and potential bleeding complication and a significant risk of thrombotic recurrences, especially in the presence of ongoing IV drug use.

## Conclusions

The ever-expanding armamentarium of healthcare practitioners to treat their patients brings along with it associated risks. The risk of iatrogenic sharp force trauma in modern procedures or treatments can be mitigated against but will never be eliminated. When these complications occur, they must be recognised and treated upon as they can significantly impact on the morbidity and mortality of patients.

With regard to the safety of healthcare practitioners, advances in protections with regard to needle and sharp standards have helped reduce the risk of NSIs; however, this problem has by no means been eradicated, partly due to a failure of adequate reporting of such incidents when they occur. Finally, the global burden of IV drug use and the myriad associated complications that are coupled to this activity is a problem that remains ever present and the modern healthcare practitioner must be cognizant to them.

# References

Aranaz Andrés, J., Aibar Remón, C., Vitaller Burillo, J., & Ruiz Lopez, P. (2006). National Study on Hospitalisation-Related Adverse Events: ENEAS 2005.

Baker, G. R., Norton, P. G., Flintoft, V., Blais, R., Brown, A., Cox, J., Etchells E., Ghali W. A., Hebert, P., Majumdar, S. R., O'Beirne, M., Palacios-Derflingher, L., Reid, R. J., Sheps, S., Tamblyn, R. (2004). The Canadian adverse events study: the incidence of adverse events among hospital patients in Canada. *CMAJ*, 170, 1678–1686.

Ball, C. G., Lord, J., Laupland, K. B., Gmora, S., Mulloy, R. H., Ng, A. K., Schieman, C., Kirkpatrick, A. W. (2007). Chest tube complications: how well are we training our residents? *Canadian Journal of Surgery (Journal canadien de chirurgie)*, 50, 450–458.

Biancari, F., Romppanen, H., Savontaus, M., Siljander, A., Mäkikallio, T., Piira, O.-P., Piuhola, J., Vilkki, V., Ylitalo, A., Vasankari, T., Airaksinen, J. K. E., Niemelä, M. (2018). MANTA versus ProGlide vascular closure devices in transfemoral transcatheter aortic valve implantation. *International Journal of Cardiology*, 263, 29–31.

Binswanger, I. A., Kral, A. H., Bluthenthal, R. N., Rybold, D. J., & Edlin, B. R. (2000). High prevalence of abscesses and cellulitis among community-recruited injection drug users in San Francisco. *Clinical Infectious Diseases*, 30, 579–581.

Borasio, P., Ardissone, F., & Chiampo, G. (1997). Post-intubation tracheal rupture. A report on ten cases. *The European Journal of Cardio-Thoracic Surgery*, 12, 98–100.

Boyd, K. D., Thomas, S. J., Gold, J., & Boyd, A. D. (1983). A prospective study of complications of pulmonary artery catheterizations in 500 consecutive patients. *Chest*, 84, 245–249.

Bruneau, J., Roy, E., Arruda, N., Zang, G., & Jutras-Aswad, D. (2012). The rising prevalence of prescription opioid injection and its association with hepatitis C incidence among street-drug users. *Addiction*, 107, 1318–1327.

Chaudhry, M. A., & Sardar, M. R. (2017). Vascular complications of transcatheter aortic valve replacement: a concise literature review. *World Journal of Cardiology*, 9, 574–582.

Colville, T., Sharma, V., & Albouaini, K. (2016). Infective endocarditis in intravenous drug users: a review article. *Postgraduate Medical Journal*, 92(1084), 105–111.

Cornford, C. S., Mason, J. M., & Inns, F. (2011). Deep vein thromboses in users of opioid drugs: incidence, prevalence, and risk factors. *The British Journal of General Practice: The Journal of the Royal College of General Practitioners*, 61, e781–e786.

Covarrubias, D. A., O'Connor, O. J., McDermott, S., & Arellano, R. S. (2013). Radiologic percutaneous gastrostomy: review of potential complications and approach to managing the unexpected outcome. *The American Journal of Roentgenology*, 200, 921–931.

Darchy, B., Le Mière, E., Figuérédo, B., Bavoux, E., & Domart, Y. (1999). Iatrogenic diseases as a reason for admission to the intensive care unit: incidence, causes, and consequences. *Archives of Internal Medicine*, 159, 71–78.

Davies, H. E., Davies, R. J. O., & Davies, C. W. H. (2010). Management of pleural infection in adults: British Thoracic Society pleural disease guideline 2010. *Thorax*, 65(Suppl 2), ii41–ii53.

Ebright, J. R., & Pieper, B. (2002). Skin and soft tissue infections in injection drug users. *Infectious Disease Clinics of North America*, 16(3), 697–712.

Ellis, M. E., Al-Abdely, H., Sandridge, A., Greer, W., & Ventura, W. (2001). Fungal endocarditis: evidence in the world literature, 1965–1995. *Clinical Infectious Diseases*, 32, 50–62.

Ellis, S. G., Ajluni, S., Arnold, A. Z., Popma, J. J., Bittl, J. A., Eigler, N. L., Cowley, M. J., Raymond, R. E., Safian, R. D., Whitlow, P. L. (1994). Increased coronary perforation in the new device era. Incidence, classification, management, and outcome. *Circulation*, 90, 2725–2730.

Evans, D., McGlashan, J., & Norris, A. (2015). Iatrogenic airway injury. *BJA Education*, 15, 184–189.

Feldman, R. (2014). Precise location of ideal common femoral artery puncture site. *JACC: Cardiovascular Interventions*, 7, 229.

Ghahremani, G. G., Turner, M. A., & Port, R. B. (1980). Iatrogenic intubation injuries of the upper gastrointestinal tract in adults. *Gastrointestinal Radiology*, 5, 1–10.

Giswold, M. E., Landry, G. J., Taylor, L. M., & Moneta, G. L. (2004). Iatrogenic arterial injury is an increasingly important cause of arterial trauma. *The American Journal of Surgery*, 187, 590–593.

Gold, K. (2011). Analysis: the impact of needle, syringe, and lancet disposal on the community. *Journal of Diabetes Science and Technology*, 5, 848–850.

Guttmann, O., Jones, D., Gulati, A., Crake, T., Ozkor, M., Wragg, A., Smith, E., Weerackody, R., Knight, C., Mathur, A., O'Mahony, C. (2016). TCT-259 Coronary artery perforation during percutaneous coronary intervention: incidence and outcomes. *Journal of the American College of Cardiology*, 68(18 Supplement), B105.

Habib, G., Lancellotti, P., Antunes, M. J., Bongiorni, M. G., Casalta, J.-P., Del Zotti, F., Dulgheru, R., El Khoury, G., Erba, P. A., Iung, B., Miro, J. M., Mulder, B. J., Plonska-Gosciniak, E., Price, S., Roos-Hesselink, J., Snygg-Martin, U., Thuny, F., Tornos Mas, P., Vilacosta, I., Zamorano, J. L., Group, E. S. D. (2015). 2015 ESC guidelines for the management of infective endocarditis: the task force for the management of infective endocarditis of the European Society of Cardiology (ESC) Endorsed by: European Association for Cardio-Thoracic Surgery (EACTS), the European Association of Nuclear Medicine (EANM). *European Heart Journal*, 36, 3075–3128.

Hasak, J. M., Novak, C. B., Patterson, J. M. M., & Mackinnon, S. E. (2018). Prevalence of needlestick injuries, attitude changes, and prevention practices over 12 years in an Urban Academic Hospital Surgery Department. *Annals of Surgery*, 267, 291–296.

Hecker, A., Schneck, E., Röhrig, R., Roller, F., Hecker, B., Holler, J., Koch, C., Hecker, M., Reichert, M., Lichtenstern, C., Krombach, G. A., Padberg, W., Weigand, M. A. (2015). The impact of early surgical intervention in free intestinal perforation: a time-to-intervention pilot study. *World Journal of Emergency Surgery*, 10, 54.

Heron, M. P. (2019). Deaths: leading causes for 2017. *National Vital Statistics Reports*, 68, 6.

Higgs, Z. C. J., Macafee, D. A. L., Braithwaite, B. D., & Maxwell-Armstrong, C. A. (2005). The Seldinger technique: 50 years on. *Lancet*, 366, 1407–1409.

Hoeper, M. M., Lee, S. H., Voswinckel, R., Palazzini, M., Jais, X., Marinelli, A., Barst, R. J., Ghofrani, H. A., Jing, Z-C., Opitz, C., Seyfarth, H-J., Halank, M., McLaughlin, V., Oudiz, R. J., Ewert, R., Wilkens, H., Kluge, S., Bremer, H-C., Baroke, E., Rubin, L. J. (2006). Complications of right heart catheterization procedures in patients with pulmonary hypertension in experienced centers. *Journal of the American College of Cardiology*, 48, 2546–2552.

Hoffmann, P., Al-Ani, A., von Lueder, T., Hoffmann, J., Majak, P., Hagen, O., Loose, H., Opdahl, A. (2018). Access site complications after transfemoral aortic valve implantation - a comparison of Manta and ProGlide. *CVIR Endovascular*, 1, 20.

Hyman, N., Manchester, T. L., Osler, T., Burns, B., & Cataldo, P. A. (2007). Anastomotic leaks after intestinal anastomosis: it's later than you think. *Annals of Surgery*, 245, 254–258.

Ippolito, G., Puro, V., Heptonstall, J., Jagger, J., De Carli, G., & Petrosillo, N. (1999). Occupational human immunodeficiency virus infection in health care workers: worldwide cases through September 1997. *Clinical Infectious Diseases*, 28, 365–383.

Jackson, T., Duckett, S., & Shepheard, J. (2006). Measurement of adverse events using 'incidence flagged' diagnosis codes. *Journal of Health Services Research & Policy*, 11(1), 21–26.

John, M., Razi, S., Sainathan, S., & Stavropoulos, C. (2014). Is the trocar technique for tube thoracostomy safe in the current era? *Interactive CardioVascular and Thoracic Surgery*, 19, 125–128.

Jougon, J., Ballester, M., Choukroun, E., Dubrez, J., Reboul, G., & Velly, J. F. (2000). Conservative treatment for postintubation tracheobronchial rupture. *The Annals of Thoracic Surgery*, 69, 216–220.

Kapoor, T., & Gutierrez, G. (2003). Air embolism as a cause of the systemic inflammatory response syndrome: a case report. Critical Care, 7, R98–R100.

Kearney, T. J., & Shabot, M. M. (1995). Pulmonary artery rupture associated with the Swan-Ganz catheter. *Chest*, 108, 1349–1352.

Kinnaird, T., Anderson, R., Ossei-Gerning, N., Cockburn, J., Sirker, A., Ludman, P., & Mamas, M. A. (2017). Coronary perforation complicating percutaneous coronary intervention in patients with a history of coronary artery bypass surgery. *Circulation: Cardiovascular Interventions*, 10(9), e005581.

Kraus, L., Augustin, R., Frischer, M., Kümmler, P., Uhl, A., & Wiessing, L. (2003). Estimating prevalence of problem drug use at national level in countries of the European Union and Norway. *Addiction*, 98, 471–485.

Kwok, C. S., Kontopantelis, E., Kinnaird, T., Potts, J., Rashid, M., Shoaib, A., Nolan, J., Bagur, R., de Belder, M. A., Ludman, P., Mamas, M. A. National Institute of Cardiovascular Outcomes, R. (2018). Retroperitoneal hemorrhage after percutaneous coronary intervention: incidence, determinants, and outcomes as recorded by the British Cardiovascular Intervention Society. *Circulation: Cardiovascular Interventions*, 11(2), e005866.

Langford, N. J. (2010). Therapeutic misadventure. *Medicine, Science and the Law*, 50, 179–182.

Laws, D., Neville, E., & Duffy, J. (2003). BTS guidelines for the insertion of a chest drain. *Thorax*, 58(suppl 2), ii53–ii59.

Leach, R.M., Rees, P.J., & Wilmshurst, P. (1998). Hyperbaric oxygen therapy. *BMJ*, 317, 1140–1143.

Lee, Y. H., Kim, T. K., Jung, Y. S., Cho, Y. J., Yoon, S., Seo, J. H., Jeon, Y., Bahk, J. H., Hong, D. M. (2015). Comparison of needle insertion and guidewire placement techniques during internal jugular vein catheterization: the thin-wall introducer needle technique versus the cannula-over-needle technique. *Critical Care Medicine*, 43, 2112–2116.

Lemmert, M. E., van Bommel, R. J., Diletti, R., Wilschut, J. M., de Jaegere, P. P., Zijlstra, F., Daemen, J., & Van Mieghem, N. M. (2017). Clinical characteristics and management of coronary artery perforations: a single-center 11–year experience and practical overview. *Journal of the American Heart Association*, 6, e007049.

Levinson, D. R. (2010). Adverse events in hospitals: national incidence among medicare beneficiaries. US Department of Health and Human Services; Office of the Inspector General; OIG. https://www.psnet.ahrq.gov/issue/adverse-events-hospitals-national-incidence-among-medicare-beneficiaries. Accessed April 2020.

Lewis, J. D., Enfield, K. B., & Sifri, C. D. (2015). Hepatitis B in healthcare workers: transmission events and guidance for management. *World Journal of Hepatology*, 7, 488–497.

Lim, H., Kim, J. H., Kim, D., Lee, J., Son, J. S., Kim, D. C., & Ko, S. (2012). Tracheal rupture after endotracheal intubation—a report of three cases. *Korean Journal of Anesthesiology*, 62, 277–280.

Lobato, E. B., Risley, W. P., III, & Stoltzfus, D. P. (1997). Intraoperative management of distal tracheal rupture with selective bronchial intubation. *The Journal of Clinical Anesthesia*, 9, 155–158.

Mack, M. J., Leon, M. B., Thourani, V. H., Makkar, R., Kodali, S. K., Russo, M., Kapadia, S. R., Malaisrie, S. C., Cohen, D. J., Pibarot, P., Leipsic, J., Hahn, R. T., Blanke, P., Williams, M. R., McCabe, J. M., Brown, D. L., Babaliaros, V., Goldman, S., Szeto, W. Y., Genereux, P., Pershad, A., Pocock, S. J., Alu, M. C., Webb, J. G., Smith, C. R. (2019). Transcatheter aortic-valve replacement with a balloon-expandable valve in low-risk patients. *New England Journal of Medicine*, 380, 1695–1705.

Makary, M. A., & Daniel, M. (2016). Medical error—the third leading cause of death in the US. *BMJ*, 353, i2139.

Maskell, N. A., Medford, A., & Gleeson, F. V. (2010). Seldinger chest drain insertion: simpler but not necessarily safer. *Thorax*, 65, 5–6.

Mathers, B. M., Degenhardt, L., Phillips, B., Wiessing, L., Hickman, M., Strathdee, S. A., Wodak, A., Panda, S., Tyndall, M., Toufik, A., Mattick, R. P., Reference Group to the UNoHIV, Injecting Drug, U. (2008). Global epidemiology of injecting drug use and HIV among people who inject drugs: a systematic review. *Lancet*, 372, 1733–1745.

McCarthy, C. J., Behravesh, S., Naidu, S. G., & Oklu, R. (2017). Air embolism: diagnosis, clinical management and outcomes. *Diagnostics (Basel)*, 17, 7.

Minambres, E., Buron, J., Ballesteros, M. A., Llorca, J., Munoz, P., & Gonzalez-Castro, A. (2009). Tracheal rupture after endotracheal intubation: a literature systematic review. *The European Journal of Cardio-Thoracic Surgery*, 35, 1056–1062.

Mirski, M. A., Lele, A. V., Fitzsimmons, L., & Toung, T. J. (2007). Diagnosis and treatment of vascular air embolism. *Anesthesiology*, 106(1):164–177.

Moore, C. L. (2014). Ultrasound first, second, and last for vascular access. *Journal of Ultrasound in Medicine*, 33, 1135–1142.

Murdoch, D. R., Corey, G. R., Hoen, B., Miró, J. M., Fowler, V. G., Jr, Bayer, A. S., Karchmer, A. W., Olaison, L., Pappas, P. A., Moreillon, P., Chambers, S. T., Chu, V. H., Falcó, V., Holland, D. J., Jones, P., Klein, J. L., Raymond, N. J., Read, K. M., Tripodi, M. F., Utili, R., Wang, A., Woods, C. W., Cabell, C. H., Investigators, I. C. o. E. P. C. S. (2009). Clinical presentation, aetiology, and outcome of infective endocarditis in the 21st century: the international collaboration on endocarditis–prospective cohort study. *Archives of Internal Medicine*, 169, 463–473.

Mussardo, M., Latib, A., Chieffo, A., Godino, C., Ielasi, A., Cioni, M., Takagi, K., Davidavicius, G., Montorfano, M., Maisano, F., Carlino, M., Franco, A., Covello, R. D., Spagnolo, P., Grimaldi, A., Alfieri, O., Colombo, A. (2011). Periprocedural and short-term outcomes of transfemoral transcatheter aortic valve implantation with the Sapien XT as compared with the Edwards Sapien valve. *JACC: Cardiovascular Intervention*, 4, 743–750.

Nassour, I., & Fang, S. H. (2015). Gastrointestinal perforation. *JAMA Surgery*, 150(2), 177–178.

Nielsen, N. E., Baranowska, J., Bramlage, P., & Baranowski, J. (2019). Minimizing the risk for left ventricular rupture during transcatheter aortic valve implantation by reducing the presence of stiff guidewires in the ventricle. *Interactive CardioVascular and Thoracic Surgery*, 29, 365–370.

Owais, T., El Garhy, M., Fuchs, J., Disha, K., Elkaffas, S., Breuer, M., Lauer, B., Kuntze, T. (2017). Pathophysiological factors associated with left ventricular perforation in transcatheter aortic valve implantation by transfemoral approach. *The Journal of Heart Valve Disease*, 26, 430–436.

Paspatis, G. A., Dumonceau, J. M., Barthet, M., Meisner, S., Repici, A., Saunders, B. P., Vezakis, A., Gonzalez, J. M., Turino, S. Y., Tsiamoulos, Z. P., Fockens, P., Hassan, C. (2014). Diagnosis and management of iatrogenic endoscopic perforations: European Society of Gastrointestinal Endoscopy (ESGE) Position Statement. *Endoscopy*, 46, 693–711.

Patel, V. G., Brayton, K. M., Tamayo, A., Mogabgab, O., Michael, T. T., Lo, N., Alomar, M., Shorrock, D., Cipher, D., Abdullah, S., Banerjee, S., Brilakis, E. S. (2013). Angiographic success and procedural complications in patients undergoing percutaneous coronary chronic total occlusion interventions: a weighted meta-analysis of 18,061 patients from 65 studies. *JACC: Cardiovascular Intervention*, 6, 128–136.

Perla, R. J., Hohmann, S. F., & Annis, K. (2013). Whole-patient measure of safety: using administrative data to assess the probability of highly undesirable events during hospitalization. *The Journal for Healthcare Quality*, 35, 20–31.

Petrovic, M., Berkow, L., & Merritt, W. (2011). Needles, needles, everywhere! *Anesthesiology: The Journal of the American Society of Anesthesiologists*, 114, 681–681.

Popma, J. J., Deeb, G. M., Yakubov, S. J., Mumtaz, M., Gada, H., O'Hair, D., Bajwa, T., Heiser, J. C., Merhi, W., Kleiman, N. S., Askew, J., Sorajja, P., Rovin, J., Chetcuti, S. J., Adams, D. H., Teirstein, P. S., Zorn, G. L., Forrest, J. K., Tchétché, D., Resar, J., Walton, A., Piazza, N., Ramlawi, B., Robinson, N., Petrossian, G., Gleason, T. G., Oh, J. K., Boulware, M. J., Qiao, H., Mugglin, A. S., Reardon, M. J. (2019). Transcatheter aortic-valve replacement with a self-expanding valve in low-risk patients. *New England Journal of Medicine*, 380, 1706–1715.

Pruss-Ustun, A., Rapiti, E., & Hutin, Y. (2005). Estimation of the global burden of disease attributable to contaminated sharps injuries among health-care workers. *The American Journal of Industrial Medicine*, 48, 482–490.

Pue, C. A., & Pacht, E. R. (1995). Complications of fiber-optic bronchoscopy at a university hospital. *Chest*, 107, 430–432.

Rogers, J. H., & Lasala, J. M. (2004). Coronary artery dissection and perforation complicating percutaneous coronary intervention. *The Journal of Invasive Cardiology*, 16, 493–499.

Rudström, H., Bergqvist, D., Ögren, M., & Björck, M. (2008). Iatrogenic Vascular Injuries in Sweden. A Nationwide Study 1987–2005. *European Journal of Vascular and Endovascular Surgery*, 35, 131–138.

Schmitz, R. J., Sharma, P., Badr, A. S., Qamar, M. T., & Weston, A. P. (2001). Incidence and management of oesophageal stricture formation, ulcer bleeding, perforation, and massive hematoma formation from sclerotherapy versus band ligation. *The American Journal of Gastroenterology*, 96(2), 437–441.

Schramm, R., Abugameh, A., Tscholl, D., & Schäfers, H.-J. (2009). Managing pulmonary artery catheter-induced pulmonary haemorrhage by bronchial occlusion. *The Annals of Thoracic Surgery*, 88, 284–287.

Schummer, W., Schummer, C., Gaser, E., & Bartunek, R. (2002). Loss of the guide wire: mishap or blunder? *The British Journal of Anaesthesia*, 88, 144–146.

Seldinger, S. I. (1953). Catheter replacement of the needle in percutaneous arteriography: a new technique. *Acta Radiologica*, 39, 368–376.

Shimony, A., Joseph, L., Mottillo, S., & Eisenberg, M. J. (2011). Coronary artery perforation during percutaneous coronary intervention: a systematic review and meta-analysis. *The Canadian Journal of Cardiology*, 27, 843–850.

Shojania, K. G., & Dixon-Woods, M. (2017). Estimating deaths due to medical error: the ongoing controversy and why it matters. *BMJ Quality & Safety*, 26, 423–428.

Sirivella, S., Gielchinsky, I., & Parsonnet, V. (2001). Management of catheter-induced pulmonary artery perforation: a rare complication in cardiovascular operations. *The Annals of Thoracic Surgery*, 72, 2056–2059.

Song, I. K., Kim, E. H., Lee, J. H., Jang, Y. E., Kim, H. S., & Kim, J. T. (2018). Seldinger vs modified Seldinger techniques for ultrasound-guided central venous catheterisation in neonates: a randomised controlled trial. *British Journal of Anaesthesia*, 121, 1332–1337.

Stone, P. A., Campbell, J. E., & AbuRahma, A. F. (2014). Femoral pseudoaneurysms after percutaneous access. *Journal of Vascular Surgery*, 60, 1359–1366.

Syed, F. F., & Beeching, N. J. (2005). Lower-limb deep-vein thrombosis in a general hospital: risk factors, outcomes and the contribution of intravenous drug use. *QJM*, 98, 139–145.

Thomas, M., Schymik, G., Walther, T., Himbert, D., Lefevre, T., Treede, H., Eggebrecht, H., Rubino, P., Michev, I., Lange, R., Anderson, W. N., Wendler, O. (2010). Thirty-day results of the SAPIEN aortic Bioprosthesis European Outcome (SOURCE) Registry: a European registry of transcatheter aortic valve implantation using the Edwards SAPIEN valve. *Circulation*, 122, 62–69.

Tullavardhana, T. (2015). Iatrogenic Esophageal Perforation. *Journal of the Medical Association of Thailand*, 98(Suppl 9), S177–183.

Warrington, W. G., Aragon Penoyer, D., Kamps, T. A., & Van Hoeck, E. H. (2012). Outcomes of using a modified Seldinger technique for long term intravenous therapy in hospitalized patients with difficult venous access. *Journal of the Association for Vascular Access*, 17, 24–30.

Wurcel, A. G., Merchant, E. A., Clark, R. P., & Stone, D. R. (2015). Emerging and Underrecognized complications of illicit drug use. *Clinical Infectious Diseases*, 61, 1840–1849.

# Chapter 14
## Presentation of Evidence and Issues Arising in Court in Sharp Force Trauma Cases

## Introduction

The presentation of sound evidence can only be achieved if the expert is accurate in his/her factual assessment of the findings and reasonable in the opinions drawn from such facts. Indeed, in the vast majority of cases, experts generally agree on the factual information gleaned from their examination but may well not agree on their views derived from their findings.

Different court systems throughout the world require an appropriate approach to comply with local legal requirements in terms of preparation and delivery of evidence by forensic practitioners. At all times, however, the forensic witness should be aware that he/she is a witness to the court, whether working in an adversarial or inquisitorial system, and especially in adversarial proceedings, not tailoring their evidence to suit the party that is engaging them. The object of a forensic investigation is to ensure that the best possible evidence is collected, its integrity protected throughout and the evidence presented in a court of law in a clear and logical manner, to enable not only the judiciary to comprehend it, but to be understood by the lay jury and others without medical or legal knowledge.

This chapter will discuss the content and other aspects of the preparation of statements for the delivery of evidence in court, in particular those areas which relate to issues which frequently arise during witness examination in sharp force trauma cases, the vast majority of which involve stabbing resulting from the use of knives.

## Preparation of Statements and Common Issues Arising in Court

In addition to the general requirements common to all statements for use in court hearings, whether in relation to autopsy or clinical examination of living subjects, there are specific aspects which need to be addressed which take into account issues relevant to sharp force trauma.

These include the following:

- Scene findings, particularly amount of blood and its distribution
- Number, location and pattern of wounds
- Direction of infliction
- Weapon characteristics (usually knife)
- Force of impact
- Whether one or more sharp weapons/assailants
- Whether more than one type of trauma is present and likelihood of more than one assailant
- Length of attack
- Length of survival after attack and physical activity
- Statement on manner of death and differentiation from accident or suicide
- Complications post-stabbing and whether there was a novus actus interveniens

- Conferences between the pathologist and prosecutors or defence advocates to assess the strength of evidence and which aspects are relevant to the case

- Production of supplementary reports to address issues at the request of the prosecution or defence.

## At the Scene

As with all forensic cases it is important to appreciate that the involvement of the pathologist or other forensic medical practitioner begins with consideration of the location or associated sites where the crime was committed, whether or not he/she has personally visited the scene (see chapter 4). The pathologist may be questioned on a number of aspects relating to the scene including whether they can state where the deceased had been attacked in relation to the position in which the body was found and the amount of blood and its distribution. Where blood is concerned, occasionally lawyers may draw the pathologist into giving a detailed opinion on blood distribution. Other than general comments, it would be wiser for pathologists to defer to the forensic scientist expert in blood distribution analysis, to give a comprehensive account.

The type of question, however, which a pathologist could properly be expected to answer in relation to blood might include its redistribution on the body as a result of moving the victim at the scene for various reasons including for necessary medical intervention, dragging from one room to another or to an entirely different location by the assailant or when the body is moved from the scene to the mortuary.

Another issue which may arise is the possible production of artefactual injury on moving the body at the scene especially when the deceased is lying in a confined space. The pathologist must be clear in their mind as to which defects or other marks are artefactual by being aware of the possibility that a post-mortem "injury" may have been caused by the deceased being inadvertently impacted against a surface by personnel, such as police or undertakers, moving the body.

In addition, medical intervention, such as the placement of chest drains, if removed by the time the body is in the mortuary, may be confused with stab wounds, particularly when dealing with a large number of injuries. Medical intervention marks should be clearly identified by examining records from ambulance personnel or from emergency admission staff. Clarifying the status of such findings will save any embarrassment in court and not raise doubts about the credibility of the rest of the evidence.

## Number of Wounds

Where there is more than one wound, the question frequently arises as to the sequence of the injuries. The pathologist, based on autopsy findings alone will in the vast majority of cases not be in a position to confidently opine on the sequence of wounding. In some cases, the pattern and distribution of wounds may assist, together with information regarding the circumstances surrounding the assault. Occasionally when there are two wounds with one being produced before death and one after death, the lack of vital reaction and yellow and dry appearance in the post-mortem wound would allow obvious differentiation between them.

In a situation where if it obvious that the first wound had been rapidly disabling, one may well be able to confidently assert that that wound was the first, before others were inflicted.

It should also be appreciated that when a pathologist numbers wounds in the autopsy report, this does not signify the sequence of wounding as might be thought but is done to facilitate reference to injuries in the statement. It is actually very difficult for the pathologist to give an accurate sequence of wounds apart from the circumstances noted above.

In cases where there are multiple wounds the pathologist may sometimes be requested to give his/her view on whether the number of injuries constitute a "frenzied attack." The motive behind this may well be to infer that the attacker was in a temporarily emotionally charged state for a number of possible reasons, including mental health issues or being under the influence of alcohol or drugs. The pathologist should refrain from giving a view on the emotional state of the attacker as it is outside his/her expertise. Such an assessment should be left to an expert in forensic psychiatry or other appropriately qualified expert.

## Which Was the Fatal Wound?

Where there is more than one wound, the pathologist may be asked which was responsible for causing death particularly if it is thought that more than one assailant was yielding a knife. The answer, however, may not be clear if there are deep wounds grouped closely together, and especially if their tracks are overlapping. The other questions which might be anticipated, are usually along the lines of "which wound was the most fatal" and "what part in causing death did other wounds play," thus seeking from the pathologist a hierarchical order of their severity.

In complex homicides, in addition to sharp force trauma, other types of injuries are seen such as blunt force or compressive neck injuries. The role of sharp force injuries in such cases in relation to other types of trauma will be explored in the court room and the pathologist needs to be prepared to assess the various types of injuries in relation to the overall effect on the victim.

## Survival and Physical Activity Following Injury

Another issue that frequently arises in court is the question of how long a person survived following infliction of the injuries. This question is very difficult to answer with any degree of certainty. Survival time and activity varies so much between individuals (Franchi et al 2016; Karger et al 1999). There are too many variables to be able to give an accurate answer and only an approximate view can be given based on consideration of factors such as severity and number of wounds, site of injury blood loss, age and state of health of the victim, witness accounts and so on (Sauvageau et al 2006).

## Intent to Injure

The pathologist or forensic physician may be asked questions regarding the intent of wounding, based on the location of the wound or wounds, believing that some locations show greater intent than others to wound the victim. For example, a stab wound to the head may be proposed by a lawyer to the witness that it indicates much more intent to kill compared to stabbing to the abdomen which, because of the direction of the thrust, is more likely to be accidental (Taff and Boglioli 1998). There is absolutely no

scientific basis for such assumptions and the notion should be rejected by the witness.

A lawyer may put to the witness the proposition that there is greater intent to kill because of the length of the wound track, i.e. the greater the length of penetration of a knife into the body, the greater is the intent to kill. This theory, which is simplistic and unscientific, does not take into account all the variables involved in stabbing scenarios such as force of thrust, clothing thickness, knife characteristics, tissue resistance and movement between victim and assailant.

In relation to intent, lawyers also frequently try to ascertain the pathologist's view on the use of force used by the assailant. In reality an accurate assessment can very rarely, if at all, be made. In order to be in a position to calculate force with any degree of accuracy, a knowledge of the biomechanics of injury is essential as well as taking into account all the various factors which are involved in each individual case. Further details in this area can be found in chapter 3. In reality, all that the court can expect from a pathologist is a subjective assessment based on the injuries seen, characteristics of the knife, its velocity just prior to impact, the intervening clothing worn and the dynamics between the assailant and the victim. Such an estimation of the degree of force is not based on any scientific calculations but rather on a crude scale of force stated as slight, moderate or severe (Nolan et al 2018). Others use a scale of 1 to 10 where 10 is the most severe force.

## Whether There Was More Than One Assailant and/or Weapon

When there is more than one person involved in a fracas with the murdered victim, the question sometimes arises whether more than one person was involved in physically injuring the deceased and in addition, the question also arises in those circumstances as to who delivered the fatal blow. The accounts of witnesses may well be unreliable and the pathologist may well be requested to give an opinion on this issue. This is frequently a difficult question to answer with any degree of accuracy. Clearly the pathologist will take into account the circumstances of the assault including the type of weapon or weapons used, the accounts of witnesses and relate this information to the findings at autopsy.

When there is more than one assailant using knives which result in wounds with similar characteristics, it is usually impossible to say whether or not more than one attacker was involved without taking into account other information as mentioned above. If, in addition to sharp force trauma, there is evidence of other types of injury, such as blunt force trauma, it becomes easier to assess whether more than one person is involved. For example, where a victim has been subjected to violent kicking from one attacker and stabbed by another.

## Interaction and the Dynamics Between the Assailant and Victim and Relationship to the Injuries Seen

An assault is a dynamic event and thus it becomes extremely difficult to calculate exact positions of assailant and victim when wounds were inflicted, although questioning in court may give the impression that reconstruction of positions of the attacker and injured person and direction of delivery of a wound are straightforward matters. One of the difficulties, however, in assessing the relative positions of the attacker and the victim and the direction from which the knife is thrust, is that the sequence of events may happen very quickly. The two individuals involved may be facing each other, side on, one behind the other, both standing, one or both lying or sitting and so on. In addition to these "snapshot" positions, various movements between them, to take avoiding action for example, will further complicate assumptions of their relative positions during the short time the knife in question, has entered and exited from the body. Handedness in relation to direction is sometimes raised in court but the pathologist, for the reasons mentioned above is not in a position to give a clear answer on this issue unless there are good eye witness accounts and the location of the wound(s) on the body and tracks are consistent.

A further interesting issue involves discussion around the cause of a wound which is notched. It is sometimes put to the pathologist that the reason that a wound has this irregular shape is because the knife had been twisted in the body. This is a very unusual thing to happen. It is much more likely that the victim and/or attacker were moving relative to

each other during the time the knife was within the victim's body. Once again, this stems from the misconception that the victim is not moving.

## Characteristics of Knife (or Other Sharp Object) and Relationship to Wound Morphology

The question of blade length and width is regularly aired in court and the pathologist is expected to be able to assess these parameters from examination of the injuries and their tracks. Equating length of a wound track with the length of a knife blade is far from an easy task. Where there is a hilt mark on the surface and the knife has terminated in bone, for example the spine, one can assume that all of the blade has entered the body. Furthermore, it is relatively easy to estimate reasonably accurately the distance of the track in those circumstances. On the other hand, where the wound has terminated in an organ or other soft tissue the length of the track can only be an approximation. It should be made clear to lawyers that when relating the length of a track to the length of a blade, not only might the length of the track be difficult to measure accurately but consideration should be given to the added variable of compressibility of the chest and particularly of the abdomen. Further, it should be made clear that knives with a short blade length are capable of producing a length of track which is significantly longer than their blade. One must also bear in mind that the full length of a blade may not have penetrated the body.

In relation to the length of the wound on the body surface because the skin is elastic and flexible the blade width when the stab wound is perpendicular to the surface is usually narrower or equal to the wound length, contracting slightly after the knife has been removed. This has been demonstrated by Barber (2009) in pig skin experiments and a retrospective survey of 40 homicide cases.

## Accidental Stabbing or Knife Used in Self-defence

Another question which frequently arises is whether the assailant was using a knife to defend himself and the victim ran on to him, or whether during a struggle the victim fell on to the knife causing him to be accidentally stabbed. There may on rare occasions be a plausible explanation, as in the case presented by Wilke and Püschel (2011) of a 14-year-old boy who apparently walked into a kitchen knife held by his mother and was fatally wounded.

This is not an infrequent question posed by defence counsel especially when a victim dies of a single stab wound. The pathologist needs to consider carefully such a situation put to him/her, taking into account the dynamics between the assailant and victim, whether there are any other wounds to the body which were not fatal such as defence wounds and other information such as from witness statements. On anatomical grounds alone, in reality the intent to stab may be difficult to resolve.

An interesting and widely reported example of a victim allegedly impaling themselves on to a knife is that of Jeffrey Locker who was found stabbed in his car in 2009. Kenneth Minor, the alleged assailant claimed that he held the knife against a steering wheel in the car while Locker thrust his body into it. In a Manhattan court in 2011 he received a 20-year sentence for second degree murder. His claim of assisted suicide as a defence was given some credence, however, when further information came to light. Apparently Locker had accumulated large debts, acquired a number of life insurance policies and examination of his computer revealed searches for funeral arrangements.

His initial conviction in New York was overturned in 2013 because the trial judge had informed the jury that assisted suicide fell into the murder category whereas in that state it is categorised as second degree manslaughter; his sentence was accordingly changed to 12 years (Bever 2014).

# Presentation of Evidence

The presentation of evidence based on statements from the autopsy examination or medical notes is frequently insufficient to explain the features and extent of injury and needs to be supplemented by visual aids such as the use of photography, video, radiographic imaging, plans and drawings, as well as aids which allow reconstruction of events such as the application of virtual reality.

It is important for the expert to present evidence to the court which is comprehensible to lay public; and at the same time avoid the use of graphic images directly from photographs which might upset the jury and be regarded as prejudicial to the defendant, unless it is absolutely essential to show them, whilst at the same time ensuring that the quality of the evidence is not diminished in any way. Wherever possible, the use of body diagram, showing injuries, which may be drawn freehand or by the use of computer graphics or 3-D reconstructions from CT and MRI scans is to be encouraged. With reconstructed 3-D imaging, the possibility of misinterpreting artefacts for injuries needs to be borne in mind and therefore reconstructions should be produced from high quality CT scans and reference also made to the corresponding 2-D scan images (Borowska-Solonynko and Solonynko 2015). In cases where evidence from such imaging including from the more usual radiographs is required, unless the forensic pathologist is experienced and has adequate training in interpretation of radiographic images, a radiologist should attend to give that aspect of the evidence.

# References

Barber LR. (2009). Matching the wound to the weapon: the correlation between the size of stab wounds on the skin and the size of weapon in homicide victims. MSc Dissertation, Queen Mary, University of London.

Bever L. (2014). 'Harlem Kevorkian' sentenced to 12 years in prison in suicide-for-hire insurance scam. *Washington Post*, Oct. 21.

Borowska-Solonynko A, Solonynko B. (2015). The use of 3D computed tomography reconstruction in medico-legal testimony regarding injuries in living victims—risks and benefits. *J Forensic Leg Med* 30, 9–13.

Franchi A, Kolopp M, Coudane H, Martrille L. (2016) Precise survival time and physical activity after fatal left ventricle injury from sharp pointed weapon: a case report and a review of the literature. *Int J Legal Med* 130, 1299–1301.

Karger B, Niemeyer J, Brinkmann B. (1999). Physical activity following fatal injury from sharp pointed weapons. *Int J Legal Med* 112, 188–191.

Nolan G, Hainsworth SV, Rutty GN. (2018). Forces generated in stabbing attacks: an evaluation of the utility of the mild, moderate and severe scale. *Int J Legal Med* 132, 229–236.

Sauvageau A, Trépanier JS, Racette S. (2006). Delayed deaths after vascular traumatism: two cases. *J Clin Forensic Med* 13, 344–248.

Taff ML, Boglioli LR. (1998). Science and politics of cutting and stabbing injuries in the USA. *J Clin Forensic Med* 5, 80–84.

Wilke N, Püschel K. (2011). Hineinlaufen in ein Messer—Schutzbehauptung oder (tragischer) Unfall? [Bumping into a knife—exculpatory statement or (tragic) accident?]. *Arch Kriminol* 228, 108–113.

# Index

Page numbers in *italics* denote Figures.

**297**